D0686105

DR. SANDY'S
TOP TO BOTTOM GUIDE
TO YOUR NEWBORN

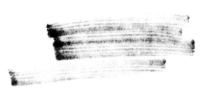

Dr. Sandy's Top to Bottom Guide to Your Newborn

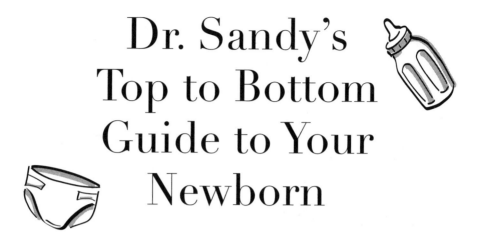

ANSWERS TO THE QUESTIONS
EVERY PARENT ASKS

SANDY L. CHUNG, MD

Illustrations by David Lee and Elizabeth Leach
Photography by Kin Y. Chung

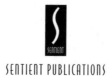

SENTIENT PUBLICATIONS

First Sentient Publications edition 2011
Copyright © 2011 by Sandy L. Chung, MD

All rights reserved. This book, or parts thereof, may not be reproduced in any form without permission, except in the case of brief quotations embodied in critical articles and reviews.

A paperback original

Cover design by Kim Johansen, Black Dog Design
Book design by Timm Bryson

Library of Congress Cataloging-in-Publication Data

Chung, Sandy L., 1971–
  Dr. Sandy's top to bottom guide to your newborn : answers to the questions every new parent asks / Sandy L. Chung. — 1st Sentient Publications ed.
    p. cm.
  ISBN 978-1-59181-168-8
  1. Newborn infants—Popular works. I. Title.
  RJ251.C48 2010
  618.92'01—dc22

                              2010032061

Printed in the United States of America

10 9 8 7 6 5 4 3 2 1

SENTIENT PUBLICATIONS
A Limited Liability Company
1113 Spruce Street
Boulder, CO 80302
www.sentientpublications.com

CONTENTS

PART II

Guide to Your Newborn's Body from Head to Toe

Chapter 29: Skin   136

Appendices

ACKNOWLEDGEMENTS

Many people have asked me, "How did you ever find time to write a book?" It has been a fun challenge trying to write, work, raise four children, be active in the physician community, and try to have some semblance of normal life. I could achieve all of these only with the love and support of my amazing husband, Kin. His talent with photography and computers made it so much easier for me to get the work done that I needed for the book. I would like to thank him for always being there for me and our children and allowing me to pursue my dreams.

I would also like to express my love for my wonderful children, Kevin, Alex, Sarah and Ryan. Thank you for being so patient with Mommy when she was working on her computer all the time. Each one of you has taught me more about how children grow and develop than any pediatric residency or textbook ever could.

Thank you to Connie Shaw, my editor at Sentient Publications, for helping me to bring this book to reality. I would also like to thank Elizabeth Leach for her great illustrations, and Bethany Bryan for her excellent copyediting on my first draft.

I am indebted to my talented brother David Lee for his amazing work with chapter logos. I want to thank him for taking time out of his busy schedule to help me with them. I would like to thank my other brother, Johnny Lee, for helping with some of the drawings as well. Thank you to my parents for all of their hard work, love, and support.

My heartfelt appreciation goes out to Christine Nwosu, who helped me with my children while I was writing this book. She helped to keep all my kids' lives in order while I worked.

Last, but not least, thank you to all my wonderful patients, their parents and my practice for inspiring me and helping me to write this book. I would especially like to thank the adorable children who are featured in the photographs in this book and their generous parents, for allowing me to take pictures of their children.

INTRODUCTION

"Does her belly button look okay? Does it hurt her? Am I supposed to *do* something to it?" asked Jennifer, questions tumbling out of her mouth. She gestured to the center of her newborn daughter's belly and looked at me anxiously. "Is it okay?"

"It looks just fine," I said to her, examining the dried little hard stump of umbilical cord. "She cannot feel it. The edges might be a bit scratchy, so just try not to press onto her skin with the diaper," I reassured her. Then, I showed Jennifer how to fold the top edge of the diaper down. "Just keep it dry, and it should fall off in seven to ten days. Once it does, you can give her a bath. Until then, just give her a sponge bath."

Then, I asked, "Do you have any other questions?"

Jennifer nodded, "Yes, I do." She reached over to her overflowing diaper bag, which was piled precariously on the exam table. After pulling out an assortment of diapers, wipes, blankets, and bibs, she took out a notebook with several questions scribbled on the first few pages. "Just a few..." she began, clicking on her pen and getting poised to write. "Ummm...how do you give a sponge bath?"

This scenario is a common routine in my daily pediatric practice. As I look back over my years in pediatrics, it has always intrigued me that the same questions come up time and time again. If new parents all want to know the same things, why is there not a resource for parents?

Well, there are...lots of them. There are almost too many. It is hard to know which ones to turn to and believe. Some parents are "type A" personalities (like me) and read about everything, take notes, make lists, and prepare for all instances. Others prefer to wait until they need to know something and then start learning about it. And then some just go with the flow and figure that everything will work itself out in due time (my husband!). For everyone, there are lots of resources out there—books, magazines, grandparents, friends, and, of course, your pediatrician. It is nearly impossible to sort through them all, and several of them seem to conflict.

What I've learned over my training and years of practice is this: The good news is that even with all the different ways to raise children, our parents figured it out—and most of us turned out just fine! There is a reason why you'll get so many different answers. Quite simply, every baby is different. Not only that, but often there is not one *right* way to do things. This is harder to accept if you are the controlling type (like me). Most babies do great despite some of the mistakes we make! People all over the world in different cultures and environments manage to successfully take care of babies. There cannot possibly be a single right way of doing things.

One of the most challenging aspects of my job is to convince parents that there is not always a right answer, but rather a range of normal behavior. For example, in reality, there is not an exact number of ounces that a baby must drink every feeding each day. The big picture is much more important—is your child growing and gaining weight? Is your child reaching milestones? Your baby did not read the child development textbook. Just because he is doing things a little bit later, it does not mean that he won't get into the Ivy League school of his choice. (It's a good thing the college applications do not ask when he took his first step!)

That being said, there are certainly guidelines for childcare. Parents often tell me how lucky it is that I'm a pediatrician, and that it must make raising children so much easier. And, yes, there are certainly aspects of having children that are less worrisome to me since I've had additional training in how children grow and develop. So, in this book, I would like to share with you the questions and concerns that thousands of other parents have shared with me. I hope that the information in this book will help you feel more comfortable and more prepared for the amazing bundle of joy that is yours.

So, how do you use this book? Use it as another guideline as you travel through the exciting journey of your child's first month of life. These chapters describe to you what I tell the parents in my everyday practice. They are not hard and fast rules. In fact, your child may not follow these rules. If you are concerned about anything, definitely bring up the subject with your child's pediatrician or family physician. I like to think of this book as your "pocket pediatrician." I'm a real life practicing pediatrician, but I'm also the mother of four children. I know firsthand how different methods are needed for each child. Hopefully, some of the information in this book will make you feel better prepared in some instances, help you sleep easier at night in other instances, and confirm what you've heard from your sources in others.

Each chapter covers the essential parts of a child's health and daily life. I recommend reading this book in its entirety before your baby arrives, if you have time. Then, after your baby is born, use it as your pocket pediatrician to help you remember how to do certain things and to decide if your newborn's behavior is normal or not. Many behaviors and habits change as your child grows, so use these guidelines to help you through one of the most physically challenging periods of your child's life.

I've helped thousands of parents with their children and raised my own four lovely children. I hope that this book will help you with your child. Best of luck to you in this exciting and challenging trip!

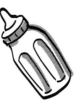

PART I

Newborn Basics

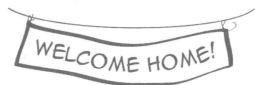

CHAPTER I

Welcome, Baby!

Sleepless Nights, Here We Come!

Okay…now the worst is over. The delivery is done. You are now a parent!

It is an amazing and incredible experience to look at this new baby and know that you are now responsible for the well-being of this little person.

So…what's next?

Well, you are going to take care of your baby. But first, you need to take care of yourself.

You are likely tired, relieved, overwhelmed, in pain (if you're mom), and did I mention tired? The first two weeks are often a big blur. The first week often feels like one long, jet-lagged day. You may have done all-nighters when you were younger…but how about fourteen all-nighters in a row? How about three months' worth? You will likely not be sleeping through the night for the first few months. Some people say that you will finally get a good night's sleep in, oh, about, eighteen *years*!

But truly, thousands of women deliver babies every day. It is amazing how well you will be able to handle the every two-to-three-hour feedings, even if you are sleep-walking through much of it! Trying to learn new skills while sleep-deprived can be very overwhelming and difficult to do.

But do not be concerned; your body and mind will adapt. There is an end to sleepless nights at some point, and then you have an adorable little person to show for all of your hard work.

I clearly remember one occasion when I woke up one night to feed my newborn baby. I was in the nursery in this big, comfy sofa chair, holding him while he nursed. My body was feeding him on autopilot, and my brain was in a hazy, half-awake fog. At some point I must have fallen asleep in the chair where I was feeding him. When I woke up, I was in a total panic as it registered in my cloudy brain that my arms were empty! I thought for certain that I had dropped my son on the floor and that he was injured. Luckily, it turns out that some part of my brain was functioning enough to put my baby back in the crib before I fell asleep. My heart rate still goes up when I think about that episode!

You may have heard the old wives' tale that you lose brain cells every time you have a baby. While scientifically that may not be true, it sure feels like it. And if you have more than one child, then just forget it! (Well, you will anyway!) I find that many parents had no idea that the first few months would be so hard. Consider it a challenge that you must rise up to meet—and one that is well worth it!

So, how can you make it through? Here are some helpful tips:

Get help…useful help. If having your parents or your in-laws over for the first two weeks will increase your stress level instead of relieving it, then tell them to come over after that time has passed. Sometimes, the most well-meaning grandparents can be a terrible burden when you are trying to get to know your baby and take care of yourself.

One mom described to me how her mother-in-law flew in from across the country to help for the first two weeks. But instead of being a help, her mother-in-law just bossed her around, constantly correcting her regarding the baby's care. Her mother-in-law still expected to be treated as a guest and have her meals cooked for her at the same time. This mom was so tired and confused, and she was resentful of her mother-in-law's presence during this stressful time. You do not need this kind of help!

Luckily, most grandparents are great. So use them while you have them. If they are willing, try to let them take over a feeding, or at least watch the baby in between feedings if you are breastfeeding. Try to sleep when they are helping you.

Let your spouse or significant other take on some of the duties. This is particularly helpful for moms who are breastfeeding. The feeding chapter will go into more detail about bottle versus breastfeeding. But realize that if you are going to do all the feedings, you will only get at most one to two hours of continuous sleep at a time in those first two weeks.

If you can, try to either pump your breast milk or give your baby one bottle of formula a least once a day so that you can get a minimum of four hours of sleep in a row. Once your baby has latched on well, you can safely use a bottle for a feeding for most babies. Your body and brain need enough time to get to deep REM sleep so that you can feel refreshed. If you are not well-rested, you are not helping yourself or your child. It is amazing how wonderful you'll feel if you can get four hours of uninterrupted sleep!

Sleep when your baby sleeps. People will tell you this often. But you'll find it is actually quite difficult to tune out your "mommy" or "daddy" sense and just go to sleep. This is especially true if your baby is in your bedroom. The best way to work around this is to have someone you trust to take care of your baby in another room in your home, preferably as far away from where you are sleeping as possible. Otherwise, if you hear your baby crying, it will be your natural instinct to go to her. Only when you cannot hear noises from your baby will your body and mind be able to relax. Also, go easy on the caffeine. Not only does it go into your breast milk, but most people are not able to sleep if they have had caffeine recently.

Write things down. I always tell my new parents, "If you have questions for the doctor, write them down. Do not feel silly coming into the office with a list of questions. We are all used to it. That way you can have all of your questions answered in one visit."

Almost every day, I have a mom start to ask me a question, then stop, stare at me blankly, and say, "I know I was going to ask you something, but now I cannot remember what it was!"

Have a plan...then plan to change it. Your baby is a person, a person with his own needs, desires, and expectations. Imagine that if when you first started dating a person, you began to dictate when everything was going to happen—when you would eat, when you would go out, what you would both wear, and when you would both go to bed! The relationship would probably not last very long.

This new baby is not just an extension of you. He is a new person. Your baby does not know what you had envisioned, what a perfect parent and perfect baby do. He doesn't understand that you think he's going to eat every three hours on a schedule from day one. He does not know that you are determined to breastfeed him for his entire first year of life. So...go with the flow. Read the cues that your baby gives you, do your best to translate them, and realize that many times there is not necessarily a "right" way to do things.

Add thirty minutes to an hour to the time it took you to doing things before. The days where you could just throw on your shoes, grab your keys, and jump into the car are gone! The process of getting out of the house and into the car takes significantly longer now. Once you have your baby fed, ready to go, and strapped into the car seat, inevitably she will poop and then start to cry to be changed. Then, once you have her changed into a clean diaper and strapped back into the car seat, she will spit up all over her clothes (and yours!). And once you change her clothes, clean yourself up, and strap her back in the car seat, she will cry again to be fed—you get the picture. Just be prepared for the normal delays that come with a baby who cannot tell time and does not know that you are already twenty minutes late for an appointment!

If you are overwhelmed, cry frequently, feel like you are not connecting with your new baby, or do not feel like you can handle the pressure of motherhood, then call your obstetrician or doctor for help. You could have symptoms of postpartum depression. This is a common problem and should not be dismissed as "normal post-baby blues." It is a real disease, like diabetes or asthma, and you should not just suffer through it or try to ignore it. Postpartum depression is treatable and can be dangerous if left untreated. Having a baby is tiring, but it should still be wonderful and enjoyable as you consider the tiny little person you have made.

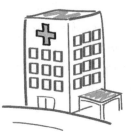

CHAPTER 2

The First Day

What's First? — Tests, Medicines, Shots, and the Doctor Visit

"What was her Apgar score?" asked Heather, when I visited her after the delivery of her new baby boy.

"8 and 9," I replied.

"Is that good?" she asked with a look of concern.

"It's the best score that most babies get!" I reassured her. And then she relaxed. Her baby's first standardized test score, and he was already a genius.

In the labor and delivery room, a flurry of activity takes place when your baby is born. Of course, the all-important weighing and measuring is done at birth. It's a great photo opportunity and an exciting moment for everyone!

Along with the weighing, several procedures are done when a baby is first born. In general, these events are universal at hospitals around the country. If you are planning a home delivery, many midwives will also perform these routine procedures. Many of these will happen without you even being aware of them since they happen quickly right after birth.

The Apgar Score—The First Test

The Apgar score was developed in the 1950's as a shorthand way to assess a baby's status in the first few minutes after delivery. This score gives physicians an idea of how your baby transitioned from being inside a uterus to being out in the world, breathing air for the first time. While it is a useful test for indicating if there were difficulties during the initial minutes of life, it is not meant to predict future outcomes or development.

There are two numbers assigned, and these numbers are the sum of five measurements added together. The total score can range from zero to ten, with higher numbers being better. The first number is the baby's status at one minute of life, and the second number is the baby's status at five minutes of life. Occasionally, if the newborn has low scores in the first five minutes, then a third number is assigned for the baby's status at ten minutes of life. This shows the progress of the baby as interventions are performed.

TABLE 1: APGAR SCORE COMPONENTS

SIGN	SCORE = 2	SCORE = 1	SCORE = 0
HEART RATE	Normal (>100 beats/min)	Slow (<100 beats/min)	No pulse
RESPIRATION	Normal, good crying	Weak, slow or irregular breaths	Absent, not breathing
MUSCLE TONE/ ACTIVITY	Well flexed, active, spontaneous movement	Some flexion of arms and legs with little movement	Flaccid, floppy tone
REFLEXES	Cough/sneezes/ pulls away with stimulation	Grimace (facial movement only to stimulation)	No response to stimulation
COLOR	Completely pink including hands and feet	Blue hands and feet, pink body	Pale/blue all over

The five measurements that make up the Apgar score are listed in Table 1.

Most babies receive an Apgar score of 8/9, meaning a sum of 8 at one minute of life, and a sum of 9 at five minutes of life. Since most newborns have bluish hands/feet, they all lose one point for color. This is normal. If your baby receives a low Apgar score, remember that the Apgar score is a measurement of the breathing and alertness status during the first few minutes of life only. It does not predict your baby's future outcome in any way.

Vitamin K Injection—The First Shot

"Why does she need a shot already?" asked Varsha's mom. "Is it safe for her to get a shot so soon?"

Some babies are born with a very low level of vitamin K. This vitamin is required to help blood to clot. Vitamin K deficiency is a rare disorder, affecting around 1 in 200,000 babies. Without enough levels of vitamin K, there is a risk of bleeding into the brain several weeks after birth and this can be fatal.

Unfortunately, there is not an easy way to identify which babies will need additional vitamin K. Therefore to prevent the risk of bleeding, all babies are routinely given extra vitamin K.

Antibiotic Eye Ointment—The First Medicine

"Why are his eyes so sticky?" Jenny asked me. "Does he have an infection?"

Some women may have bacteria in the vaginal canal that may not cause symptoms for the mom, but may affect the baby. The bacteria that cause sexually-transmitted diseases such as chlamydia, gonorrhea, and syphilis can get into the baby's eyes. This can cause eye infections and severe vision problems including blindness. Therefore, as a precaution, all babies are routinely given one dose of antibiotic eye ointment or drops at birth to reduce the risk of eye infection. This is safe and should not harm your baby as long as he is not allergic to the medication.

Bloodwork—The First Blood Test

"What's my baby's blood type?" is a common question that parents ask. The blood type of your baby is not routinely checked. Sometimes it is obtained because of potential cross-reactions between the baby's blood and mom's blood. If mom has blood type O or if mom is Rh negative (A-, B-, AB- or O-), then the baby's blood type may be checked.

Other blood tests that might be performed include a complete blood count, which will screen for infections and some blood disorders. This is especially important if mom has a bacterium called Group B Streptococcus ("Group B Strep") in her vaginal canal. A screening for this bacterium is done by your ob/gyn during the last trimester of pregnancy.

If a baby does not have any risk factors, no specific blood work may be needed. So, if your baby does not need any lab tests done, that's okay!

Cord Blood Banking—The First Bank

"I want to do cord blood banking," Addison told her obstetrician. "How do we get the cord blood?'

It has become very popular to participate in cord blood banking programs. Essentially, it is a process where blood from the umbilical cord or placenta is stored in a frozen repository for future use. Many diseases, such as some leukemias, lymphomas, and immune deficiencies, that were previously thought to be incurable, have been successfully treated with stem cell therapy using cord blood. In the future there may be many more diseases that could be cured using cord blood. Therefore, many parents are storing their child's cord blood for future use if needed.

There are public and private cord blood banks available. Participation in a public bank is usually free. However, your child's cord blood is made available to anyone who might be a match to use. There are no guarantees that it will still be available for your child to use later.

Private cord blood banks charge a fee, usually an annual fee, for as long as you want them to keep the blood stored. However, the benefit is that your child's cord blood will always be available for your use in the future.

If you are donating to a cord blood bank, public or private, the blood needs to be collected from the cord at the time of delivery, after the cord has been cut. This is blood that is normally thrown away so there is no risk to your baby during the collection process.

Generally, banks will send you a collection kit that you will need to give to your obstetrician or midwife prior to delivery. If your hospital participates in a public blood bank, they may not give you a kit, but will have you sign a consent form before the blood is collected.

Hepatitis B Vaccine—The First Immunization

Many hospitals around the country will offer the first Hepatitis B vaccine for your baby. Hepatitis B is a serious liver disease that is caused by a virus. This virus is transmitted by contact with infected blood or body fluids. Contact with infected blood can occur through blood transfusions, sexual activity, using contaminated needles, or transmission from an infected mother to a baby.

If mom has Hepatitis B, then the baby receives the vaccine, as well as another medication called Hepatitis B Immunoglobulin, to help protect him. If mom does not have Hepatitis B, the baby is still vaccinated to protect him if he gets exposed to the Hepatitis B virus.

The vaccine has been approved for use by the FDA since 1981 and has a good safety profile. Children who are very sick, who are allergic to baker's yeast, or have reacted to previous doses of Hepatitis B should not get the vaccine. Obviously, with a newborn, you will not know if your baby is allergic to yeast, and she would not have received any previous doses. Therefore, the main medical reason for which your baby should not receive the vaccine during the first two days is if she is sick. Premature babies who are very small may not be given the vaccine until they weigh more than five pounds as long as mom does not have Hepatitis B. Mild side effects from the vaccine are possible, but rare. These include redness or soreness at the site of injection or low grade fever. Severe reactions generally are not seen, but may occur if the baby is allergic to the vaccine or its components.

What's Up, Doc?—The First Exam

"I wanted to find a pediatrician that I could call on anytime for help," said Wendy. "I love the pediatrician that I chose. They have advice nurses who will answer my questions at any time! It gives me peace of mind knowing that someone can help me if I'm not sure what to do."

"My son's doctor has Saturday appointments available," commented Timothy. "It's great for working parents!"

Hopefully, you've already chosen a pediatrician or family doctor for your child before you deliver your baby. Depending on your physician's practice, either your baby's doctor or a doctor working with the practice, or a hospital doctor will examine your baby during your stay in the hospital. Either way, a doctor should examine your baby in the first 24 hours of life.

This exam is important to reassure everyone that your baby is healthy and doing well.

Finding a Doctor for Your Baby

If you haven't chosen a doctor yet, you will need to find someone before you are discharged from the hospital. If you have not delivered yet, you would ideally like to decide on your doctor by the 36th week of pregnancy. That way, if you deliver early, you will already know whom to call. Most babies need to have an appointment to be seen by a doctor within one to two days after leaving the hospital.

There are many guides on the web that help parents choose a doctor. The first step is to decide what kind of doctor you want—a pediatrician, or a family practitioner. Pediatricians are trained specially in the care of children. After medical school, they spend at least three years in residency learning children's health and how to treat their medical issues. Most pediatricians will care for children from birth until adulthood (ages 18-21). Family practitioners take care of people of all ages. They spend three years after medical school in residency learning about the medical care of children and adults, with only a portion of the time for learning about children. Some parents prefer to go to someone who can treat the entire family, so they choose a family doctor. Other parents prefer to take their children to someone who is expertly trained in the care in children, so they choose a pediatrician.

Regardless of which type of doctor you choose for your child, it is a good idea to visit potential practices before you decide. Meeting the doctors and seeing the office will give you a good feel for whether or not the practice fits your needs. Ask your friends, family, neighbors, and obstetrician or midwife who they recommend. Generally, you want to find one who is close to your home or where your baby will be (if in daycare later). You will be seeing the doctor at least six times just during the first year for well visits, not to mention the number of times you'll be there when your child is sick!

Most practices have a pre-natal visit or expectant parent visit that you can schedule. This is your chance to interview potential practices. Some questions you may want to ask include the following:

- Are all the doctors board-certified?
- How many years has the practice been in business?
- What are your hours? Do you have weekend or evening hours?
- Do you have same day appointments for sick visits?
- Will I see different doctors each time, or do I have an assigned doctor?
- Are there multiple locations? Am I required to go to a particular office?
- Do you have advice nurses available for parents?
- Do you use electronic medical records?
- Do you offer online access for patients?
- Are lactation consultant services available?
- What do I do if I have an emergency? Who do I call?
- What's your policy on vaccines?
- Do you support breastfeeding? (if you are planning on breastfeeding)
- Do you do circumcisions? (If not, then your obstetrician is usually who performs the procedure.)
- How much time do you allow for appointments?
- What's the average wait time to be seen?
- Does the office have a laboratory on-site?

And here are some factors you'll want to observe about the practice:

- Is the waiting room divided to separate sick children from well children?

- Are there enough toys and books around to occupy children while they are waiting to be seen?
- Is the office child-friendly?
- Does the staff seem helpful and accommodating?

These are just some of the questions to consider and they are included in a convenient interview form for you at the end of the book (Appendix A). The most important thing is that you feel comfortable with the doctor and the practice. Your child's doctor will be an integral part of your child's health and well-being, and you want to feel confident that you are getting great care.

CHAPTER 3

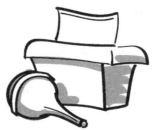

Behavior

Hiccups, Sneezing, and Gas…Oh My!

Sometimes your newborn may seem like she does not do a whole lot except sleep, eat, pee, poop, and cry—and that's basically true. There simply is not a whole lot of variety in behaviors at this age. But let that reassure you since that's what a healthy newborn should do. They sleep almost twenty hours a day. Basically, they are awake long enough to eat and get changed. Then, they go back to sleep. There may be one to two hours when she'll be awake—and of course, it will most likely be at night when you are trying to sleep!

There are few things that your newborn may do that may disturb or worry you. The ones below are behaviors that parents most commonly ask about.

Hiccups

For the first few months of life, hiccups are a common newborn behavior. You may have frequently felt your baby hiccup in utero. This does not change when your baby is born, except that now you can hear them! There is no need to try to stop the hiccups. Do not give your baby water as a remedy. Hiccups occur because the newborn nervous system is still very immature, and hiccups are triggered very easily. They will also disappear spontaneously. Hiccups do not bother babies; they only bother us!

Sneezing

Sneezing for a newborn is different from sneezing for older children or adults. For adults, sneezes may indicate illness or allergies. However, in a baby, they usually do not mean anything at all. The nervous system is still very immature, so this behavior is just triggered more easily. If your baby seems congested, then you can try to clear the nose (see Congestion). However, if he's not congested, that immature newborn nervous system is to blame. No need to do anything. It will stop.

Gassiness

"My baby is so gassy," reports Allison. "He sounds like a full-grown man sometimes...and boy, sometimes he smells like one too!"

No matter how properly you feed your baby, all babies are gassy. The way they feed, from either a bottle or a breast, results in air swallowing. If they are good burpers, most of it will be expelled. But the air that is left in the stomach has to come out the other end and is passed as gas. The gas may also include the normal by-products of digestion, so there is no reason to expect good-smelling gas from your little one!

If your baby is acting really fussy, but seems much happier after passing gas, then some anti-gas relief drops, such as Mylicon, may be the answer. These can be purchased over the counter at your local drug store or grocery store. These are safe to use starting during the newborn period. Just follow the dosing instructions on the bottle and give the drops to your baby directly into his mouth. If the drops do not help, then there may be other issues, such as formula intolerance or gastroesophageal reflux. Call your baby's doctor to discuss it further.

Noises While Sleeping

Newborns are not quiet sleepers. They grunt, make noises, and move a lot when they sleep. There is no need to intervene with every noise. If your baby is hungry or uncomfortable, he will wake up and cry. Only then do you need to check to see what is wrong. Otherwise, you will go crazy if you check on every noise and movement that your newborn makes while sleeping. This can be hard to do when your baby is sleeping in the same room as you. Try not to worry if he is making noises but is not fully awake and crying.

Rapid Breathing

Sometimes newborns have this special breathing pattern called "periodic breathing." This type of breathing occurs when they are asleep and only lasts for a few seconds. When a baby is doing this, she will take several very shallow, very rapid breaths in a row, and then take one large, almost gasping breath at the end of the episode. Then, your baby should resume normal, regular breaths. These episodes of periodic breathing should be infrequent and should not bother her. She should not experience any change to her skin tone. She should also breathe normally when awake. If your baby actually pauses between breaths for more than three to five seconds or changes color, then call 911 or your emergency services.

Congestion

"I think she's sick," worries John, father of a two-day-old newborn. "She is so congested and is always sneezing." When I asked him about other symptoms, the baby was otherwise well. No coughing, vomiting, or fever. She was feeding normally and pooping and making wet diapers.

As previously described, sneezing is normal and is not a sign of illness. Congestion can also be very normal. However, too much congestion may interfere with feeding since babies need to breathe through their nostrils during that time. Congestion with fever or significant cough is not normal, and you should immediately consult your child's doctor.

If there is no fever or other signs of illness, the congestion may be just the normal result of newborn breathing. Newborns prefer to breathe through their noses. As a result of this, the mucus dries and builds up very easily in their little nostrils. They will still try to breathe through their noses even with these secretions, so they may sound congested. To clean your baby's nostrils, use the nasal suction bulb most hospitals provide.

Many parents worry that the size of this hospital-grade bulb will hurt the baby because it looks so large in comparison to the baby's nose. This is not the case. The end of the device should be too big to go inside. It is when you start sticking smaller things into the nose that you may harm the tissues. You just want to press the end of the large suction bulb up against the nostril to create a good seal. See the instructions for suctioning the nose at the end of this section.

Smaller over-the-counter suction bulbs may not work very well. The size of the bulb is directly related to how much suction power is created. The little bulbs can be too small. Therefore, they do not produce enough suction power to pull out the mucus. The three ounce suction bulb that is given to you in the hospital works much better! You can order these online or ask your doctor if he or she can provide you with one.

Then you can squeeze the bulb out onto a tissue to empty out the secretions. Do not expect your baby to enjoy the process of having his nose suctioned. But he will feel much better afterward and will be able to breathe and eat more easily. He cannot blow his nose, so you must do it for him!

If you try this method, but you do not get much out, because the mucus is too dry or too far back in the nose, you can loosen the mucus. Do this by putting one to two drops of plain nasal saline into each nostril and then suctioning out whatever might be in there. You can buy non-medicated nasal saline for children in most drug stores and stores that carry baby supplies. This is safe to do several times a day as needed. If your baby has a true cold, you might end up doing this five to six times a day. Be careful to become overzealous though; sometimes you may end up causing a nosebleed or swelling of the nasal tissues from irritation.

HOW TO SUCTION THE NOSE

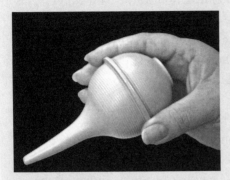

1. Hold the bulb in your hand.

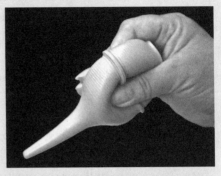

2. Squeeze the bulb BEFORE you put it on your baby's nostril.

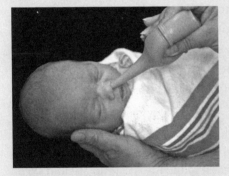

3. Put it onto your baby's nostril and make sure that you get a good seal.

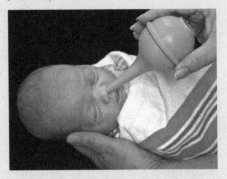

4. Release the bulb to draw the nasal secretions up into the bulb.

Then you can squeeze the bulb out onto a tissue to empty out the secretions. Do not expect your baby to enjoy the process of having his nose suctioned. But he will feel much better afterward and will be able to breathe and eat more easily. He cannot blow his nose, so you must do it for him!

If you try this method, but you do not get much out, because the mucus is too dry or too far back in the nose, you can loosen the mucus. Do this by putting one to two drops of plain nasal saline into each nostril and then suctioning out whatever might be in there. You can buy non-medicated nasal saline for children in most drug stores and stores that carry baby supplies. This is safe to do several times a day as needed. If your baby has a true cold, you might end up doing this five to six times a day. Be careful to become overzealous though; sometimes you may end up causing a nosebleed or swelling of the nasal tissues from irritation.

CHAPTER 4

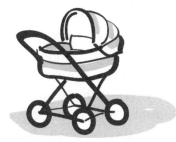

Staying Home, Going Out, and Traveling Safely

Staying Safe at Home

Home is the place where your baby is going to spend the majority of her day. Therefore, it is very important that you make your home environment safe and comfortable.

Room Temperature—Some Like It Hot!

"My wife loves to have the house cold—especially since she got pregnant," says Michael. "I'm wearing a sweater and a hat in bed every night because she has it so cold in our bedroom!"

What temperature should your house be for your baby? Many couples have thermostat battles, especially during the strange hormonal cycles of pregnancy. However, once the baby is born, the decision maker often becomes the baby, not the parents.

In general, mid-70s is a reasonable temperature for your house. If you prefer it warmer or cooler, then dress your newborn accordingly. A good rule of thumb is to have the baby wear one more layer than you do. If you are in shorts and a T-shirt, then the baby could be in a short-sleeve onesie and a thin receiving blanket. If you are in a sweater, turtleneck, and jeans, then your baby should be in two layers of clothing and a warmer blanket. She should not sleep with a thick blanket because of the risk of SIDS (Sudden Infant Death Syndrome). A zip-up fleece wearable blanket would be a safer choice.

In the first few weeks, many babies prefer to be swaddled. This is safe as long as the baby is not kicking free of the blanket. Many of the zip-up blankets include a swaddling piece that is attached with Velcro to the blanket so that it will not come loose. These are a great investment.

Be careful that you do not overheat the baby by wrapping him too warmly. Studies have shown an increase in the incidence of SIDS when babies are overheated. So, it is better not to overdress them. There are many cultures that believe that babies may get sick if they get cold. However, this is not true. Babies get sick from viruses and bacteria, not from how hot or cold they are.

How will you know if they are too hot or too cold? Usually, babies will cry if they are uncomfortable. If you've tried all the usual things, like changing diapers and feeding, and your baby is still unhappy, think about the possibility of him being too hot or cold.

If your baby's hands and feet are purplish or feel cold, you might want to put baby mittens or socks on him. When infants are cold, the first place they will often shunt blood away from is their hands and feet. This will make their hands or feet appear purplish. If this discoloration does not improve after you warm them, then call your doctor. If your baby's face or body appears blue, this may be a sign of a more serious heart or breathing problem. Call for help immediately.

Hot Water Temperature—Ouch!

Set your hot water heater to a maximum of 120 ºF (49 ºC). This allows the water to be hot enough for showers and cleaning, but will not be hot enough to result in accidental burns if skin is exposed briefly. A thirty-second exposure to hot water that is 130 ºF (54 ºC) will result in third-degree burns! By reducing the temperature to 120 ºF (49 ºC), a third-degree burn will not occur unless the exposure is at least ten minutes long.

Over four thousand children are scalded each year, primarily in bathtubs. While you may think that you would never let the water get that hot, accidents are never planned. Ninety-five percent of these injuries occur at home. A babysitter or visitor may be unaware of how hot your water gets and could accidentally leave the faucet on too hot. Also, when your child is older, she will start to wash her hands by herself, and you do not want to risk her burning herself. Change the water temperature now, and you won't have to remember to change it later!

If you live in an apartment or condominium where you do not have the ability to change the temperature setting for the hot water heater, consider installing commercially available anti-scald devices on your faucets. Also, try talking to your building manager or checking with local laws. Regulations that require apartment buildings in your area to set hot water heaters at lower temperatures to meet safety recommendations may already exist.

Pets—Baby's Best Friend?

"Do you have any pets?" I ask every new parent. Why would I ask this? Two reasons: one for safety, and the other to see if advice on bringing home a new member of the family is needed.

Many people will ask me about allergies and pets. Your newborn is too young to have allergies at birth, but she may develop allergies as she gets older. Some studies have shown that early exposure to animals prevents allergies, while other studies have shown that early exposure can cause allergies! So, no one really knows the answer right now. It is best to minimize exposure initially and then increase accordingly as your baby ages and your pet becomes more tolerant.

Your newborn should have limited exposure to animals for safety reasons. Your normally docile dog or cat may be offended that there is a new "baby" in the house and try to do things to get your attention. This could involve more aggressive behavior, or a pet might just want to "play" with the new baby—and that could lead to injury.

After coming home from the hospital, you may want to give your cat or dog an item of clothing that the newborn has already worn so that the pet can get used to the baby's scent.

Dogs are usually enthusiastic when you come home from the hospital, and you should be especially careful around large dogs. Therefore, it is best if the parent who is not holding the baby enters the house first. That way your pet can devote most of its energy to the first person. Afterward, the person holding the baby can enter.

Cats tend to not be very interested in touching the baby, but rather enjoy exploring where the baby has been. Take care to block the bassinet or crib so that the cat is not able to get into the baby's bed.

As your baby gets older, your pet will be more accustomed to her presence, and then they can be safely introduced to each other!

Other pets may not be as much of an issue. But be aware that certain birds and reptiles can carry diseases such as salmonella, which can make children sick. Wash your hands well between caring for your pets and holding your baby.

Smoking—A Good Reason to Quit!

Secondhand tobacco exposure has been shown to increase the chances of your child developing asthma, allergies, and ear infection. Being exposed to tobacco smoke also increases the chances of SIDS (Sudden Infant Death Syndrome).

According to the American Lung Association, exposure to secondhand smoke causes over 202,000 asthma episodes per year in children, results in middle ear fluid buildup, and increases frequency of lower respiratory infections, such as pneumonia and bronchitis. Babies exposed to smoke have weaker lungs after birth and are 20 percent more likely to have a low birth weight if mom was exposed during pregnancy.

If you must smoke, then smoke outside. To decrease the amount of secondhand smoke that your baby may inhale, it is best to wear a piece of clothing that you wear while you are smoking (such as a jacket or shirt), which you can remove once you are done. Infants can still breathe secondhand smoke from clothing.

If you ever needed a reason to quit smoking, your baby's health is a great one! There are many medications and patches that are now available to help people fight smoking cravings. See your doctor for more information.

Going Outside into the Big, Bad World

"When can we take the baby out?" asked Martha, cradling her two-week-old son in her arms. She and her husband looked at each other. "We want to take him for a walk—is that okay?"

Parents always ask me when it is okay to take the baby out. Quite frankly, it is not going out into the environment that is usually the problem, but rather all those germ-covered people who are out there. People can harbor viruses and bacteria on their bodies. Adults do not get sick all of the time because our immune systems are usually able to fight off these constant threats. Newborns, however, are still developing their immune systems and are more susceptible to illness.

For the most part, going out for a walk in your neighborhood to get some fresh air is a great idea, as long as the weather is good. If it is sunny, keep your baby in the shade and covered. Do not stay out too long, because your baby could get dehydrated and overheated. While you can use sunblock, the newborn's sensitive skin may react more easily to creams and could possibly develop a rash. Generally, you may want to wait until the baby is one to two months old before considering using sunblock on her skin. It is best just to keep your baby out of direct sunlight and use protective clothing such as hats and sunshades.

If it is cool or windy, keep your baby bundled appropriately, put a hat on her head, and protect her from the wind.

The bigger problem comes with taking your newborn near other people. We humans are walking germ factories! By going out into large crowds (such as the mall) or gatherings (like weddings or reunions), you are potentially exposing your newborn to diseases. In their happiness for you, other people tend to want to hold your baby, or at least touch the baby—and this is how disease can be transmitted.

While there are different schools of thought on what the actual age should be, most pediatricians will agree that you should limit a newborn's exposure to many people until he is at least four to six weeks of age. Others will advocate that babies should have limited exposure until up to three to six months.

Of course, your family and close friends will want to visit and wish you well. However, make sure that they all wash their hands before holding the baby. If they are sick, they should stay away until they are symptom free.

"How do I tell my sister-in-law to keep her little kids away from our baby?" asks Nina. "They are always so snotty and always seem to be sick. I'm worried that they will get my baby sick."

"That's a good question," I say to Nina. "Tell your sister that the doctor said that it was best to limit a newborn's exposure to other people, even though she may think you are being overly paranoid. Tell her that you really do not want to expose your baby to other kids right now."

I added, "If you think that will really make her mad and you are okay with the kids being at your house, then announce as soon as they arrive that they can *look* at the baby, but they cannot *touch* the baby. Also, have them wash their hands as soon as they arrive since they will be touching things in the house."

Remember that, while your family members' feelings are important, your top priority is the health of your child. At worst, people will think that you are being a super-paranoid first-time parent—but as long as your child is healthy, who cares?

If your baby gets sick and develops a fever at under four to six weeks of age, many times it is just a viral illness and the infant will recover. But do NOT assume this without calling your baby's doctor first! The consequences of missing a bacterial infection in a newborn or young infant could be very serious, even fatal.

Although there is some variation in physician practices, almost all doctors will admit young babies under four weeks of age with a fever to the hospital for lab tests, including a spinal tap to check for meningitis, and give the baby intravenous (I.V.) antibiotics to rule out serious illness. *A fever in a young infant is considered a rectal temperature greater than 100.4 ºF (38 ºC).*

It is in your baby's best interest for you to work hard to minimize the chance of him getting sick and having a fever during those first few weeks of life.

While you do not need to seclude your baby in a bubble, you should do the following:

1. Limit taking your baby to places where there are many people (such as malls, restaurants, and stores).
2. Anyone (including yourself) who touches your baby needs to wash his or her hands first.
3. Anyone who is ill should just stay away for now. That person can always see your baby later.
4. If someone in your household is ill and coughing, has a runny nose, or is sneezing, try to have that person use a mask in order to decrease airborne spread of viruses. You can buy simple masks at most drug stores. At the very least, that person should cover every cough and sneeze with a tissue.
5. Siblings who are ill should be separated from the newborn as much as possible. If you can separate the caregivers so that one adult takes care of the sick child and one adult takes care of the newborn, then that will help to minimize sharing of germs.
6. If mom is sick, most of the time it is still okay to breastfeed. The baby will get the protective antibodies that mom is making to fight the illness through the breast milk. The only exception to this is if mom is on certain medications. In this case, check with the doctor to see if it is still okay to nurse.
7. Again, strict hand washing should be done at all times! (Can I say it enough?)

Travel Safety — Walking, Driving and Flying

"I'm planning on taking Johnny to see my parents in Florida," said Marilyn nervously. "We have to fly about two hours on a plane. When is it safe to go? Do I need to do anything special?"

Traveling with a baby requires a lot of gear, a lot of planning, and a lot of patience. Whether you are traveling to another state or just down the street, there are many issues to consider, such as choosing strollers for walking, car seats for driving, and plans for flying.

Going for a Walk—Choosing a Stroller

Many times I try to go into an exam room to see one of my new parents and I cannot even open the door because of the humongous, super-deluxe travel system with car seat, sunshade, cup holders, rain cover, and all-terrain wheels blocking the door. It is amazing how many gadgets and convenience items strollers have now!

Shopping for baby equipment is almost as hard as buying a car. Who knew how many kinds of strollers and car seats there are? The latest model is constantly touted as better than the one before—lighter, easier to push, roomier, safer, and more convenient. We've come a long way from the simple umbrella stroller. So, now there are options such as walking strollers, jogging strollers, double strollers, and travel systems. Now, if only they could develop strollers that could feed and change the baby, too!

You want to look for a stroller that meets your daily needs, will fit in your car, can carry your stuff, and will last longer than a few months if possible. Babies grow so fast, and many babies will outgrow their infant carriers before a year of life. So, keep that in mind as you shop. You will likely have more than one stroller for different situations. Over the years, we have collected seven strollers, and I have only four kids!

Driving—Going on a Road Trip!

Driving is probably the easiest way to travel with a newborn, simply because you have the option to pull over and stop. I know of one family who took six hours to make a trip that would normally take two hours! Why? Because the baby was fussy much of the way, and they had to stop repeatedly to feed him, change him, etc. While this may not always be the case, plan on extra time for your travels. It is a safe bet that you will have to stop every two to three hours since that is usually how often a young infant needs to eat. If you plan accordingly, it will be much less stressful for all involved.

Choosing a Car Seat

Your newborn should be in an appropriate infant restraint when riding in a car. Usually this is a car seat approved for newborns and infants. There are a number of different types of car seats, and the infant ones may come with stroller systems. Each type of seat is designed for children of different weights, heights, and ages. Types of car seats include infant car seats, car beds, convertible car seats, and booster seats (see Figures 1 through 4).

Generally, an infant carrier is convenient because you can take the baby in and out of the car without having to wake her up. Many babies will outgrow the infant carrier before the first year of life, so you will then need a larger car seat that stays installed in the vehicle. Check with your state's laws

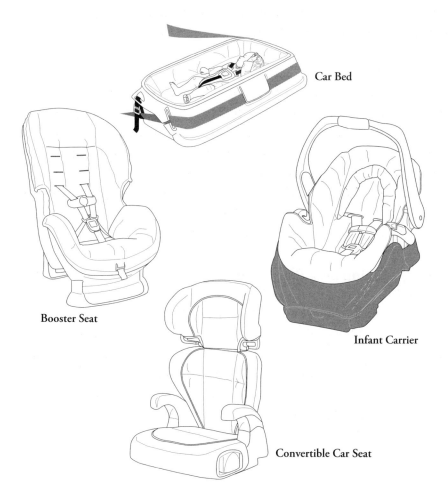

Car Bed

Booster Seat

Infant Carrier

Convertible Car Seat

to see requirements. Most states require that infants remain in rear-facing car seats until one year of age or until they weigh at least 20 pounds (9 kg).

Some low-birth-weight babies require an infant car bed (see Figure 1). If your baby is very small at birth, your hospital may perform a car seat challenge. This is a test to see whether or not the baby has adequate head and neck support to keep his head upright enough to breathe while in a car seat. If the baby is unable to do this, they will recommend a car bed, which looks a bit like a little bassinet that is buckled into the car. The baby will stay in this until he grows big enough to be in a regular infant seat.

Regardless of the type of car seat you have, it is best to have your car seat installation inspected at a safety station. This may be your local fire department or police department. You may be able to check the National Highway Traffic Safety Administration's web site for locations near you doing car seat inspections. While you may end up moving your car seat from car to car later on, it is a good idea to see what a certified car seat installer checks for in a safe installation.

If you get a hand-me-down or used car seat, make sure that it has never been in a car during an accident and has never been subject to a recall. A car seat that has been in an accident may have damage or undue stress placed upon the restraints. Also, make sure to check for consumer recalls on car seats. You can go online to the U.S. Consumer Product Safety Commission web site, and search for the brand and model of your car seat to see if there have been any recalls. This site is useful for all baby and children's products. There are frequently safety recalls on any number of items.

Flying—Going on a Plane with a Newborn

Flying with a baby is always a stressful situation. It is amazing how much stuff a tiny little baby needs and how bulky it is. All the bottles, milk, diapers, wipes, clothes, and not to mention all the gear! I remember flying with one of our children when he was a baby, and he had his own huge suitcase full of stuff, a car seat, and a portable crib! My husband and I just had our stuff crammed into one small suitcase—mostly because we couldn't carry anything else!

To reduce some of the items that you need to bring on an airplane, consider buying bulky items such as diapers and wipes once you arrive at your destination. Also, many hotels will provide a crib for you by request. If you are traveling for a longer period of time, baby equipment rental agencies may be a good option for items such as high chairs, portable cribs, and swings.

Usually, newborns make reasonable traveling companions when flying. As long as you feed them on time and change them, they are happy. Of note, they won't be able to "pop" their ears to equalize the ear pressure while in flight, but you can help them. When a baby is swallowing, he will naturally pop his ears. So during take-off, landing, and whenever your ears need to pop, try to have him swallow. A bottle, breast, or pacifier in the mouth will help to encourage this.

The main concern with air travel is that the re-circulation of air in the airplane may enhance the spread of viruses. Also, for the length of the flight, you might be in close proximity to people who are sick. Airborne viruses may travel more easily in an airplane. Once again, newborns are more susceptible than we are to catching colds and getting sick since their immune systems are not yet fully developed. If at all possible, try to put off flying until your baby is older than four to six weeks of age.

Sometimes that is not feasible, so you can help prevent illness by washing your hands often and keeping your baby away from anyone obviously coughing, sneezing, or sick who might be seated near you on the plane.

Traveling Abroad

"We are going to Africa in four weeks. Is that okay?" asks Christine. "My family is there, and I am planning to take the baby there for a few months."

The precautions to take when traveling abroad vary from region to region. The Center for Disease Control (CDC) has a web site that allows you to select your destination country to see what the latest recommendations for vaccines and medicines are for that country. For newborns and young infants, there are very few travel vaccines that can be given, other than the routine ones. For many countries, malaria prevention medications may be necessary. Your child may need these if he is old enough to be given the medication. See your baby's doctor or go to a travel clinic.

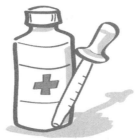

CHAPTER 5

Getting Sick— When to Worry

"Aa-choo, aa-choo, aa-choo!" sneezes a newborn in one exam room.

"Waahhhhhhhhhh!" complains another one in the room next door.

"Zzzzzzzzzzzzz…" sleeps another baby soundly in the third room.

Which one is sick? Well, the answer is that any of them might be sick, and it very much depends on whether or not each baby is showing other symptoms.

Newborns can get colds and minor illnesses just like adults and older children. However, they are more susceptible to serious illnesses, such as bacterial bloodstream infections or meningitis, because of their immature immune systems. Luckily, there are usually signs when significant illness is present, but often it takes someone with experience with treating young babies to diagnose the illness with lab tests and other studies.

So, how will you know when to seek help?

Newborns can show signs of illness by being lethargic and sleeping a lot. So, with a newborn, the concept of "sleeping through the night" is not necessarily a good thing—it often means that the baby is ill or dehydrated. They can have very low body temperatures instead of running a fever.

Some newborns are very irritable when they are sick, and despite your best efforts, you cannot make your baby happy.

Some babies are born with metabolic or anatomical problems that cannot be diagnosed until the baby is born. With the improvements in ultrasound technology and newborn state screening tests, many problems can be found before the baby is born or shortly after birth, and treatment can be planned ahead of time.

Following are some red flags that indicate serious illness in newborns. Read these carefully and memorize them if you can. Some are obvious; others are more subtle. If your baby shows any of these signs, call your child's doctor immediately. Your baby still may have only a minor illness, but it is important to be extra careful with young infants. This list is also included at the end of the book so that you can refer to it easily (Appendix B).

These red flags primarily apply to newborns and very young infants (babies under three months of age). As your baby gets older, her immune system

CALL YOUR DOCTOR IF ANY OF THE
FOLLOWING OCCUR WITH YOUR NEWBORN

1. Rectal temperature less than 97.0 ºF (36 ºC), or greater than 100.4 ºF (38 ºC). (See later in the section for how to take a rectal temperature.)
2. Difficulty breathing, flaring nostrils, or persistent cough. Call 911 if there is blueness of the face or body.
3. Difficulty with feeding for several feeds.
4. Less than three to four wet diapers in 24 hours.
5. Lethargic, difficult to wake up, or sleeping more than six hours straight, despite your best efforts to wake your baby.
6. Inconsolable fussiness or crankiness that lasts for more than two hours.
7. Projectile vomiting after most or all feeds.
8. Blood in stools, or frequent watery stools (more than five per day).
9. Bulging soft spot on the top of the head and fussiness.
10. White-colored stools.
11. No stools during the first three days of life.
12. Yellow-colored skin (jaundice) of the entire body, including the legs.

will become stronger and can fight off many more germs and diseases. This does not mean that you can stop being vigilant, but it does mean that after three months of age, every fever is not necessarily an emergency. Ask your doctor for guidance on when to call.

Taking Rectal Temperatures: You want me to put that where?

"Is that really the only way?" John looked at me with an "Are-you-for-real?" expression on his face. His wife Michelle looked at me in horror and asked, "Are you sure it won't hurt her?"

"No, it won't hurt, but she won't really enjoy the process," I reassured them. "Let me show you how to do it safely."

Up until at least six months of age, the most accurate way to take your baby's temperature is rectally. Many parents get squeamish at the thought of putting a thermometer "down there," but it is not as bad as it sounds. Your baby may cry, but it is because something is different and feels strange—not because it hurts.

Rectal temperatures are the only way to get an accurate temperature in a newborn. Ear thermometers are fine after six months of age. Before then, it is difficult to get an accurate ear temperature because of the small size of babies' ear canals. Oral temperatures cannot be done accurately until the child can hold a thermometer still under the tongue (typically seven years of age or older). Pacifier thermometers and forehead strip thermometers are not accurate and should not be used.

Taking axillary, or under-the-armpit, temperatures is a common method, but again, rectal temperatures are the most accurate. If you get an elevated or low temperature when measuring under the arm, you should take a rectal temperature to confirm high or low readings in a young infant. Do not rely on adding a degree to the axillary measurement to estimate your newborn's actual temperature.

Temporal artery thermometers, which are digital thermometers that you slide over the temporal artery in the forehead, are reasonable to use for an estimate as well. But these can be difficult to use on a squirming, fussy infant. Again, take a rectal temperature to confirm your readings.

Your child's doctor will make important treatment decisions based on the rectal temperature of your child, so you need to be able to do this comfortably.

How to Take a Rectal Temperature
Coat the tip of a digital thermometer with a lubricant, such as petroleum jelly.

Place your child...

a) belly-down on a firm, flat surface and keep your palm along the lower back.

or

b) face-up with legs bent toward the chest, with your hand against the back of the thighs.

With your other hand, insert the lubricated thermometer into the anal opening about ½ inch to one inch (about 1.25 to 2.5 centimeters)—just until the metal tip is no longer visible. Stop if you feel any resistance.

Steady the thermometer between your second and third fingers as you cup your hand against your baby's bottom. Soothe your child and speak quietly as you hold the thermometer in place.

Wait until you hear the appropriate number of beeps or other signal that the temperature is ready to be read. Write down the number displayed on the screen, noting the time of day that you took the reading.

If your thermometer does not use a disposable cover, clean the thermometer as directed by the manufacturer's instructions. Many thermometers can be cleaned by rinsing in warm soapy water. Once a thermometer has been used for rectal temperature, it should not be used for other methods for sanitary reasons—especially oral temperatures!

When should you take your baby's temperature? There's no need to do so constantly. Generally, if your baby is sick, he will act sick. If your baby feels warm, if he is fussy and you cannot figure out why, or if he is lethargic, then take your child's temperature to rule out a fever or very low body temperature.

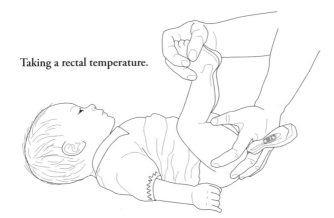

Taking a rectal temperature.

As mentioned in previous chapters, newborns are also unique in that sometimes instead of getting hot or having a fever when they are sick, they actually get cold. Their regulatory system for temperature is still immature, and sometimes they have low temperatures and get hypothermic instead. So, if your newborn's temperature is **less than 97.0 ºF (36 ºC)**, call your doctor immediately.

A temperature in an infant under three months of age that is **above 100.4 ºF (38.0 ºC)** is considered a fever. If this occurs, then you need to call your doctor, whether it is day or night, or go to the emergency room.

Infants under three months of age should not be given any medication for fever without being evaluated by a doctor. Medications will not treat the underlying reason for the fever. It may also mask a high temperature if you give fever reducing medication, such as acetaminophen (like Tylenol) or ibuprofen (like Motrin or Advil). If your infant is under three months of age, do not use these medicines without the guidance of a physician.

Thermometers: Which One to Buy?

There are many different types of thermometers available on the market. Here is a brief description of what is available:

Digital thermometers tend to provide the quickest, most accurate readings. They are available at most supermarkets and pharmacies in a range of prices. Digital thermometers usually can be used for rectal, oral, or axillary measurements.

For rectal temperatures, I recommend getting one that beeps and gives you a reading within a few seconds. It would be very difficult to hold a newborn still for a full minute. Digital thermometers usually have a plastic, flexible probe with a temperature sensor at the tip. Some use disposable plastic sleeves or covers

Electronic ear thermometers measure the tympanic temperature—the temperature inside the ear canal. Although they're quick and easy to use in older babies and kids, when used on infants three months or younger, they aren't as accurate. Readings can be inaccurate because of the way you are pointing the tip into the ear. They can also be affected by the presence of a lot of ear wax, as well as the size of the ear canal. This type of thermometer is also more expensive. While they are easy to use, they should not be used in newborns.

Temporal artery thermometers are not accurate for newborns. They are digital and can be somewhat expensive. You use a temporal artery thermometer by sliding it across the forehead over the temporal artery to measure temperature. They can be difficult to use on a squirmy, feverish newborn and are not as accurate as a rectal temperature.

Plastic strip thermometers (small plastic strips that you press against the forehead) are not accurate.

Pacifier thermometers may seem easiest, but they are not accurate for measuring temperatures and many require kids to keep the pacifier in their mouth for several minutes without moving, which is not possible for most babies.

Glass mercury thermometers were once common, but should not be used because of concerns about possible exposure to mercury, which is an environmental toxin. These need to be disposed of in a special way, so do not just throw them in the trash.

CHAPTER 6

Crying—What Does It Mean?

Crying is your baby's primary way of communicating. If your baby is tired, hungry, cold, sick, hurt, lonely, bored, upset, or just wants to be changed, you will generally know because your baby will cry. Over time you may be able to tell what your baby wants based on the type of cry.

If you aren't sure why your baby is crying, just go through a routine and try things that commonly cause discomfort. Trying changing, feeding, holding, rocking, burping, re-wrapping, and walking with your baby.

Some parents say they are able to tell from the beginning what their baby is trying to say with the crying. However, most people learn over time what the different pitches and types of crying mean. Some parents never actually figure it out, but they establish a routine of things to check when their baby cries, and usually one of them will solve the problem.

Baby Cry Translator
"Feed me! I'm hungry!"
This is the most frequent cause for crying. Look for signs like rooting (moving the mouth and turning the head to the side looking to nurse),

sucking on his fingers or hands, and the amount of time since the last feeding. Most babies need to suck on something to relax. So, if you know that you just fed your baby, give him something to suck on, such as a pacifier or a clean finger.

"My diaper is dirty—it's yucky!"
After being hungry, a dirty diaper is the second most common cause for crying. Most babies are uncomfortable if their diapers are soiled.

"I'm tired!"
When babies are over tired, they cry. Rocking, vibrations, holding, and singing or humming can help an over tired baby fall asleep.

"There's too much noise!" or "It is too bright!"
Overstimulation can make a baby feel overwhelmed to the point where she will cry. Taking your baby to a quiet, darker environment may help to soothe her.

"It is cold!" or "It is hot!"
If your baby's hands or feet feel cold, or if he is sweating, then it is likely that a change in clothing or wrapping can fix the problem.

"Hold me…I'm lonely!"
Babies like to be held. Sometimes that's all that they want. That's how they know you are there. If you cannot get to her right away, sometimes just talking will help since she can hear that you are nearby. You cannot "spoil" a baby by holding her too much during the first two months.

"My tummy hurts!"
The most common bodily discomforts that newborns have revolve around the digestive system. If they are overly full, need to burp, or are especially gassy, they will feel bloated and uncomfortable. Try to burp your baby. Sometimes rubbing the belly gently in circles or laying her face down so that her tummy is across your lap will help. This gentle pressure on the belly can relieve the pressure. Anti-gas relief drops, such as Mylicon, may also be helpful and can be used safely from birth.

Colic should not be considered as a cause of fussiness in a newborn. In general, colic does not start until three weeks of age and tends to end by three months of age. Even if your baby has colic, it is important to rule out other causes of fussiness first, such as milk allergy, reflux, constipation, or illness.

"My finger/toe hurts!"

Sometimes there really is something painful to cry about. Check fingers, toes, and other body parts to make sure that nothing is caught on a piece of thread, or hair, or is injured. Look for swelling, redness, scratches, or bleeding. You may be able to treat minor injuries at home, but it is always safer to check with your doctor since your newborn is so young.

"I'm sick and feel lousy!"

If working through all of the items above does not solve the problem, then take your baby's temperature. If you get a rectal temperature of more than 100.4 ºF (38 ºC), or less than 97 ºF (36 ºC), call your doctor immediately. Even if the temperature is normal and your baby has been crying for more than two hours without being consolable, call your doctor. Your baby may be sick and will need to be checked.

CHAPTER 7

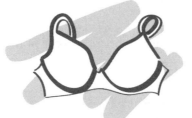

Breastfeeding— Breast is Best!

Breastfeeding 101

Breastfeeding is recommended for the first year of life by the American Academy of Pediatrics. In reality, a year can be a long time for many women in today's busy society, and breastfeeding for this long is often not feasible or practical. There are many benefits to breastfeeding, including improved immunity, protection against asthma and allergies, and increased immunity against many diseases, such as ear infections. However, many babies are successfully given formula for most or all of their infancy and have no difficulty.

There are many factors that determine how your baby ends up feeding. Of course, it starts with your plan. But, once your baby arrives, be prepared to adjust your plan if needed.

Some common factors that determine what a baby is fed include:

Maternal health, in particular just after the delivery. If mom has had a tough delivery or has complications, she may not be able to nurse the baby immediately. Breastfeeding may not be recommended if mom is taking certain medications.

Breast condition. If mom has had breast surgery or has flat or inverted nipples, breastfeeding can be challenging. If mom has large breasts and the baby's mouth is small, latching on effectively can be difficult. Nipple shields can be helpful in many cases. Working with a lactation consultant may be needed in these situations.

Baby's health. If your baby has signs of jaundice or has too much weight loss in the first few days, you may need to supplement your breast milk with some formula. If your baby is ill, has a syndrome, or was born prematurely, you may be instructed to feed your baby using different formulas or methods.

Baby's preference. Strange but true, some babies seem to be born with a preference. Most can adapt as needed. Some prefer breastfeeding only (which can be a challenge later when you try to wean). Others just do not seem to be able to breastfeed easily and need to be bottle-fed. Sometimes this is due to anatomical issues with the baby's mouth or tongue. Bottle-feeding requires less effort on the baby's part, so they will sometimes opt for the easier method and prefer bottle-feeding.

Mom's preference. Notice how low this is on the list of factors. While it is perfectly reasonable to have a plan when you start this process, be prepared to adjust it if needed!

Working need. Depending on if and when you go to work, the accessibility to areas at work where you can pump, your stress levels at work, and the time you have available at work, your ability to produce breast milk can be affected and will likely contribute to your feeding plans.

Even with all of these issues, millions of women throughout the world breastfeed very successfully. If you are breastfeeding, do not be surprised if it does not quite work out perfectly at first. It can take two weeks or more to establish breastfeeding. In the beginning, it can be very painful until your nipples get used to the force of suction, and this deters many mothers. It is also a little more exhausting since only the mother can do the feedings every two to three hours. Bottle-fed infants can be fed by other people, such as the father or grandparents. If you are breastfeeding and having trouble, I highly recommend that you work with a lactation consultant to find solutions that may help you.

How do I hold the baby to breastfeed?

There are four breastfeeding positions that have been shown to be most beneficial for mom. You may need to experiment with all of them to find the one that is most comfortable for you. Also, you may need to change position based on the situation.

"I was in so much pain after my C-section, breastfeeding just seemed impossible. Just finding a comfortable position was the hardest part!" proclaimed Heather. "I worked with the lactation consultant in the hospital. In the end, the football hold worked best for me. Later, after my incisions healed, I changed to more traditional holds."

Elizabeth described, "I was sure that I was going to breastfeed my baby from day one. However, I went into labor four weeks early, and my baby weighed only five pounds, one ounce. He was just too small to get onto my breast. So, instead I pumped and gave him breast milk without actually breastfeeding. This way he was able to get all the benefits of breast milk. Later, I was able to actually have him nurse, but I had to wait until he was big enough."

Cradle Hold

This is a commonly used position and works best for term babies, older babies, and moms who delivered vaginally. This hold puts too much pressure on the abdomen for moms who had Caesarian sections.

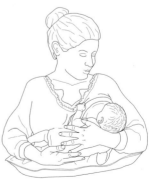

To do this hold, sit in a chair that has armrests or put pillows under your arms to provide extra support so your arms do not get tired.

Rest your feet on a stool or other raised surface so that you are not leaning down toward the baby.

If the baby is feeding on the right breast, then put the baby's head in the crook of your right arm. His mouth should be directly in front of your nipple.

Use your right arm to support the baby's head, back, and bottom.

Tuck the baby's right arm around your waist so it is out of the way.

Turn the baby so that you are belly-to-belly. He should be facing you. His knees should be folded close into your body just under or on your left breast. His body should be horizontal or at a very slight angle.

Cross-cradle Hold

This hold is very helpful for many during the newborn phase or for smaller, premature infants. You have better control over the baby's head and can see the latch easier. It is very similar to the cradle hold, but using the opposite arm.

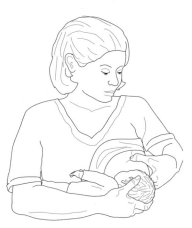

To do this hold, sit in a chair that has armrests or put pillows under your arms to provide extra support so your arms do not get tired.

Rest your feet on a stool or other raised surface so that you are not leaning down toward the baby.

If the baby is feeding on the right breast, then put the baby's head in the crook of your left arm. Her mouth should be directly in front of your nipple.

Use your left forearm to support the baby's back and the crook of your arm to support her bottom. Use your palm to support the head. Spread your thumb and first finger to create a U-shape around your baby's upper head.

Turn the baby so that you are belly-to-belly. She should be facing you.

Use your other hand (the right hand in this case) to lift your breast to guide it toward your baby's mouth. Do not lean forward; instead cradle your baby in toward your breast. Again, her body should be horizontal or at a very slight angle.

Football Hold

This hold works well for moms who cannot do the cradle or cross-cradle hold comfortably. This includes mothers who have had C-sections; moms with small babies, twins, or babies who have trouble latching on; moms who have difficulty with one side; or those with large or flat nipples.

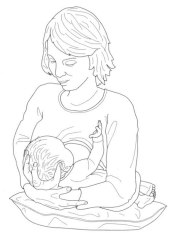

You are essentially holding the baby under your arm on the same side that you are feeding from, kind of like you would tuck a football under your arm.

Start by having the baby lie beside you on some pillows to raise her up a little. She should be facing you with her nose at your nipple level and her feet sticking out behind you.

If you are feeding on the right side, you should "scoop" her body up a little by putting your inner forearm underneath her body, back, and neck.

Use your palm to support her head. Use your first finger and thumb in a U-shape to support the head.

Guide her mouth to your nipple. Try to lean the head back very slightly, chin first, while you guide her to the breast.

Lying Down

This position is helpful if sitting up is uncomfortable, or you're nursing in bed and would rather lie down than sit up. Be careful that you will not fall asleep while lying down so that you do not accidentally roll onto your baby!

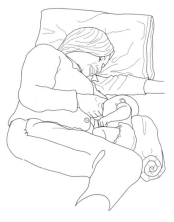

Lie on one side and support your head and back with pillows.

Lay the baby beside you facing toward you, belly-to-belly. If needed, you can put a rolled-up blanket behind his body to prevent him from rolling backward.

At first, use the hand on the side you are lying on to support the baby's head. Once a latch has been established, you can bend your arm under your own head for support.

His mouth should be opposite your nipple. Use the arm opposite the side you are lying on to guide your breast to his mouth. He should be at the level of your nipple. If needed, raise him up on a small pillow or folded blanket.

To feed on the other side, you can reposition yourself and the baby by turning over onto the other side. Some women can just lean farther over to put the other nipple into the baby's mouth. However, make sure the baby is in good position and is not straining to reach the nipple.

Supplementation–Do I need to do this?

"I really only wanted to just breastfeed, and I was determined to breastfeed successfully," explained Anne. "But then Mikayla became very jaundiced, wouldn't nurse well, and stopped making wet diapers. My doctor told me that I had to supplement with formula or Mikayla would be dehydrated and might need phototherapy for the jaundice. I was devastated and felt like a total failure of a mother already. I must have cried for hours."

"Luckily, my doctor and the lactation consultant worked with me closely. I still was able to breastfeed her and gave her formula supplementation after each nursing until my breast milk came in on the fourth day. We avoided having to give Mikayla the light therapy, and she was able to come home with me when I was discharged on the third day after delivery." Anne said proudly, "She has been breastfeeding fine ever since then and she's ten months old now!"

Supplementing along with breastfeeding is an option for many babies. In particular, if there are medical issues such as jaundice, weight loss, or dehydration in the first few days of life, supplementing is not only an option, but is needed to prevent further problems for your newborn. Supplementation can be done with formula or with pumped breast milk, if you have any. Many times this has to be done just because the breast milk supply is not adequate until three to four days after delivery.

Supplementation can be given to the baby using various methods including a bottle, finger feeding, or syringe feeding. The last two methods do not involve a bottle nipple and can be used for those moms concerned about "nipple confusion." Many babies do not have any trouble feeding from both bottle and breast for the first few days. However, there are certainly some moms who swear that their baby never took to the breast again after taking a bottle. Drinking from a bottle is certainly easier than from a breast and this may be the reason why some babies resist going back to the breast.

Remember that if your baby has jaundice or has lost too much weight, supplementing is not a bad thing and may be preventing further health complications. If you are really concerned about using a bottle, then ask about finger feeding or syringe feeding. This is a way to provide supplementation without having to use a bottle. Essentially, the baby "nurses" on your finger while you inject formula with a syringe beside your finger. This emulates breastfeeding and generally eliminates chances of nipple confusion.

How do I pump breast milk?

"I wanted to pump my breast milk since I knew I would be going back to work," explained Nicole. "It really hurt when I started to do it and it felt so weird being hooked up to a machine. I felt like a cow!"

Pumping breast milk is very common. This is a great way to store breast milk for future use, and allows other people to feed your baby while still giving him the benefits of breast milk. Most women end up using a pump if they go back to work while still nursing their baby.

Breast pumps come in various styles. Hospital–grade pumps have stronger motors and are very useful in the first few days when you are trying to stimulate your body to produce breast milk. These are very expensive to buy. Many hospitals or lactation programs will rent this type of pump.

HOW TO FINGER/SYRINGE FEED

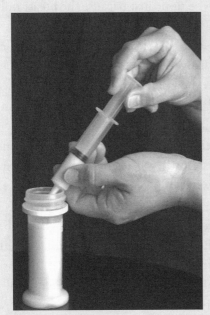

Draw up formula or pumped breast milk into a clean syringe.

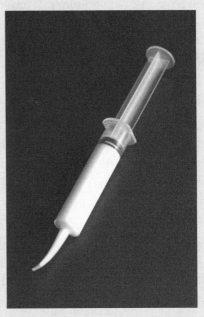

Fill the syringe until it is almost full.

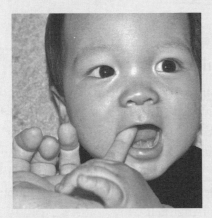

Put your clean pinky finger into your baby's mouth up to the first knuckle.

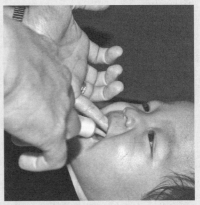

Insert the syringe next to your finger and slowly push the plunger to release formula/breast milk into your baby's mouth while he is sucking on your finger. Push it fast enough so that he has enough to drink, but not so fast that it dribbles out of his mouth.

Personal–use electric pumps, such as Medela or Ameda, are well suited for mothers who will be returning to work or who wish to pump on a regular basis. Most electric pumps allow you to pump from both breasts at the same time and mimic true nursing, which helps you to maintain your milk supply.

Manual pumps are operated by hand and can be very tiring to use. These can be useful for very occasional use. They do not provide as much power as electric pumps. The benefit of manual pumps is that they are inexpensive.

Be careful if considering buying a used or borrowed pump. Certain diseases, such as HIV, hepatitis, and other serious viruses, can be transmitted through breast milk. Only re-use a pump if it is approved for multiple users and buy a new set of attachments, including tubing, breast shields, valves, and collection bottles.

Pumped breast milk can be stored according to the "Rule of Three's." It can be kept at room temperature for three hours, in the refrigerator for three days, and in the freezer for three months.

Can I take medicines while breastfeeding?

"My doctor gave me codeine for pain after my C-section," said Donna. "But I was afraid to take it while I was nursing."

If mom is breastfeeding and taking medications, it is important to make sure that it is safe to continue breastfeeding while taking those medicines. Just as in pregnancy, certain medications should be avoided. If the medicine that mom is taking is not compatible with breastfeeding, then the milk can be pumped and discarded until mom is done taking the medication. Each medicine is metabolized at a different speed, so it may be several hours to a day before the last traces of medicine are out of the breast milk.

Unfortunately, many medications have not been tested to see if they are fully safe for breastfeeding. Several good references exist that rank medications as safe, likely safe, moderately safe, moderately unsafe, or definitely unsafe. Since new medications are invented and new studies are constantly being performed, the best thing to do is to check with your pediatrician or family doctor to see if breastfeeding can continue while taking the medication.

Vitamin D for Your Baby

Breast milk is loaded with great health benefits for your baby, including antibodies, fats, proteins, vitamins and minerals. However, it is lacking in sufficient vitamin D. The American Academy of Pediatrics recommended that babies who are breastfed be given vitamin D supplements to prevent a bone disease called rickets. Your baby needs 400 IU of vitamin D per day. This can be purchased over the counter in either a pure vitamin D liquid vitamin or as part of a multi-vitamin liquid, such as Poly-Vi-Sol or Tri-Vi-Sol.

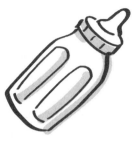

CHAPTER 8

Bottle-feeding—
The Essentials

If you choose to bottle-feed, or if you do a combination of breast- and bottle-feeding, it can be overwhelming at first when you look at all the types and brands of bottles on the market.

Sarah lamented, "When my baby was born, he didn't want to latch on, so we ended up having to use a bottle to supplement during the first few weeks to make sure he would gain weight. I had completely planned on breastfeeding, so I didn't have any bottles in the house. I wasn't feeling well enough to go to the store, so I sent my husband. He was absolutely stunned into immobility when he went to the baby store and saw the bottle selection! He called me from the store for help, and I had no idea what to tell him! Wide bottles, thin bottles, straight nipples, cross-cut nipples... So, I told him to just get a few different kinds. Now we have at least six different kinds of bottles and even more kinds of nipples in the house!"

Bottles, Bottles, Everywhere!

Which one to buy? Well, quite frankly, the one that your baby will take! Babies tend to be picky over not so much the bottle, but rather the nipple that is used. The nipples are designed to have various levels of flow, and many try to simulate the breast nipple shape. Many babies do not seem to have any issues over it. Here's a quick guide to the various kinds of nipple shapes and flows and which babies may benefit from them.

Nipples: What Shape?

Straight nipple: As its name suggests, this nipple is straight and narrow. This is a common type of nipple that many babies tolerate well.

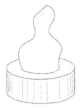 *Orthodontic nipple:* This type of nipple is curved and is meant to simulate the shape of a breast nipple inside the mouth. Many babies who are both breast-fed and bottle-fed do well with this type of nipple. One example of this is Gerber's NUK nipple.

Cross-cut nipple: The opening to this nipple is a small X-shape. This X-shaped opening allows thicker formula to flow freely. Babies who are receiving thickened formula for certain conditions, such as gastroesophageal reflux, may need this type of nipple.

Premature nipples: These nipples are smaller and have a slower flow. They are designed for premature infants. They also work for very small term babies who need a slower flow.

Nipple Flow Rate

Nipples are rated by their level of flow: slow, medium, or fast.

Slow flow: In general, newborns and young infants need the slower flow nipple. This prevents the fluid from coming out too quickly and gagging them.

Medium flow: While the age range on changing to this nipple may vary, I would recommend changing to a medium flow nipple when your baby is a little older (around six months) and is drinking fairly quickly. If your baby gags and sputters when you switch to this one, then he may not be ready for it yet.

Fast flow: As the name implies, fast flow nipples allow quicker fluid flow. This is best suited for older infants, usually around nine months of age.

Bottles: Which Type?

Each brand of bottle touts its own design. Many claim to decrease gas ingestion. Some babies may not benefit from the elaborate designs. Some bottles are free of plastic additives, while others are made of glass or plastic, and may use plastic bag inserts. I would recommend choosing one or two kinds, and buying just a few of each (so that you can have at least one clean one when the others are dirty). Then, try them out on your baby. Once you have settled on a certain type, buy many, many more so that you do not have keep washing them all day! If you are bottle-feeding only, you will be using at minimum six to eight bottles per day. When your baby is young, the last thing you need to be doing while you're exhausted is washing dishes! Start with the smaller sized bottles (usually two to four ounces). As your baby grows, you will need the larger bottles.

"Now I have the bottle...What do I put in it?"

If buying the bottle and nipple weren't challenging enough, now you have to pick a formula! All one has to do is to stroll through the baby section of the grocery store to realize that there are a *lot* of formula types out there! And they keep coming up with new ones.

For the most part, you will start with a cow's milk based formula. Generally, I recommend a brand-name formula when your baby is a newborn, since these formulas have been time-tested and most babies have no trouble with them. As your baby gets older, you can switch to a store-brand formula if you desire. Unless your baby is premature or has a medical condition, you won't know if your child needs a special or different formula. So, it is best to start with one that most babies can tolerate.

All formula has to meet basic federal nutrition standards. However, they are not all identical. Many have extra supplements or different proteins with claims to enhance growth, development, aid digestion, reduce colic, etc. It is up to you which one you want to use. Often, you will receive samples of the most popular formulas at the hospital when you deliver or at prenatal visits. It is fine to start with one of these. If your child has a reaction, or seems unhappy with a particular formula, your doctor can guide you on switching to another formula.

"I had breast surgery, so I couldn't breastfeed," stated one mom. "So, I started Jack on a regular formula that they gave me in the hospital. Immediately, he began spitting up with each feeding, even though it was only half an ounce per feeding. He was gassy and clearly uncomfortable. So, my doctor suggested that I try a soy formula. It was like night and day, he settled down nicely after I switched him."

What are some signs of formula intolerance? Gassiness is not particularly reliable since every baby is gassy. However, blood in the stool is the most common sign of a cow's milk allergy. If you see this, call your child's doctor.

Sometimes spitting up can be a sign, but sometimes it is a normal spit-up. And sometimes it can be more significant if it results from gastroesophageal reflux disease. If you think the formula is the culprit, you might try changing it to see if there is any improvement. Inconsolable fussiness for more than two hours can be a sign of a more serious condition so you should see your child's doctor.

Of note, if your baby is gassy or spitty in the first two days, I generally do not recommend switching formulas at this early stage. Sometimes babies are just settling into being a newborn and then they are fine after a few days. If the problems still continue after the first week, then a formula change may be advised.

TABLE 2: A QUICK GUIDE TO THE MAJOR TYPES OF FORMULAS

TYPE	EXAMPLES
Cow's milk based	Enfamil Premium Newborn, Enfamil Premium Infant, Similac Advanced
Soy milk based	Prosobee, Isomil
Lactose-free	LactoFree, Similac Lactose-free
Thickened formula	Enfamil AR, Similac Sensitive RS
Hypoallergenic	Nutramigen, Alimentum
Premature/ High calorie	Enfacare, NeoSure
Toddler	Enfamil Premium Toddler, GrowN'Go
Toddler/ High calorie	Pediasure, Boost

CHAPTER 9

Feeding Amounts and Feeding Problems

Hungry All the Time!

Your newborn will need to eat on average every two to three hours. Notice that I say "on average." This means that sometimes it will be every hour, and sometimes it may stretch to four hours. Until your baby regains his or her birth weight, you should probably wake her up for feedings every two to three hours. A four-hour stretch (hopefully at night) would be fine as long as there are no medical issues such as jaundice, prematurity, or significant weight loss.

If you are breastfeeding, you may be feeding your baby every one to two hours in the first few days. This is due in part to the fact that most women do not start producing breast milk until three to four days after delivery. Up until that point you have colostrum, which is a rich fluid filled with protective antibodies, but is only a few drops of fluid. Your baby will likely still be hungry after nursing and will want to eat again soon. Once your breast milk comes in, the time between feedings should stretch out to two to three hours on average. If you are still nursing every hour and your milk has come in, you may want to discuss this with your pediatrician or lactation consultant.

When you measure frequency of feedings, the timing is from the start of one feeding to the start of another feeding. This surprises many parents because it really seems like one long feeding. Generally, a feeding will take 30-45 minutes, so you really only get about an hour break in between feeds.

After your baby regains birth weight, then you are more safely able to let the baby set his own schedule. Most babies will wake up for feeds every two to three hours. By four months of age, most can sleep "though the night" for six to eight hours at night.

For your convenience, a sample tracking sheet for your baby's feeding and stooling/voiding pattern is included in the back of this book in Appendix C. This tool is a useful reference for you and your child's doctor when discussing your baby's habits.

Do You Have a Piggy or a Snacker?

Parents always ask me how much their baby should be eating. This is actually a difficult question because there is a different answer for every baby. While guidelines exist that pertain to most babies, pediatricians generally gauge whether or not your baby is eating enough by whether or not your baby is gaining weight appropriately.

We have the luxury of knowing exactly how much your baby weighs that day, and thus, we can answer that question more easily. Weight is a measure of adequate feeding. That being said, unless your baby has health issues, I do not usually recommend that you get a baby scale. Just as you would if you weighed yourself every day, you'll drive yourself crazy if you watch your baby's weight fluctuate on a daily basis.

General guidelines for newborns and infants are listed below. I would start with following these rules, but if your doctor tells you something different, it is usually for a good reason.

First things first: you will quickly learn that newborns drink in metric measurements, such as cc's or ml's (milliliters). Then, after the first week or two, you will start measuring in the English measurement system of ounces (oz.). For your conversion, 30 cc = 30 ml = 1 oz. I have no idea why doctors do it this way, but we do. Your doctor will want to know how much the baby is taking at every feeding, as well as the number of times he has urinated and has passed stools.

In the hospital, you will usually be given a chart on which to write this information. Just continue it when you go home for the first week or so. After that, you'll get the hang of what your baby's feeding and output pattern is and will be able to answer the questions when asked by your doctor.

In the first three to four days of life, most babies will take 15 cc (ml) to 45 cc (ml) per feeding. This is very much dependent on the size of your baby's stomach. It is approximately the size of a golf ball. If the amount of fluid does not fit, then your baby will spit it up. If you give 45 cc each time, and each time there is spit-up, then you may want to cut back a little. However, if you give only 15 cc each time and your baby still keeps spitting up, then your baby may have a stomach condition, such as reflux, and you need to discuss this with your doctor.

If you are giving formula, then you are able to measure the amount that the baby is taking. If you are breastfeeding, you won't know how much your baby is drinking. Aim for about 15-20 minutes per breast each feeding. Your body produces breast milk based on demand. So, if your baby (or a breast pump) is on your breast for 15-20 minutes every two to three hours, then usually your body will eventually make enough milk. Remember that during the first three to four days of breastfeeding, you will not have much more than a few drops of colostrum.

So, how do you know if your newborn is getting enough? There are a few clues. Your newborn should have about four wet diapers in a 24-hour period, and at least one stool per 24 hours. All newborns lose weight in the beginning, so do not take this as a sign of breastfeeding failure.

Loss of Weight (For Your Baby, Not You!): When to Get Concerned

If your baby has lost more than 10 percent of his birth weight, then he is getting too dehydrated. How do you tell if your baby has lost too much weight? Below is an example calculation. Remember to convert the pounds to ounces before making this calculation.

- Baby Ryan weighs 7 lbs. 10 oz. at birth. First, convert the pounds to ounces. There are 16 ounces in a pound.
  - 7 lbs. = 7 x 16 oz./lb. = 112 oz.
  - Then, add the ounces <u>+ 10 oz.</u>
  - Total ounces = 122 oz.
- If Baby Ryan can lose 10 percent of his birth weight, which we just calculated to be 122 oz., then he can lose 122 oz. x 0.10 = 12.2 oz., or approximately 12 oz.
- Thus, Baby Ryan can lose 12 oz. before we would get concerned. Since his birth weight was 7 lbs. 10 oz., we would not worry unless his weight dropped to below 6 lbs. 14 oz. (remember that there are 16 oz. in a pound). If he dropped below this weight, then formula supplementation would be in order until he started to gain weight again.

Do not get too concerned about memorizing or learning how to do this calculation. Your doctor and most postpartum nurses know to watch for this and will calculate it for you.

If your baby loses more than 10 percent of his birth weight, you will usually be instructed to supplement either with formula or pumped breast milk (if you have any). Do not give up breastfeeding at this point though. This is a very common issue and is usually temporary. You usually need to supplement with formula until your baby starts to regain weight and you start to produce true breast milk.

Wet Burps, Spit Up, Vomiting, and Projectile Vomiting: What's the Difference?

As silly as it sounds, there are actually medical implications regarding whether or not your baby is having wet burps, spitting up, vomiting, or projectile vomiting. So, how do you tell? Spit-ups and wet burps are little dribbles out of the mouth. These usually occur just after a feed, especially if the baby is too full, or just with a burp. They do not happen very often, and the baby is not uncomfortable with them.

Vomiting has more volume—sometimes up to what seems like the entire feeding—and is not always right after eating. It could be one to two hours after a feeding. Projectile vomiting is the same, but comes out so forcefully, it would hit the floor a foot or two away if you were holding your baby upright. Both vomiting and projectile vomiting can come out of the nose and the mouth. If there is milk in the nose, you may want to use a bulb syringe to suction out the nose. Do not try to suction the throat as this may cause your baby to gag and hold his breath. If your baby is vomiting more than twice in a row, is fussy with the vomiting, or having any projectile vomiting, call your doctor.

Repeated projectile vomiting may be a sign of obstruction of the stomach called pyloric stenosis, which is an emergency condition that requires surgery to repair. If your baby has projectile vomiting more than twice in a row, call your baby's doctor.

Gastroesophageal Reflux Disease (GERD)—A Common Problem

Vomiting can occur with gastroesophageal reflux disease (GERD) and often results in the need for medications to prevent heartburn for the baby. Severe GERD can cause babies to stop feeding, or requires limiting their feedings, and eventually may cause growth problems.

Mild GERD is much more common and does not always require medication. If your baby tends to be a spitty baby or has an occasional vomiting episode (without pain or fussiness), then you can try a few home treatments before seeking medical help.

To help mild GERD, try the following:

Keep your baby upright after feeds for up to one hour. You do not need to hold him upright for the entire time, but you can use a car seat or bouncy seat with adequate head support (do not turn on the vibrating mechanism). You can also elevate the mattress of your baby's crib or bassinet. Use something firm underneath the mattress to keep it stable. Do NOT put pillows under the baby's head, because it is a suffocation risk. The baby's body should be elevated about the same as it would in a car seat to be effective (around 30 degrees of elevation).

Burp frequently. Extra gas takes up volume in the stomach and can make the reflux worse.

Do not overfeed. If your baby's belly is too full, then he is more likely to spit up. You may need to give smaller, more frequent feeds to provide enough calories for your baby to grow.

Consider thickening feeds as your baby gets older (one to two months of age). You can use one to two teaspoons of baby rice cereal in each ounce of formula or breast milk. There are also commercially available thickening agents, such as Thick-It. These can be used safely from birth and are often used for premature infants with GERD.

If you do all of these things, but it does not help, or if your baby seems fussy, arches, and cries with feeds, or has projectile vomiting, then call your baby's doctor.

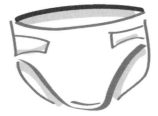

CHAPTER 10

Pee and Poop

What Goes In, Must Come Out...

You will never be so obsessed with pee and poop as you will be as the parent of a new baby. It is amazing how much we focus on these bodily functions for our little ones! This begins from day one when the hospital staff asks you to track every little thing that comes out of your child's body, from pee to poop to spit-up.

At every checkup, your doctor will want to know how your child is doing with each of these functions. Generally, this topic is not normally part of your daily discussions ("Could you please pass the salt, and, oh, by the way, how much did little Brian poop today?") However, knowing how much a baby is voiding (peeing) and stooling (pooping) gives your doctor a lot of information about the health and well-being of your baby.

As with feeding, there can be a wide range of what is considered normal for every child. There are some standards that most newborns will follow. If this is not occurring, you should let your doctor know.

To help you keep track of the number of pees and poops, you should write down when they occur, as well as each feeding. You will start tracking this on a chart in the hospital, and you should continue to do so for the first week of life or so. This will help your doctor to determine if the feeding pattern and voiding and stooling patterns are normal. It will also help you to see what your baby is doing since it can be hard to keep track of all of this when you are sleep-deprived. To help you with this, there is a tracking sheet at the end of the book (Appendix C).

Pee: The Sign of Hydration

A normal newborn should urinate at least once in the first 24 hours of life. After that, your baby should make two to three wet diapers per day for the first two to three days. Then, finally there should be at least four to six wet diapers per day for the rest of your baby's infancy. If your baby is not urinating enough, it can be a sign of dehydration. This, along with loss of weight, is the best way to tell if a baby is drinking enough, especially in the first few days of life.

"Matthew keeps spraying up and out of the diaper. Is this normal?" asked Chris. "Is he peeing too much?"

I reassure him, "It is really rare to have a condition where a baby pees too much. It is actually a sign of good hydration. For some reason, boys tend to leak out of their diapers more than girls, especially during the first few months. You may want to point his penis in a downward direction when you put his diaper on and make sure that the top is snug so that you reduce the chance of leakage."

In the first few weeks, some babies have urine that appears orange in color. These are from crystals in the urine, which are harmless. In the first few days, these orange crystals can be a sign of mild dehydration or concentrated urine. This should improve as your baby begins to feed better. However, if the urine continues to be orange or if it looks like blood, then call your doctor immediately.

Poop Happens

For the first few days, your baby will be getting rid of a dark, tarry material called meconium from his or her bowels. It is very sticky and a mess to clean up. But the fact that it is coming out is a good sign! That means that your baby is getting nourishment and the bowels are working. If your baby does not pass any stool in the first two days of life, then there may be an intestinal blockage.

After the first few days, the dark, tarry meconium will turn into greenish-brown transitional stools, and then finally to the normal loose, yellow, seedy stools of a young infant. Call your doctor if the stool is white in color, has blood, or contains a lot of mucus.

"Julie's poops are so watery," describes her mother. "It will even leak out onto her back. I think she is having diarrhea."

Watery stools with bits of digested material or seeds are normal. As long as there is a little substance to it, then it is likely normal. If your baby is producing pure liquid stools multiple times a day, it may be considered diarrhea, and you should call your doctor. Another sign of a problem is if there is blood in the stools.

The number of stools per day varies for each baby and is not an accurate indicator of problems. Most babies will poop multiple times a day—some with every feeding!

"William is always straining when he poops," worries his father. "He turns purple in the face, pushes, and grunts. Then, after he does, he feels much better. He must be so constipated!"

Newborns tend to poop every day—usually several times a day. However, some older babies will go much longer, up to three to five days, between stools. This is common after the first few months of life, especially in breastfed babies. Newborns should poop daily or go every other day between stools. If they do not, then it can be a sign of an intestinal problem.

If your baby is pooping regularly (daily or every other day), and as long as the final product is soft, then it is not likely to be constipation. Many babies will grunt and push and turn red in the face when trying to poop. This can be very normal as long as the final result is a soft stool.

Your baby does not do a whole lot of activities, so making a bowel movement is probably the most strenuous activity that he does! To help your baby, try to prevent tightening of the buttocks by moving his legs in a bicycling motion. Or hold your baby in an upright sitting position since we poop sitting up, not lying down. Sometimes giving your baby a bath to relax the muscles, including the anal sphincter, will help.

HOW TO CHANGE A DIAPER: STEP-BY-STEP INSTRUCTIONS

Before you take off the dirty diaper, have your clean diaper ready and several wipes pulled out. Keep diaper creams or powders within reach. Place the baby on a surface that is soft. It may get soiled, so a washable surface, such as a changing pad with a cover, is best. Often you will get poop leakage as the baby kicks and moves. Always keep one hand on your baby at all times to prevent falls from changing tables.

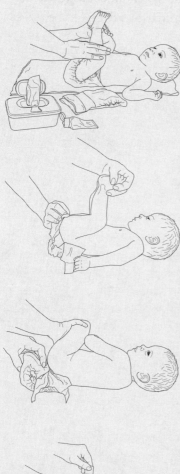

1. Lay the baby down on a changing pad and have wipes, a new diaper and diaper cream available.

2. Unfasten the dirty diaper, but do not take it away yet. Just open the front half to see what's inside. Hold your baby's ankles to lift his bottom off the changing surface. If there is poop, then you can use the front half of the diaper to help to wipe the poop away. You should always wipe from front to back. If you have a boy, you may want to put a wipe on the penis so he does not spray you while you are cleaning.

3. Tuck the front part of the soiled diaper under his bottom so that the clean outside of the diaper is under him. Finish wiping any pee or poop off the skin from the front using diaper wipes while still holding the legs. Clean any poop out from the vaginal area, if you have a girl, being careful to wipe from front to back. Clean any poop from the penis, if you have a boy. Lift the legs up higher to wipe the buttocks clean. Remove the soiled diaper and fold in any used wipes.

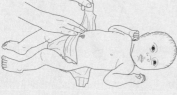

4. Put the clean diaper opened up underneath the bottom. Apply any creams or Vaseline at this time if needed. Fold up the front half of the diaper, and fasten the side strips to the front. You want to make it secure so there won't be leakage, but not so tight as to cause constriction or rubbing. If you have a boy, you may want to position the penis downward so that he does not pee up and out of the diaper.

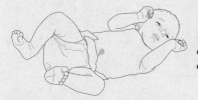

5. If your baby still has the umbilical stump, then fold down the top edge of the diaper so that it does not rub or push on the stump.

If your baby is producing a hard, formed stool, then he is considered constipated, and you should call your doctor for advice. Interventions include rectal stimulation with a thermometer, glycerin suppositories, formula changes, water by mouth, or Karo syrup by mouth. However, the proper intervention varies on a case by case scenario and should be done under a physician's guidance.

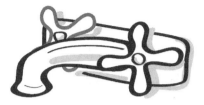

CHAPTER 11

Bathing

Newborns do not require frequent bathing. They are not out playing and getting dirty and sweaty. Newborn skin is so sensitive that frequent bathing may actually dry the skin out. Until the umbilical cord falls off, you will need to give sponge baths every other day. Shampooing the hair once or twice a week is sufficient. Use mostly water for cleaning and a mild baby soap or shampoo for areas that require it.

Once the cord falls off and appears dry, you can now get the belly button area wet. A "regular" bath for a young infant still involves using only about one to two inches of lukewarm water in a small bathtub or sink.

NEVER leave your baby unattended in water. It takes only one to two inches of water to drown a baby!

Regular baths are still required only every other day, with a shampoo every few days. Again, mostly use water for cleaning and use mild baby soap for the soiled areas, such as the diaper region. After the first two weeks of life, if your baby has really dry skin, then you may want to use an adult hypoallergenic soap instead of the perfumed baby soaps.

All newborn skin has to peel. It has been in a liquid environment for nine months, and it dries out once the baby is born and out in the environment. The top layer of your newborn's skin will peel and be nice and soft after

HOW TO GIVE A SPONGE BATH

Before you undress your baby, get all your supplies together and get the bath water ready. You'll need a towel, washcloths, mild baby soap, baby shampoo, cotton balls, a clean diaper, and clean clothes. Many newborns will cry during their first baths because they do not like being naked or wet. You can minimize their discomfort by keeping them mostly covered by a towel until you are ready to wash that body part. For safety purposes, always keep at least one hand on your baby when bathing him.

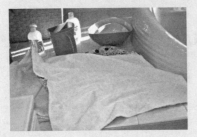

1. Lay the towel flat on a soft surface. Fill a nearby sink or a small bowl with lukewarm water. It should be a little cooler than what you would bathe in.

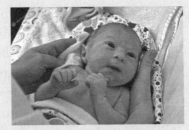

2. Undress the baby and wrap him in the towel. Keep the diaper on until you are ready to wash the diaper area to minimize the chance of a mess.

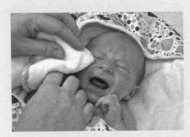

3. Work your way from the head down to the toes. Start with wiping your baby's closed eyes with a damp cotton ball or washcloth. Wipe gently outward from the bridge of the nose out toward the ears.

4. Support your baby's head with one hand while you dampen the washcloth in the water in the sink or bowl. Squeeze out excess water so that the washcloth is just damp, not dripping. Wash the rest of your baby's face, including the ears. Focus on cleaning behind the ears and within the folds of the outer ear. Just use plain water. No soap is needed for the face.

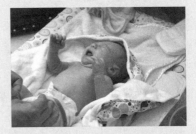

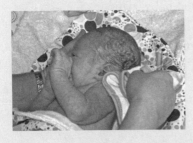

5. Next, wash his hair. This only needs to be done once or twice a week. Put a little baby shampoo on a damp washcloth and rub it into his hair. Then use a second washcloth that has water on it to rinse the soap out. If you have too much shampoo on your baby's head, you can hold his head just over the end of the sink or over the bowl and pour small amounts of water on the scalp to rinse it. Avoid pouring water on the face and into his eyes. Hold him tight so that he does not fall or hit his head.

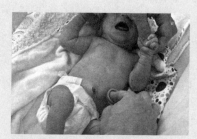

6. Continue cleaning him with just water on a washcloth, focusing on his neck, chest, and belly. Avoid the umbilical stump area. Focus on cleaning the little creases, like under the arms and between fat folds.

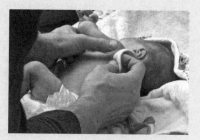

7. To wash his back, roll your baby onto his side and clean one side of his back at a time. Rinse his back with a damp washcloth. Then, roll him back over so that he is lying flat again.

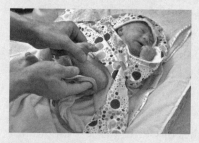

8. Cover the upper part of his body with a towel to keep him warm and dry. Next, clean his legs and feet with the washcloth.

9. Now, remove the diaper. Wash the genitals with a little baby soap:

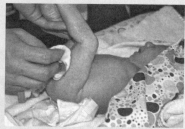

- If you have a boy who is not circumcised, pull the foreskin back gently just as far as it goes. It may not pull back very far at all; this is normal. If your son is circumcised, clean the area gently since it is likely still to be healing during the first week of life.
- If you have a girl, gently clean between the labia (folds of skin in the vaginal area) to remove any stool or mucus that may be trapped there. No need to remove all the mucus. Girls produce a fair amount of vaginal mucus in the first week.
- Clean the buttocks last. You can do this just as you would during a diaper change. Lift the legs and clean around the anus and buttocks with some mild soap on a washcloth and rinse with a clean damp washcloth.

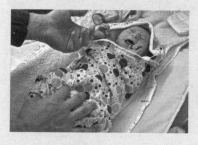

10. Pat the baby completely dry and then dress her in a clean diaper and clothes. No lotions or oils should be applied during the first two weeks of life.

the first two weeks of life. No need to put lotion on the skin until after two weeks of age.

If your baby has very dry skin or is diagnosed with eczema, use a thick, greasy lotion on her skin after the bath. Try the lotion on a small spot on the baby before slathering it all over just in case she gets a rash from the lotion itself.

How to Give a Regular Tub Bath

Do this only once the cord has fallen off and the belly button appears dry.

Use a baby bathtub designed for newborns, or you can use a clean kitchen sink lined with a big baby bath sponge or thick towel. Just as with the sponge bath, gather all of your supplies before you undress your baby. You'll need washcloths, towel, mild baby soap, shampoo, cotton balls, a clean diaper, and clean clothes.

Fill the sink or tub with about two inches of warm water. It should just be lukewarm—approximately 90 °F (32 °C). Use a bath thermometer, if you have one, to test the temperature.

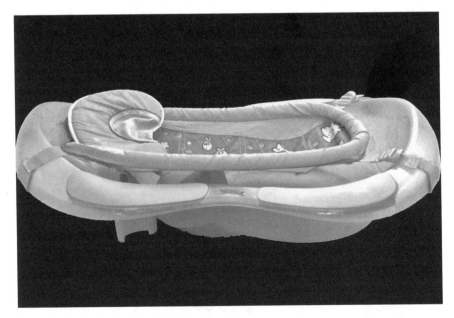

Infant bathtub with a newborn sling attachment

Gently lower your baby into the water, feet first. Make sure that she has complete head and body support throughout the bath and that her head is well above the water level. Always keep one hand on her while bathing. NEVER leave a baby alone in a bathtub—this is a drowning risk.

Wash your baby the same way that you did for the sponge bath. Only now you can also clean the belly button area.

Rinse soap and shampoo away promptly to avoid drying or irritating her skin. Avoid giving prolonged baths and letting your baby sit in soapy water for long periods of time.

When done, make sure that the towel is close to the tub. Lift her out of the tub using good head support. Wrap her in the towel, pat her dry, and then apply lotions if needed (after two weeks of age). Put on her diaper and dress her in clean clothes.

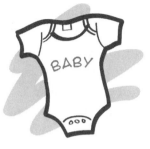

CHAPTER 12

Dressing

If you've had a baby shower or have friends or siblings who have baby clothes to give you, then you probably have lots of new clothes for your newborn! It is so much fun looking at the cute little outfits displayed at the stores. However, the clothing that a newborn requires is pretty basic. You can certainly have some cute outfits for photos, but in general, you will want to keep it simple since you will be changing diapers and cleaning up messes from burps and spit-ups pretty frequently. The last thing you'll want to do at the 2 AM feeding is deal with lots of snaps and buttons while you are exhausted!

Be sure to wash all new clothing in a mild hypoallergenic laundry detergent (such as Dreft) before putting them on your baby. New clothes can frequently have trace chemicals from the clothing factory. These substances may cause a rash on your newborn's sensitive skin. Also, wash any hand-me-downs before putting them on your newborn.

In general, your baby should be in one more layer of clothing than you. Be aware that there is an increased risk of Sudden Infant Death Syndrome (SIDS) if you overdress and overheat your baby.

In the hospital, your baby was probably put in a hat and swaddled tightly by the nurses. This, for most babies, is the most soothing position and keeps them from losing too much body heat, especially from their heads (the largest exposed surface area). After the first 24-48 hours, your baby no longer needs a hat indoors.

Swaddling is the process of wrapping a baby snugly in a blanket so that the arms are held closely to the body and have limited range of motion. Most newborns tend to sleep better when they are swaddled. They've been curled up tightly in a nice warm environment in the uterus, and it can be disconcerting to a newborn to suddenly be out in the real world.

There are also commercial swaddling wraps that you can buy. These are safer since they are usually attached by Velcro and cannot come free and suffocate the baby. In general though, it is safe to use a light, small newborn blanket for swaddling until your baby begins to kick or flail its arms to be free of it. A loose blanket in the crib or bassinet is a SIDS risk, so once your baby starts to reject the swaddling, then you need to remove it. You can then use the zip-up sleeper outfits to keep your baby warm while sleeping.

The Baby Layette—What Is It?

A baby's layette is the complete set of clothing and equipment for a newborn infant. The basics of a layette include onesies, sleepers, bibs, socks, hats, blankets, bedding, diapers, and toiletries. Below is a description of what you need for a basic layette. Always buy baby clothes based on your child's weight, not the age. Clothes are designed to fit a particular size body based on weight.

"My baby was huge!" exclaimed Margaret. "He was in six-month clothing by the time he was two months old. I had to give away all the little clothes that all my friends gave me."

Until you see how big your baby is going to be, do not go too crazy with clothing purchases. You may end up with a stockpile of adorable winter clothes that your summer baby will outgrow by August! Also, buy clothes that are easily washable. Babies are very messy. I did more laundry during my babies' newborn periods than I had ever done before!

HOW TO SWADDLE YOUR BABY

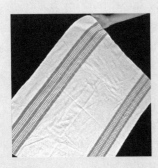

1. Lay your blanket flat diagonally.

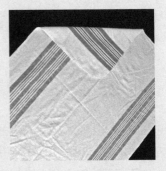

2. Fold the top point of the blanket down.

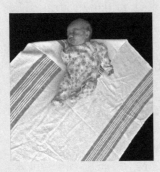

3. Put your baby on her back on the blanket with her head just above the folded part of the blanket.

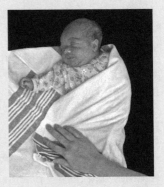

4. Take one side of the blanket and wrap it across her body toward the opposite side.

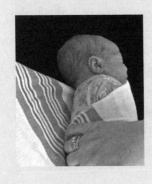

5. Roll her to the side and tuck the end of the corner snugly under your baby's back. Position her arms so that they are by her side.

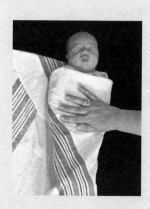

6. Roll her back so she is flat on her back again.

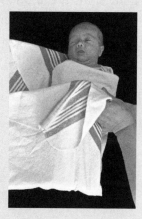

7. Lift the bottom point of the blanket and bring it to the top toward your baby's head. Fold the top part of the blanket down so that it does not cover your baby's face.

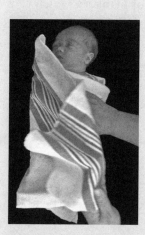

8. Lift the remaining side of the blanket and wrap it across your baby's body toward the opposite side.

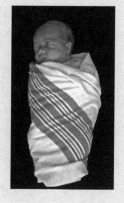

9. Tuck the edge of the blanket under your baby's back to complete the swaddle.

Onesies, Twosies, Threesies…What Are These Things?

Onesies or bodysuits: This is a one-piece, thin baby shirt that snaps at the crotch to keep it from sliding upward. These are usually short-sleeved and do not cover the baby's legs, but some can be long sleeved with leg coverings. Think of the onesie as a T-shirt or undershirt. It can provide an extra layer of clothing, or it can serve as a T-shirt when it is warm. You need around five to ten of these, more if you want to do laundry less frequently.

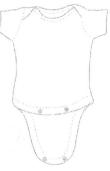

Onesie

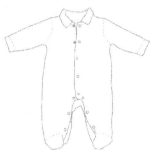

Sleeper

Sleepers: This is a one-piece outfit that is long sleeved with long leg coverings or a gown at the bottom. These are designed to keep the baby warm without the use of blankets, which can increase the incidence of SIDS. Thin versions are called bodysuits or stretch suits.

Thick versions are made of blanket-like material, cotton, fleece, or velboa. Halo Sleep-Sacks are a brand of these. These wearable blankets keep the baby warm, but zip up and cannot come free and cover the baby's face. Many baby supply stores also sell a Velcro swaddling attachment. This is a good way to swaddle your newborn without worrying that the blanket will come loose.

You will need four to five sleepers—some thin, some thick, depending on the time of year.

Gowns: A baby gown is a garment that resembles a long T-shirt that has elastic at the bottom to keep it mostly closed. This is a convenient outfit, especially at night, making changing diapers easier since you do not have to deal with putting together snaps when you are sleep-deprived.

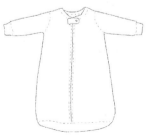

Gown

For newborns that still have their umbilical cord attached, gowns are nice because they fit more loosely and put less pressure on the stump. You should have four or five of these if you want to use them.

Mittens: Some people like to put little cotton mittens on their baby's hands to keep him from scratching his own face. However, I do not recommend these after the first few weeks, because we want your baby to be able to explore and find his hands.

Socks: Newborn socks are adorable because they are so tiny, but they tend to slide off very easily as your newborn kicks his feet around. Try to find ones that are a little longer or have more hold at the top of the sock to keep it from sliding off. You'll need five to seven pairs of socks. You can also use booties to keep your newborn's feet warm.

Hats: Your newborn will need to wear a hat for the first 24-48 hours while in the hospital. After the first two days of life, your baby needs a hat only when traveling outdoors or if you are somewhere that is particularly chilly. Hats are also important for shading the face and eyes when it is sunny outside.

Outerwear: If you live in a cold climate, then a heavy one-piece garment called a bunting is useful to have. It is like a heavier version of a zip-up blanket that is designed for outdoors. It usually snaps or zips up, covering the baby completely, except for the face, and has a hood attached. In warmer climates, a light sweater or blanket to wrap the baby in may be sufficient.

Clothing Safety

Here are some tips for safety when deciding what clothes to purchase:

- Avoid buttons. They can come off and be a choking hazard.
- Sleepwear should be comfortable, but snug enough so that there is not a lot of loose fabric.

- Stay away from drawstrings, ties, and ribbons. The baby can become tangled in these, which becomes a choking hazard.
- Avoid lacy frills. Little fingers can get stuck in the lace.
- Cotton is the most hypoallergenic fabric and usually a safe bet for comfort.

CHAPTER 13

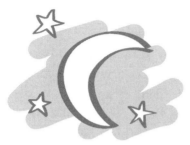

Sleeping

"Joseph is not a good sleeper," lamented his mother. "I spend most of the night checking on him. He keeps making noises and moving around. I'm so worried that he's uncomfortable or that he is having trouble breathing!"

Newborns are noisy sleepers. They will grunt, make noises, flail their arms and legs, and move around. If your baby is not actually awake and crying, you do not need to intervene. You will go crazy if you keep checking on your baby all night. It is natural to be anxious, but if you do not get some sleep for yourself, you will not be a productive or useful parent for the rest of the day.

All babies should be placed on their backs to sleep. The risk of Sudden Infant Death Syndrome is dramatically reduced when babies sleep on their backs. Try to alternate the side of the head that the baby is sleeping on to prevent flattening of one side of the skull over time.

The baby's crib or bassinet should have a firm mattress and tight fitting sheets and should be free of all other objects, such as quilts, bumpers, and toys. Most newborns sleep approximately 20 to 22 hours, waking up just to eat and be changed. They will also often have their days and nights mixed up for the first two weeks. Many mothers experience a phenomenon during the last trimester where the baby keeps kicking inside her at night just as she's trying to sleep. That's because the fetus has many of its awake periods in the middle of the night. This does not change when the baby is first born, so the baby may be more alert and awake at night for a while.

To help to adjust his sleep cycle, wake him up to feed every two to three hours during the day. If there are no medical issues, such as weight loss, prematurity, or jaundice, then you can allow up to four hours of sleep at night. After the baby regains his birth weight, you can allow longer periods of continuous sleep at night. Most babies will not go longer than four hours without eating at this age.

Until four months of age, you cannot really spoil a baby. So, if your baby will sleep only when being held, it is okay. Make sure that you remain awake if you are holding your baby. There have been many cases of newborns being smothered by the bodies of sleeping parents.

Time to Sleep—But Where?

Choosing a place for your baby to sleep is an important decision. First, decide on which room—yours or a nursery? Even if you have a nursery set up, many parents find it easier to have the baby sleep in their room for the first month or so. This is due to the frequency of feedings that are required and the general desire to not be far from the baby while she's asleep in case there is a problem.

If you have the baby sleep in your room, there are several options for places for her to sleep. The most common choice is to start with the baby sleeping in a bassinet in the parents' room and then transition her to a crib in the nursery once she is a little older.

Bassinets

A bassinet, or bassinette, is a bed designed for babies from the newborn period until about four months of age or when a baby starts to be able to roll over. It is smaller than a crib and can make a baby feel more snug and comfortable without being unsafe.

To prevent SIDS, the mattress should be firm and the sheet tightly fitted. The bassinet should be free of any other materials, such as pillows, stuffed animals, toys, or blankets.

Bassinets are useful if you want to have the baby in your room for the first few months and you do not have a lot of space. However, you may choose not to get a bassinet if you do not want to spend money on a bed that your baby will outgrow in three to four months. Keep that in mind when you are shopping for one so that you do not spend too much money on it.

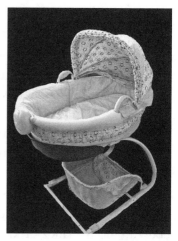

Bassinet

Cribs

One of the most important pieces of baby furniture you will buy is the crib. Most likely, your baby will spend more hours here than anywhere else. You will be using your crib until your baby is around eighteen months to two years of age. Comfort, design, safety, cost, and sturdiness are key aspects to focus on when you buy your crib. Whether you end up using a hand-me-down crib or buy a new one, be sure to check for recalls with the Consumer Product Safety Commission (CPSC).

There are mandatory federal safety standards for cribs as well as voluntary safety standards. Cribs that meet or exceed these safety standards are certified by the Juvenile Products Manufacturers Association (JPMA). You should be able to tell if a crib is JPMA certified by the seal that is displayed on the crib or carton.

Safety standards that meet current guidelines include the following:

- Slats should be no more than 2-3/8 inches (6.032 cm) apart. If you can pass a soda can between the slats, then they are too wide.
- There should be no missing, loose, damaged, or improperly installed hardware, such as screws, bolts, or brackets.
- Corner posts should not be higher than 1/16 inch (1.5 mm) above the panels at the end of the crib. This prevents your baby's clothes from being caught on the posts.
- Mattress support hangers should be secured to the crib frame with closed hooks or bolts. This prevents the mattress support from coming loose.

- Drop-side cribs have been banned by the Consumer Product Safety Commission as of 2010 because of several reports of deaths due to the drop-sides. Drop-side cribs make it easier to get babies in and out, but can also trap children, especially when the cribs have broken pieces or missing hardware. Do not use cribs with drop-sides.

The crib mattress should fit snugly with no more than two finger widths between the edge of the mattress and the crib frame. The mattress should be firm.

You should use the highest setting of your crib mattress support for a newborn. Then, lower it to the middle level when the baby can raise his body up on his hands or knees (around four to six months). The lowest setting should be used when your baby is starting to pull up to stand (around eight to twelve months).

Keep your baby's crib at least three inches (7 cm) away from drapes, blind cords, and wall hangings. Never have strings, ropes, or ribbons in or near the crib since they could strangle the baby. Also, beware of things that the baby can hang onto and pull down onto himself. Avoid decorative cutouts in the end boards of the crib that could trap your baby's body parts.

Crib Designs

Design and color of cribs are personal choices, but there are a few features that you should decide on before buying a crib.

Standard or Convertible? Standard cribs have drop-down railings on one or both sides. There are several different mechanisms that cribs have to lower the sides. Try them before you decide to buy. Try to lower the crib side with only one hand since you are likely to be holding a baby with your other hand.

Convertible cribs can be changed from a standard crib to a toddler bed, and then to a day or full-sized bed. These are more expensive, but can last a lot longer since they can change as the child grows. However, if you plan on having another child in the next few years, it may not be as useful, since you'll need the crib for the next baby.

Mattress Supports These connect the crib sides securely and hold up the mattress. Metal supports are sturdier than wooden ones. Adjustable supports allow you to lower the mattress height as your baby is growing and developing. Supports should be secure, attached with bolts or closed hooks to keep them from loosening when you are changing the sheets.

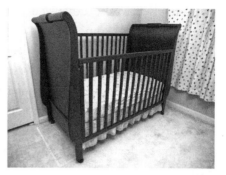

Convertible Crib

Wheels or Casters Wheels are useful for moving the crib when necessary. It can make changing the sheets a little easier and cleaning underneath simpler. The wheels should have some type of locking device to keep the crib from rolling when you are not moving it.

Teething Rail A plastic covering on a wooden rail can protect your baby and the railing when she is able to stand and chew on it. These should be securely attached to the railing.

Drawers Some cribs have a drawer underneath the mattress support. Some are free standing and can roll out from under the crib. Others have drawers that are attached. Check for sturdy construction and durability.

Finish If you are using a second-hand crib, beware that some older cribs (especially ones from before 1975) may have lead-based paint on them. Verify the absence of lead or buy a newer crib. Painting over lead-based paint is not an effective way to protect your baby, since she may chew through the top layer of paint as she starts biting on objects when teething. Lead is toxic to the nervous system and developing brain.

Co-sleeping, or Family Bed

"I tried to put Henry in the bassinet, but he just wouldn't have it!" confessed Diane. "He cried constantly unless he was near me or I was holding him. Finally, I was so exhausted I just had to put him in our bed so that we could both get some rest!"

Some parents choose to co-sleep with their baby and have what is known as a "family bed." This is not recommended, due to the risk of SIDS. There are also several reports of suffocation from a parent rolling over onto the baby. That being said, many parents report that they have had to bring their baby into their beds at least once during infancy to get their baby to sleep. Also, people in many cultures traditionally sleep with their babies.

If you need to co-sleep, there are some ways to make it safer. There are side-cribs that can be attached snugly to the side of the parents' bed. This allows the parent to reach the baby easily, but each person has his own sleeping space. This is a nice compromise that lets you have the baby nearby without placing her at risk.

If the baby is in your bed, make sure that there are no pillows or excess blankets where she will sleep. The mattress should be firm and the sheets tightly fitted so that they won't come loose. There are sleep nests and other devices that are designed to give a baby her own space within your bed. None of these have been proven to be completely safe. However, they are likely to be better than just having the baby freely sleeping in your bed.

Monitors—I Can Hear You!

Many parents invest in monitors as a way to keep tabs on their sleeping baby. As with every baby product, there are many choices of types on the market. For the most part, monitors are a useful way to see or hear your baby when she's sleeping in another room.

"I had to turn off the monitor after a few weeks," said Allison. "Every little noise Brian made during his sleep would keep me awake and I would have to check on him. I would strain to hear his little breaths to make sure that he was breathing. I couldn't sleep at all because I was so nervous. After the first few weeks, I turned it off. I just left the nursery door open so that I could hear him if he was crying."

John said, "We had just the opposite experience. Our baby monitor let us sleep with some peace of mind knowing that we could hear her if she cried. Also, it was so much easier to be able to work around the house knowing that we could hear her even though she was at the other end of the house."

Monitors can be very reassuring, but for some, they can be anxiety-provoking since every little noise is amplified. Buy one that appeals to you and try it. See what works for you. Do not rely on it as a way to monitor your baby's breathing—you still need to take all precautions to keep soft things and extra items, such as blankets, animals, toys, or bumpers, out of your baby's bassinet or crib to prevent SIDS.

What Type of Monitor?

There are two basic types of monitors: audio and audio/video. These come in analog (using radio frequencies) or digital (using encoded transmissions). Monitors consist of two parts: a transmitter and receiver or receivers. The base unit or transmitter is placed near the child. This sends signals (sound and/or video) to the receiver units, which the parents can carry or wear. Video units have a small camera than sends images to a video monitor.

Some monitors light up when your baby cries. This feature can be helpful if visual cues are needed more than sounds. This is useful for parents who are hearing impaired, or if you need to turn the volume down for some reason.

The biggest problem with monitors is usually interference with the signal transmission. This is especially true for analog models that rely just on radio frequency transmission. If you have a lot of electronic devices in your home, especially cordless phones, large appliances, lights, or microwaves, you should consider a digital model. However, digital models tend to be more expensive.

Interference may result in static or buzzing, or you might be able to hear conversations on phone lines. For video, it can mean fuzzy or incomplete images. If you have a cordless phone system in your house, try to pick a monitor that uses a different frequency. For example, if you have

a phone system that operates at 2.4 Ghz, try to buy a monitor that operates at 900 mHz or 1.9 Ghz.

Digital models are not as likely to experience interference, since they
use encrypted signals that allow for more secure transmissions. Some digital
models can also transmit video to your computer. These signals are much
less likely to be received by your neighbors since you would need the appropriate receiver to decode the signal. It is a more private connection and
will likely have much clearer reception.

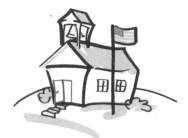

CHAPTER 14

Daycare or Childcare

Only one in four mothers is a stay-at-home mom. Even fewer fathers are stay-at-home dads. This means that at least 75 percent of the mothers in the U.S. are working. Some mothers may be working from home, working part-time or full-time. In any case, childcare is needed. So rest assured, if you end up needing childcare, you are certainly not alone.

"Emily's been coughing and has had a runny nose for three days. She has had low-grade fever since Saturday," says one mother. "And she just started daycare last week!"

This is a common scenario. When babies are enrolled in daycare for the first time and they are exposed to all the viruses and germs that kids bring to daycare, they are susceptible to getting sick. Every virus is new to your child and she will catch that virus. This is how we build up our immunity.

It is best to allow minimal exposure to other kids (and their germs) during the newborn period. The immune system will continue to mature as your child grows. As a general guideline, I tell parents to try to minimize exposure to large groups of people until at least six weeks of age—the longer the better in this case. If you are able to keep your child out of a daycare environment until three to six months of age, then it would be more ideal. Do not be surprised if your child gets sick that first week that he is in childcare.

Often, children seem to be sick all of the time when they first start child-care, especially if they start during the winter season, when viruses are more prevalent. Once they recover from one virus, they are likely to then become victim to another one. Usually, these are mild and involve minor illness; however, there are some reasons to be concerned. Call your doctor if your child has any of the warning flags listed under the section "Getting Sick—When to Worry."

"If Emily seems like she's getting sick all the time, but each time it is mild and she recovers, then it is unlikely that she has an immune problem. Instead, she's actually making her immune system stronger," I reassure Emily's mom.

"The first two years of daycare are usually the hardest. After that, it will get better and better. She won't get sick nearly as much as she gets to school. Other kids that stay out of daycare for the first several years end up getting sick later instead."

If you have to go back to work during the first three months of your child's life, then have a trusted family member or friend take care of your child, or perhaps enroll her in a small daycare.

Going back to work and leaving your infant in the care of another person can be a very stressful ordeal. However, most working mothers and fathers are able to do this successfully. The first time I left my son in someone else's care, I felt like a horrible mother who was abandoning my child and my responsibilities. But when I checked on him later by phone, he was happy, feeding, and sleeping as usual. When I picked him up, I found that I treasured the time we spent together even more. He was happy and cared for, and I was able to use my brain and focus on grown-up things at work for a few hours.

Stay-at-home parents need a break as well. Even if it is to run a few needed errands or just talk to grown-ups for a little while. Finding a babysitter or childcare provider for even just a few hours can be vital to recharging your system.

TABLE 3: COMPARISON OF TYPES OF CHILDCARE

	FAMILY	NANNY	HOME DAYCARE	DAYCARE CENTER
COST	$	$$$-$$$$	$$	$$$
SICK CARE	Not an issue	Not an issue	Depends	Will not take sick children
PRIOR PERSONAL KNOWLEDGE OF CAREGIVER	Yes	Not usually	No	No
CPR CERTIFICATION	Less likely	Some	Some	Most have CPR certification
LICENSURE/ INSPECTIONS	None	None	Some	Yes
EXPERIENCE	Varies	Varies	Varies	Varies
# OF OTHER KIDS	None	None	Few	Many
RATIO OF CARE	1:1	1:1	Depends	Usually 1:2 to 1:4 for infants
BACKUP CARE (IF CAREGIVER IS SICK)	None	None	Usually none	Yes

"I was on a waitlist for my son to get into that daycare as soon as I found out I was pregnant," exclaimed Samantha. "And I still had to wait six months after he was born to get a spot!"

Getting a child into a good daycare can sometimes be harder than getting into college for some areas of the country. The demand for high-quality childcare with structured curricula for future success is growing. It takes time to do your homework and scout out the best options for you and your child. Check with your friends, neighbors, and trusted resources to find childcare in your area. Many childcare centers have long waiting lists for infant care, so plan in advance. Hopefully, you've already researched childcare before this point. If not, it is time to start looking!

There are several types of non-parent childcare available. These vary based on ratio of children to adults, cost of care, place of care, and policies. Babies who are exposed to other children tend to get colds and illnesses earlier, so pay attention to the "sick care" policy of the place where your child will be staying.

It is best to canvas your area and visit multiple locations. If possible, ask other parents. They are often the best source of inside information about the various childcare facilities in your area. Read online reviews and check your state board for licensing and inspection information for licensed childcare providers. Check with Child Protective Services to make sure there have not been any complaints lodged against the daycare. Which ones are located conveniently for you? Would you prefer that it be closer to work or to home (or to the doctor)?

Narrow your choices to a handful and then take a tour of each facility. Usually, you can get a gut feeling about a place when you visit to know if it makes you comfortable.

What should I ask when looking for childcare?

There are many questions you could ask when choosing childcare. Make sure you do your homework. This can be a very difficult process, but once you find quality childcare, you and your baby will thrive there! These are samples of some of the important questions to ask. All of these questions have been compiled in a convenient checklist for you at the end of this book (Appendix D).

- What is the staff-to-child ratio?
- Are there different rooms for infants and toddlers?
- What are the policies on illness? What are the criteria for not allowing a sick child to come in?
- What are the facility's hours and holiday schedule?
- What happens if you are late picking up your child?

- What is their certification status?
- What kind of background check do they conduct on employees?
- What would disqualify someone from employment?
- How are their employees trained? Is infant and child CPR included?
- Does the same caregiver take care of your child every day?
- What is their employee turnover rate? How long have the teachers (especially the infant teachers) been there?
- Have they ever been the subject of an investigation? If so, what was the outcome?
- What are their hours? Do they provide care on holidays, weekends, or during early morning or evening hours?
- What is included in the fees? What must you supply?
- What types of meals and/or snacks do they provide? What is the feeding schedule?
- How often do they change diapers?
- How do they communicate back to you about the day? Do they give you a daily report?
- Do they currently have openings, or how long is the waiting list?
- Are parents encouraged to drop in to check on their children at any time?
- Do they provide closed-circuit monitoring via the web for parents?
- How do they verify the identity of the person picking up the child?
- What are their policies for handling accidents?
- How do they handle administering medications (prescription or over-the-counter)?
- Does the center have a policy of releasing children only to people whom the parents have authorized, in writing, to pick them up?

Observations to make while you are there:

- Does the staff seem flustered at being observed, or do they seem comfortable?
- Is the facility clean and neat? Are there age-appropriate toys and activities in each area?
- Is it easy for a person to enter the daycare center, or is there some barrier to prevent unauthorized entry?

- Do the children seem engaged with the caregivers? Or are the babies all sitting in swings and left to entertain themselves?
- How do the caregivers respond to unhappy children?
- How do you feel when you interact with the staff?
- Do children at the center appear to be secure and comfortable there?
- Is the facility well ventilated, well lit, and kept at a comfortable temperature?
- Is the childcare environment (both indoors and outdoors) safe and well maintained?
- Are they organized?
- Is there enough open space to allow children to move around and explore their surroundings?
- Do the parents seem happy with the care that their children are receiving?

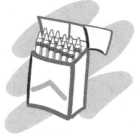

CHAPTER 15

Developmental/ Playing/Learning— Milestones for Growth

"When Thomas starting rolling over early, we just knew that he was going to be a star athlete. Then, he started to sing along with us, so we thought he was going to be a musical genius. After that, he was so in love with trains, we thought he was going to be a train conductor. Now, he climbs everything and has no fear, so we are worried that he will be a daredevil," laughs his mother.

Every parent wonders what their children will be like as they grow up— what will they be good at and will they succeed? While we cannot predict your child's future, your child's doctor will assess for normal development. When examining your child's development, there are four basic areas that we look at: gross motor skills, fine motor skills, social skills, and language development. In each of these areas, there are certain milestones that most full term babies should achieve by a certain age.

While there are certainly normal variations, these milestones are used as a screen to detect developmental disorders, such as low muscle tone, hearing or vision problems; communication disorders, such as autism; as well as a host of other diseases. If your child has not met the milestones listed below for her age group, do not panic. Call your physician to further discuss development and to see if more detailed evaluation needs to be done.

If your child was born premature (at less than 37 weeks gestation), the doctor will correct the age that milestones should generally be reached at by subtracting how many weeks early your baby was from his age. For example, if your baby was born two months early, subtract two months from his age to see what developmental milestone he should have reached. For those children with syndromes such as Down's Syndrome, the milestones also vary. Please discuss any concerns with your physician.

Developmental Milestones for Your Newborn

Newborns have only a few milestones that are assessed. At this age, the focus is the physical exam and behaviors such as feeding and sleeping. Developmental assessments are outlined as follows.

Gross Motor Skills

Your baby should be kicking his legs and moving his arms equally. There will be no particular purpose to the movement just yet since your baby is not quite aware that these body parts belong to him. If he does not move a particular limb as well as the others, there could be an injury or weak area that may need help or physical therapy.

Fine Motor Skills

Since the newborn nervous system is still very immature and developing, doctors do not expect any particular achievement regarding fine motor skills at this age. By two months of age, they should start to find their hands. You'll see this because she will start to put her hands in her mouth on purpose.

Social Skills

You should start seeing your baby smile spontaneously. She may smile during sleep or sometimes when awake. While it would be nice for her to smile at you, you really won't see your baby smile on purpose until two months of age.

Language Skills

Your baby should be making some cooing noises, like oohs and aahs. She is trying out the vocal cords and will make various noises. You should expect to hear some noises other than just crying. This is just the beginning of language.

Recommended Learning Activities (or How to Get Your Child into the Super Bowl/Harvard/ Hollywood)

Vision, hearing, and touch are some of the important ways that your newborn is learning about the world. Spend lots of time talking and singing to and holding your baby. Use high contrast toys (black and white) to stimulate vision. Babies cannot see color very well and cannot see very far. However, the contrast of sharp lines and dark and light colors attracts their attention. There are many videos that are designed to enhance brain development. These are not recommended for newborns. The American Academy of Pediatrics recommends no television prior to two years of age.

PART II

Guide to Your Newborn's Body from Head to Toe

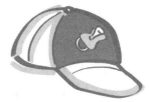

CHAPTER 16

Hair and Head

Hair Color

"Can you tell what color her hair is going to be?" asked Samantha. "I would love for her to have red hair like her dad."

Some babies are born bald; others have a head full of hair. Do not despair if yours lacks hair though, because this does not indicate what his hair will be like in the future. Much of the hair on your baby's head will fall out in the first six to nine months. Then, his real hair will start to grow in. By nine months of age, the baby's hair will usually be the color that his hair will be during toddlerhood.

Body Hair

"When Miranda was born, I was so worried that all of that hair on her back and arms was permanent," said her mother. "She was so hairy—she looked like her dad!"

When your baby is born, the body is often covered with a fine, downy hair called lanugo. This is normal newborn hair and will gradually be shed over the next several months of life. Even some of the hair on your baby's head is lanugo and may be lost during the first several months. If your baby's skin tone is darker, then her body hair will also be darker in color.

Head—Shape, Bumps, and Soft Spots

A newborn's head can be pretty oddly-shaped when he is first born. The skull of a newborn is made up of five separate plates of bone that fuse over the first two years of life to become a complete, solid skull like what you and I have. Because the bones are not completely fused at birth, they can create bumps, gaps, and ridges that concern many parents.

Soft Spots

"Can I touch his head there?" asked Jeff, pointing to his baby's soft spot. "I'm worried that I'm going to hurt him."

Your baby's scalp actually has several soft spots at birth. These spots are where the plates of bones do not completely meet yet. This space gives the baby's skull room to grow.

The biggest soft spot will be in the middle of the front top part of your baby's head and is called the anterior fontanelle. Underneath the skin, there are several layers of protective tissue and fluid to protect your baby's brain. Unless there is direct trauma

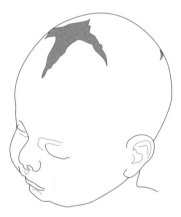

Soft spots (fontanelles) on a baby's skull

to this part of the head, it is difficult to hurt your baby through his soft spot.

Molding

Because babies' skull bones are moveable, they will "mold" into whatever shape they need to in utero and during the delivery process. This is why many babies who have spent a lot of time in the birth canal have a "cone head" after delivery. Even babies delivered via Caesarian delivery can have molding if their position in utero was spent head down and the head was compressed in the pelvic bones for a period of time.

Many babies will have hard bumps or ridges on the skulls where the plates of bone are overlapping slightly. This is normal, and the bones will gradually shift back into place, making the bumps less prominent. This may take several months to a year to occur.

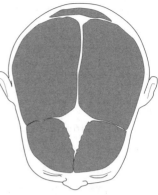

The bony plates of the skull

Swelling

The soft tissues of the head swell easily during the birthing process. This is especially true if mechanical manipulation, such as forceps or vacuum, was needed to complete the delivery process. Just being "squished" into the vaginal canal for a prolonged period of time can result in swelling of the presenting area of the scalp. There can be bruising or bleeding into the swollen area as well.

Local areas of swelling after the delivery do not usually become a problem. The swelling will go down two to three weeks after delivery. Some babies are tender in that area and will be fussy if you put pressure on it. Many babies do not seem to be bothered by it.

Because there is usually a little blood or bruising inside the swollen area, some babies get more jaundiced (see "Jaundice" section) as the blood gets reabsorbed. As this happens, there may be calcium deposits left behind in the scalp. If this occurs, the baby will end up with a hard, small lump in the area after the swelling has gone down. Your doctor can verify this. Any swelling that gets *larger* after the day of delivery should be examined by your doctor immediately.

Preventing a Flat Head

Since the "Back to Sleep" campaign, many babies' lives have been saved from Sudden Infant Death Syndrome (SIDS). However, as a result of lying on their backs for long periods of time, many babies now have flattening of the backs of their heads.

To prevent this, there are a few things you can do. First, once your baby's umbilical cord has fallen off, you can start "Tummy Time." This is where you put your baby on her belly while awake and give her a chance to practice lifting her head. This will strengthen the neck muscles, as well as prevent flatness of the back of the head since she's spending time not lying on her back.

Second, alternate the side of the head on which your baby rests. She may prefer a certain side due to tightness of a neck muscle, or she may just like a particular side. It is important to try to alternate the side of the head that has pressure on it. If there is significant neck tightness, your baby may need additional stretching exercises (see "Neck" section) or physical therapy. See your doctor.

To tell if your baby's head shape is getting flat, look at her from the top of her head. The head shape should be roughly circular and even all around. If you see that one side is getting flatter or that the head shape is very oval (either front-to-back or side-to-side), see your pediatrician for further evaluation and advice. There may be a medical reason for the unevenness that requires surgical intervention. If there is not, there are devices such as helmets that can be specially customized to your baby to help even out the shape of the head.

Positioning Tips to Prevent Flat Spots on the Head

Once the umbilical cord has fallen out, it is important to give tummy time when your baby is awake. Several times a day, have your baby lie on her belly while awake. This will strengthen her neck muscles as she tries to hold up her head and will reduce the amount of time that she is lying on the back of the head.

Whenever possible, try to have your baby rest on alternate sides of her head. This will help to even out the pressure on the back of the head and prevent one side from being flatter than the other.

Put toys on the both sides of her body so she will want to look in both directions.

When putting her down to sleep, if the bassinet or crib is against a wall, alternate the direction she is lying in the bed. This way when she looks

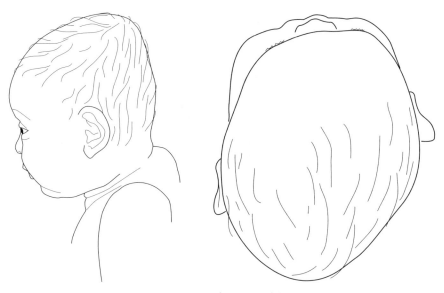

Flattening of the head—view from the side

Flattening of the head—view from the top

out into the room, she will be resting on different sides of her head each time.

If your child is getting a flat spot, it is also important to alternate which arm you use when you carry or feed your baby. We tend to always carry or hold them in the same way so that one side of the head gets more pressure than the other.

Sometimes, a flattening of the head occurs because a baby prefers to turn his neck in one direction over the other. This may be due to a tightening of the neck muscles. See the section on the neck to learn how you can help prevent this condition at home.

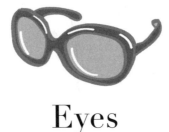

CHAPTER 17

Eyes

Color — Blue, Green, Brown?

What color will your baby's eyes be? Well, you cannot tell when your baby is a newborn. Most babies are born with grayish-blue eyes. Darker pigmented children will have a darker version of this. Your baby's true eye color won't be clear until around nine months of age.

Crossed Eyes

"There's a family history of crossed eyes, and I've noticed that Owen's eyes cross sometimes. Is there a problem with his eyes?" asked a worried mother.

You may notice that your baby appears cross-eyed sometimes. While this looks disturbing, it does not indicate a problem at this age. The muscles and nerves that control eye movement are still very immature, and thus your baby's eyes may appear crossed or even look in totally different directions sometimes. This should last only a few seconds and then return back to normal.

If your baby's eyes continue to look crossed sometimes after he is six months old, then it may indicate a real problem with strabismus or "lazy eye." At this point, you may need to take your baby to a pediatric ophthalmologist.

Vision—Can she see me?

Your baby can only see about six to eight inches (15 to 20 cm) away and can only really see contrast (such as black and white) well at this age. Color vision is not fully developed. Babies are near-sighted at birth. Do not worry if she does not seem to be looking at anything in particular for very long. This is normal.

To stimulate vision development, get close to her face so that you are in her focus range. Also, toys and books that use contrasting colors like black and white will attract her attention for longer.

Eye Goop or Drainage

"I think he has pink eye," stated Jonah's mom. "He's got this yellow drainage from his left eye, and it is so much that I have to use a wet washcloth to clean it so that he can open his eye in the mornings."

Most newborns are given antibiotic eye ointment at birth to prevent serious eye infections. However, this is not 100 percent curative. If your baby has continued eye drainage after birth, you should call your doctor. Very often, the eye drainage is not a sign of infection, but is a sign of a blocked tear duct.

Many babies have blocked tear ducts that can result in buildup of mucus, which then results in a gooey discharge. The tear duct drains tears that our bodies make to lubricate our eyeballs. The tear duct in a newborn is extremely small and can get clogged easily. This results in a buildup of tears and mucus.

If there is just a little drainage from the eye, clean the eye with a washcloth as needed. If a lot of mucus is present, sticking the eyelids together, sometimes an antibiotic ointment is needed to prevent or treat infection.

Massaging the tear duct may help to remove any mucous that is blocking the tear duct. To massage the tear duct, do the following:

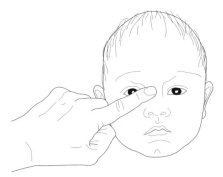

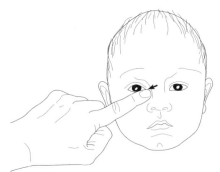

1. Put the tip of your clean index finger on the bridge of your baby's nose.

2. Rub gently with a slight amount of pressure outward from the bridge of the nose toward the inside corner of the eye that has discharge. Repeat this three times as you try to "milk" out the material that is blocking the tear duct.

Red Spots on the Eyeball

As your baby is born, there is a lot of pressure applied to the head and body. This can sometimes cause small blood vessels in the whites of the eyes to burst, resulting in a small red spot on the whites of your baby's eyes. This will not hurt the baby and will usually disappear in one to two weeks. Occasionally, after the red spot disappears, a light purple or gray spot is left on the eye and will remain there. There is nothing that needs to be done for this. If the red spot is getting larger instead of disappearing, call your doctor.

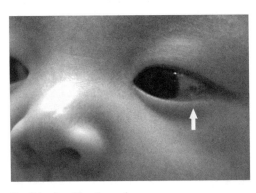

Small broken blood vessel on eye

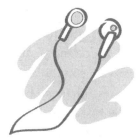

CHAPTER 18

Ears

Shape

"Her right ear looks different than her left ear," said Cynthia, pointing to her daughter's squished right ear. "Is it going to stay that way?"

Your baby's ears may come out folded or squished in appearance. This is due to the way that the ears were compressed in the uterus. Over the first month, this should straighten out on its own. Your baby's ears may never be identical on both sides; this is normal. We are not symmetric, and chances are that your ears are different too!

Hearing

"When there's a loud noise, he sleeps right through, but sometimes just the smallest sound will startle him. I'm worried that Ryan cannot hear," explained his father.

Many hospitals do newborn hearing tests in the hospital during the first two days of life. While this does not guarantee that your child can hear, it is a good screening test. It will pick up some congenital hearing problems and allows these children to get intervention and treatment early on.

Most hospitals perform a test called an Otoacoustic Emissions test (OAE) to screen newborns for hearing. For this test, the baby has special earplugs put into the ear that measure the acoustic response of the inner ear to clicks or bursts of noise. It does not truly measure hearing, but will measure if the inner ear is receiving sounds correctly. If there are concerns, then there are more definitive tests that can be done.

Many newborns will fail the first hearing test, due to the fact that the test requires that the baby's ear canals be completely clear. Many babies have vernix in the ear canal. When your baby was first born, he was covered in a sticky substance called vernix. If there is any of this in the ear canal, the hearing test may not work. Often a repeated OAE test after a few days will be normal once the vernix has been reabsorbed. Do not panic if your baby fails the first test. Most times a repeat test or a more detailed test will show normal hearing responses.

True hearing can only be tested when a baby can respond. If language is developing appropriately, that's usually a good indicator of normal hearing. Humans need to be able to hear to learn how to form words. If your baby has a delay in speech development, a hearing test is appropriate.

Extra Holes or Skin Around the Ears

When a baby's ears are forming in utero, they start off as tubes in the fetal development very early on in the pregnancy. As the fetus is developing, these tubes close up and take the shape of various parts of the body, such as ears. However, sometimes there are left-over residuals of these tubes after the baby is born that look like holes or tags.

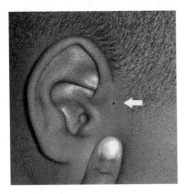

If there is a little hole in the front of the ear, this may be an ear pit. If the hole is still connected internally, then this may need to be repaired. If it is just a shallow hole or "pit," then nothing else needs to be done. Additional hearing tests may be recommended by your doctor to check for normal hearing.

Ear pit

In the same way, extra pieces of skin or cartilage may be left. In the case of this, your baby may have a little skin tag present near the ear. Again, nothing needs to be done about this, but your doctor may recommend additional hearing tests. If you want to have it removed, this can be done as an elective procedure later on.

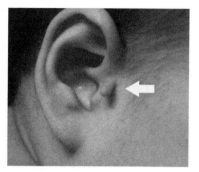

Skin tag near ear

Cleaning Ears/Ear Wax

"He makes SO much wax! How am I supposed to clean it out?" asks Philip's mom.

Your baby will have ear wax in the canals. This is normal. If you can see wax on the outside, then you can clean it with a washcloth or cotton ball. However, do not use Q-tips or cotton swabs inside the ear canal. Cotton swabs are too big for baby ears. By using these in the canals, you can end up pushing the wax farther in and impacting it instead. Do not worry about wax since your baby's body will naturally expel it. Occasionally, your doctor may need to clean out the wax, but this is usually because it is blocking the view of the eardrum—not because there is a problem.

There are ear wax removal drops and systems available over the counter. These are not safe for newborns and should be avoided.

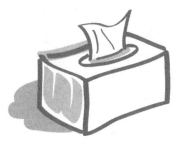

CHAPTER 19

Nose

Aa-choo! Sneezing

Sneezing, like hiccupping, is a reflexive action, which is the result of an immature nervous system. This is normal in newborns and is not a sign of illness. Sometimes it can indicate that there is some mucus in the nose that is irritating the nasal passageway. If your baby sounds congested, then clear the nose out as described in the next section.

Sniff, Snort! Congestion and Noisy Breathing

If your baby sounds congested, then use the large suction bulb that most hospitals give you when the baby is born to remove the mucus. The large size of these nasal suction bulbs provides much better suction for removing mucus. The smaller ones that can be purchased at most retail stores do not provide enough suction power.

Do not be afraid that you will hurt your baby's nose. The end of the large suction bulb is too big to go inside. Just press it gently up against the skin of the nostrils to create a good seal. If the mucus is too dry, use one to two drops of non-medicated nasal saline in each nostril to loosen the mucus. Then, use the suction bulb to clear the nostrils. See "How to Suction the Nose" in Part I of this book for more information.

If your baby is very congested or has a cold, then using a humidifier where the baby sleeps will help. There are generally three types of humidifiers: cool mist, warm mist, and vaporizers.

Cool mist humidifiers can humidify larger areas and are safe to use with children. There are several different methods by which cool mist humidifiers evaporate the water. Evaporation wicks pull water up and a fan blows the moisture into the air. Impeller models use a spinning disk in the water to make a mist. Ultrasonic models use ultrasonic waves to vibrate the air to create a mist and are generally quieter since there are no fans. It is important to keep filters clean to prevent mold growth.

Warm mist humidifiers provide warmer air, and they use a heating element to heat the water. Be careful of possible burn risks. As with cool mist, it is important to keep the filters clean.

Vaporizers boil the water and send steam into the air. Because the water is boiled, most mold and bacteria is killed. However, they have the highest burn risk because of the steam and should not be used around children.

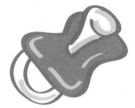

CHAPTER 20

Mouth

White Tongue—Milk or Thrush?

The two most common reasons for a whitish coating on your baby's tongue is milk residue or thrush. To tell the difference, try to wipe the tongue gently clean with a washcloth. If it comes off, then it is milk residue, and there is nothing else to do. If it does not come off, or if it is also on the inside of your baby's cheek, then it is more likely to be thrush, or yeast overgrowth.

Yeast is a normal fungus that is present in almost all mouths naturally. However, adults do not get overgrowth because we brush our teeth, and our normal immune system keeps the yeast in check. A baby's mouth is a prime spot for yeast to flourish because it is dark and warm. The sugar from the milk that is in the baby's mouth provides food for the yeast to grow.

To prevent thrush, wipe the tongue down once or twice a day with a damp washcloth. If a small amount of thrush occurs, it does not usually bother the baby. However, if it is not treated, mom can get a yeast infection of her nipples from the yeast in the baby's mouth if she is breastfeeding. The infection for mom is usually a red, painful, spotty rash around the nipples. Call your baby's doctor for further information and treatment if needed.

White Bumps—Does my baby have teeth already?

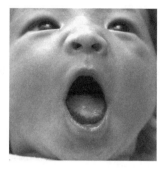

Thrush on tongue

Some babies are born with tiny hard white nodules on the gums or on the roof of the mouth. These are not teeth, but are called Epstein's pearls. These are calcium deposits that will eventually disappear. No treatment is needed.

If the nodule is bigger than a large grain of sand and is on the gum line, it may not be an Epstein's pearl and could be a premature tooth. These are not true teeth and are not usually securely attached to the gums. This can pose a choking risk if the tooth comes loose and should be removed. See your doctor if you are unsure.

Peeling Lips—Are they chapped?

The skin on your newborn has been in a liquid environment for nine months. The top layer of this skin will peel off during the first two to three weeks of life. This includes the skin on his lips. It does not necessarily indicate dryness. Also, a small blister may be present from when he was sucking on his lips in the womb. No treatment is needed as long as there is no bleeding, drainage, pus, swelling, or tenderness, and he can feed normally.

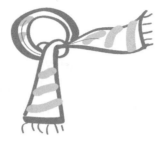

CHAPTER 21

Neck

Holding Up That Heavy Head — Can she get whiplash?

John worried, "I was holding Sarah and I reached over to get something from the table. All the sudden, she arched back and her head fell backward kind of hard. Is she hurt? She seems okay now. She cried at first, but I think it just scared her."

Your newborn's neck muscles are not strong enough to hold up the head yet. By four months of age, the neck should be strong enough to support the head alone. Until then, you will have to provide that head support. Despite how awful it looks for your baby's head to fall forward or backward, it is rare that any true damage can be caused if it was just a matter of not providing quick enough head support while holding your baby.

However, you should NEVER SHAKE YOUR BABY. This can cause brain damage if her head is forcefully shaken back and forth. Rapid back and forth movements of her head can cause internal blood vessels to break, and significant brain damage can occur. This is child abuse and is called Shaken Baby Syndrome or Abusive Head Trauma.

A single drop forward or backward that was not forceful is likely to be just fine. She should behave and feed normally. If you are concerned or if she is very fussy, call your doctor.

While your baby is seated in a car seat, bouncy seat, or swing, it is important to provide adequate head support. You can use commercial head support devices that look like an upside down letter "U." Or you can fashion one by rolling up a small blanket and securing it with some tape so that it does not unravel, and then putting it around her head. (See photo)

Tightness of the Neck

Some babies are born with a tight neck muscle on one side. How do you know if your baby has this problem? Your baby will strongly prefer to turn her head in one direction over the other. It will always be the same side. The condition is called torticollis and results in the inability to fully turn the head in one direction. While most cases are mild and resolve themselves as babies gets older, some are significant enough to require physical therapy. In either case, your baby's head can get very flat on one side since the baby always prefers to lie on one side. (See the chapter "Head").

If you suspect that your baby is not able to fully turn her neck, try some simple stretching exercises. If she is very fussy or has pain when you try these exercises, stop them immediately and call your physician for further advice and evaluation.

These exercises should be done slowly and gently. Your baby may be uncomfortable during the stretches since it will be difficult for her. Massaging the muscles may help to loosen the muscles before performing the exercises.

If your baby has difficulty turning to the left (her left side), then she prefers to look to the right and may eventually get a flat spot on her head on the right. To guide you, the instructions that follow are written for a baby who has trouble turning to the LEFT.

If, instead, your baby has difficulty turning to the other side (her right side) then just reverse the directions of each step. For example, if the instruction says "turn to the left," then change it to "turn to the right."

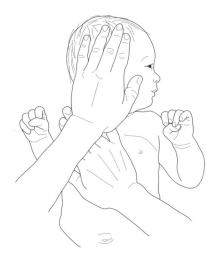

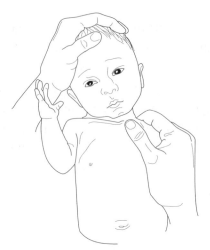

Rotation neck stretch for tight neck muscle (torticollis)

Side bend neck stretch for tight neck muscle (torticollis)

Rotation Neck Stretch (perform five times a day)

With your baby lying on her back, hold her right shoulder down with your left hand and gently turn her head with your right hand until her chin is over the left shoulder.

Hold this position for 10-15 seconds, then release.

Repeat three times.

Side Bend Neck Stretch (perform five times a day)

With your baby lying on her back, hold her left shoulder down with your right hand and hold her head with your left hand.

Gently bend your baby's head down sideways toward her right shoulder (ear to shoulder). Keep her face looking forward toward you. Stop when you start to feel resistance.

Hold this position for 10-15 seconds.

Repeat this three times.

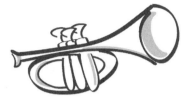

CHAPTER 22

Lungs and Chest

Breathing Fast and Shallowly

"Simon does this strange breathing where all the sudden he will breathe really fast and shallowly, then he's almost gasping for air—is this okay?" asks an anxious dad hovering over his baby boy, who was brightly looking around the room.

When your baby is sleeping, you may notice that he will occasionally have these episodes where he is breathing fast and shallowly. Then, at the end of the episode, he will take a deep breath. Then, he should go back to breathing regularly again. This is called periodic breathing and is normal for newborns. If your baby continues to breathe fast when awake, is coughing, has blue coloring of the skin, or is struggling to take a breath, call your doctor immediately.

Chest Wall — Bumps Poking Out or Divots Poking In

"What is that thing sticking out of his chest?" asked Maura, pointing to the hard lump in the middle of her son's chest. "Is it a deformity?"

In the middle of the bottom of the rib cage, there is a bone called the xiphoid, which is at the end of the sternum. On many people, this sticks out a little. This is a normal variation and can be prominent in a little

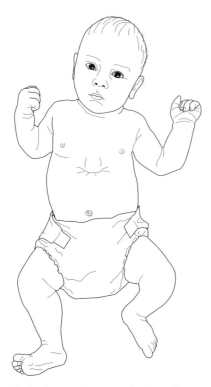

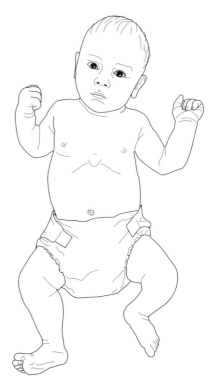

Xiphoid bone that protrudes inward

Xiphoid bone that protrudes outward

baby's chest. For some babies, this bone can either stick up and out, or be recessed and leave a depression that is visible in the middle of the chest. Mild versions of this do not require intervention and may improve a little as the child grows up and develops more muscle and fat tissue over the bone. Severe cases may interfere with the lungs and heart and may need surgical repair when the child is older.

Extra Nipples or Spots on the Chest

When nipples are developing in a fetus, they actually form lower on the belly and then travel upward to the chest as the fetus develops. When the nipples make this trip upward, sometimes remnants can be left behind. When the baby is fully formed, the remnants may take the shape of a small spot, like a mole, or can develop into an actual nipple. These are called supernumerary nipples and do not require intervention. These are usually just superficial marks and never fully develop breast tissue.

Breast Buds—She's not a teenager yet!

Both newborn girls and boys can have slightly swollen areas under the nipples at birth. These are actually little breast buds and come from the extra estrogen hormones that mom had circulating in the bloodstream. Some breast buds are so developed that they can even secrete a breast milk-like substance from the nipples!

But not to worry, your baby girl is not hitting puberty and your little boy won't have breasts. As the hormone levels settle down, the breast buds gradually go flat. This may take up to nine months to a year to happen. The breast should not get bigger in size or appear red or tender. This could be a sign of infection.

CHAPTER 23

Heart

Rapid Heart Beats

"I can feel her heart beating so fast!" said Jacklyn's mom. "It is like her heart is beating out of her chest!"

A newborn's normal heart rate is around 100-140 beats per minute. This is much faster than an adult's heart rate. Since babies are small, you may sometimes be able to feel the heart beating through the chest wall. If your baby is otherwise well, has no fever, is eating well, is not fussy, is breathing comfortably, and does not have blueness of the skin, then this is normal. When she is sleeping, the heart rate will slow down to about 100 beats per minute. This is also normal. If she is having trouble breathing, eating, is fussy or has a fever, then call your doctor immediately.

Heart Murmurs—The doctor said he had a murmur!

When your baby is examined by a doctor or nurse, they may mention to you that he has a heart murmur. A heart murmur is an extra sound that they can hear with a stethoscope. It comes from the turbulence of blood flow through the heart, which produces a noise. Depending on what is generating the noise, a murmur can be innocent or may be the result of a heart problem.

The sound of a murmur is similar to the sound of the water in the house when someone runs a hose or turns on the shower. You can hear the water (blood) rushing through the pipes (heart) because of the turbulence. The pipes (heart) are usually normal. Only by examining the pipes can one be sure. For the heart, this means doing a special type of ultrasound called an echocardiogram to look at the anatomy.

Murmurs can be a normal variation or, rarely, can indicate a more serious heart condition. The sound of the murmur and other symptoms that your baby has will help your doctor determine if the murmur is a worrisome one. Most murmurs are innocent and can just be monitored. Many murmurs can be normal during the newborn period and disappear in one to two days. Some will last up to a year of age and then disappear. If the murmur persists or changes, or if there are other symptoms, such as blue color to the face or body, difficulty breathing, or sweating while feeding, your doctor may consult a pediatric cardiologist.

CHAPTER 24

Belly

Umbilical Cord

The umbilical cord will usually fall off between seven to ten days after birth. Until then, you should keep the cord dry. It will dry up from a soft yellow-white tissue to a dry hard material (similar to how a fingernail feels). Then, it will fall off. Most practitioners no longer recommend that you apply alcohol to the cord, because it actually seems to prolong the length of time before the cord falls off. Generally, it is a good idea to fold down the top of the diaper while your baby's cord is still present. This will prevent the diaper from pressing the cord onto the baby's sensitive skin.

Once the cord falls off, it may bleed or ooze a little for a day. As long as it does not continuously bleed, have pus or swelling, you can just keep it dry until it finishes healing. If the bleeding or oozing does not go away in one or two days, your doctor may need to treat it with medication.

If the belly button still has some healing tissue at the base, it may continue to ooze a clear, yellow liquid. This is called a granuloma and will need to be treated by your doctor. Do not submerge the belly button under water until it is fully healed and dry.

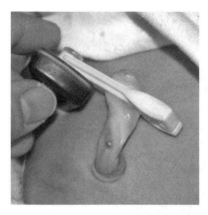

Soft umbilical cord present at birth

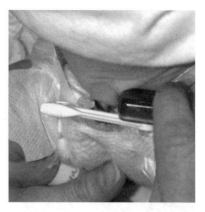

Hospital security clamp on drying cord at day 2 of life

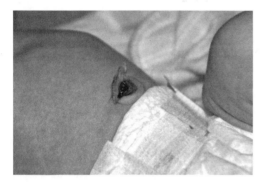

Dried umbilical cord at day 4 of life

Belly Button — Innie or Outie?

"I have a lot of parents ask me to make the belly button an innie," laughs one obstetrician. "I have to tell them that it is not up to me. The way you cut the cord does not determine innie or outie."

Once the cord falls off, you will get a better idea if your baby will have an "innie" belly button, or an "outie" one. More than 90 percent of the population has an innie. That means that about 10 percent of people have belly buttons that stick out a little.

Umbilical Hernia

Some babies have a little umbilical hernia, which makes the belly button stick out even farther. This is the result of a small gap in the muscles

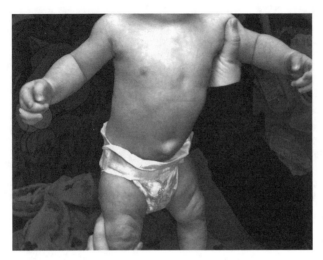

Umbilical hernia in an infant

underneath the belly button. When the baby strains or pushes out the stomach, then abdominal contents can poke through the gap. While it can look odd and may distress people who have never seen one before, there is no need to do anything about this.

Taping down a hernia, putting a coin over it, or any other home remedy does not treat a hernia. In time, the muscles will finish fusing, and then the hernia will be gone. If the hernia does not disappear by around four years of age, then surgical closure may be needed.

The only potential risk of an umbilical hernia is that the abdominal contents could get stuck in the gap. This is called an incarcerated hernia and could cut off the blood supply to those tissues, which would be an emergency. This is an extremely rare event. Millions of babies have umbilical hernias and do not have any problems.

How do you know if an umbilical hernia has gotten incarcerated? An incarcerated hernia would cause a great deal of pain. The overlying skin would turn dark purple like a bruise and be very tense and firm. Your baby would be extremely fussy and irritable. If your baby has an umbilical hernia and acts as if she is in a great deal of pain, check her hernia. If you suspect an incarcerated hernia, push the hernia down immediately and call your doctor. If you cannot get the hernia to go down, call 911 or go immediately to the emergency room for care.

What's That Noise?

Many parents get concerned because they can hear bubbly noises from their babies' bellies. These are normal digestive noises and do not indicate any problems. Because babies are so small, it's much easier to hear noises that their bodies make.

If you suspect that your baby is gassy, especially if she is uncomfortable, then you can try some gas relief drops. One brand is called Mylicon drops, which can be purchased over the counter at most drug and grocery stores. These are safe to use from birth and help to dissolve the gas bubbles. If your baby still seems extra gassy, it is reasonable to try a lactose-free formula to see if lactose intolerance may be adding to the gassiness.

His Belly is SO Big!

"Is his stomach supposed to be that big?" asked John pointing to his new-born baby's round belly. "Or is he really bloated?"

Newborns have larger bellies in proportion to the rest of their bodies. The abdominal area is supposed to be more rounded and will look disproportionately big. However, it should be soft. If it is very hard and your baby seems uncomfortable, consult your doctor.

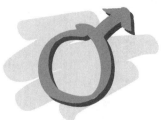

CHAPTER 25

Genitals (Boys)

Circumcision

"Can you check his circumcision?" This is the most common request at the newborn visit from parents of boys who have had a circumcision.

The choice to do a circumcision is a personal one. Frequently it is done for cultural, social, or religious reasons. This is the most common pediatric surgery and has a relatively low rate of complications. The American Academy of Pediatrics states that there is not enough evidence to support recommending a circumcision for medical reasons. Some studies show that circumcision slightly reduces the risks of penile cancer, urinary tract infections, and sexually transmitted diseases.

Whether the circumcision in done in the hospital or in the first two weeks at home (for religious reasons), the care is the same. For the first 24-48 hours, you should put Vaseline on a gauze pad and put it onto the penis with every diaper change. After that, you should continue to put Vaseline on the penis until the foreskin has completely healed.

The foreskin usually takes five to seven days to heal completely. While it heals, do not be surprised to see a whitish discoloration in some areas.

This is healing tissue and is normal. If there is an oozing discharge, increased swelling, persistent bleeding, or worsening redness, you should consult your child's doctor.

Swollen Scrotum

"Your son has a little extra fluid in his scrotum. That's why it is so puffy on this side," I explain, showing Liam's mother what I was talking about. "Oh!" she exclaimed, "I was wondering if that was supposed to be so big!"

Many newborn boys have a little extra fluid in the scrotum. This is called a hydrocele. It results from body fluid being trapped in the scrotum as the testicles make their de-

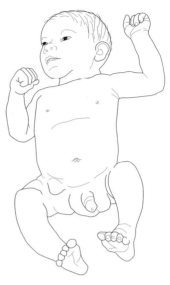

Inguinal hernia

scent from the abdomen into the scrotum. Generally, the fluid goes away in the first year of life. If not, it may need to be surgically corrected.

It is important for your doctor to differentiate a hydrocele from a hernia. A hernia will not go away and needs to be surgically corrected more immediately.

What is a Hernia?

There are many types, but the one that occurs in little boys in the genital area is called an inguinal hernia. When a baby boy's testicles are formed in the uterus, they start off located in the abdomen. During gestation, they travel down through a canal near where the legs join the body, called the inguinal canal. Once the testicles descend into the scrotum, this canal is supposed to close. If it does not close, then there remains a path from the abdomen into the scrotum. This is more common in premature infants.

Abdominal contents can be pushed into this open canal, especially when the baby is straining (as when making a bowel movement). You will then see a bulge appear anywhere along this canal. It may come and go as the contents of the canal go back up into the belly.

The danger of an inguinal hernia is that it can become incarcerated. This occurs when the contents of the abdomen get stuck in the canal and it twists and loses blood supply. This is an emergency. The bulge will generally be very painful, and you will see discoloration of the skin over it. Unlike an umbilical hernia, you cannot usually just push this back in. This is a medical emergency, and you should call your local 911 or go to your nearest emergency room immediately for help.

CHAPTER 26

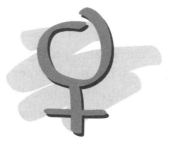

Genitals (Girls)

Vaginal Discharge (Mucus and Maybe Some Blood)

"I keep wiping her down there," said Diane. "But I cannot seem to get her clean. Am I doing something wrong?"

Newborn girls make a lot of vaginal mucus. This is in response to maternal hormones that are circulating in the baby's body. It is important to keep the vaginal area clear of stool and to wipe from front to back to avoid bringing stool to the front. This will help to prevent urinary tract infections.

You do not need to remove every last bit of mucus as long as the stool has been cleaned out. The skin in the vaginal area is sensitive. No need to rub too hard, or you may irritate her there.

Some newborn girls even have a "mini-period" and have vaginal spotting. Again, this is a result of excess estrogen that came from mom. It should only be a few spots of blood, and should disappear by two weeks of age. If you see a large amount of blood (more than a few drops), or it does not go away after two weeks, you should consult your baby's doctor.

Labial Adhesions

The opening to a newborn girl's vagina is usually open at birth. However, the labia, the tissue just outside the opening, can be fused closed or partially closed on some girls. This usually is not a problem as long as the baby can pee without difficulty. Once the child is older, her own natural estrogen will help the labia to open. Sometimes, physicians will prescribe an estrogen cream to help the labia to open sooner, especially if there is complete fusion.

Vaginal Skin Tags

Sometimes when the vaginal area is forming there can be extra skin or tags present. These are normal, and nothing needs to be done about them unless they are very large and will bother the child.

Hernias

Just as with boys, hernias can develop in the area just next to the genitals, called the inguinal area. Hernias are rarer in girls, but they can still have them. Premature infants are at a higher risk for developing hernias. These types of hernias need to be repaired.

CHAPTER 27

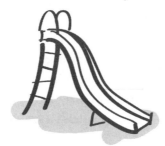

Movements

Reflexes/Startle Response

A newborn has multiple reflexes that are normal, but may appear strange to you. There is one called a moro, or startle reflex, that involves the arms and upper body. It will look like a "startle" to you, where your baby's arms flail out as if the baby is falling backward and then the arms return back in again to normal. Your baby's eyes may be open, and he may look surprised. This can be triggered by sudden movement or loud sounds. This is a normal sign of a developing nervous system.

A baby also has a sucking and rooting reflex. When something is put near his mouth, he will turn toward it and will try to suck on it. This may be a hand, a breast, a bottle nipple, pacifier, or anything else placed near the mouth!

Babies need to suck on things to relax and calm down. It does not always indicate that your baby is hungry. If he is actually hungry, he will usually cry or be fussy if no milk is produced by the object.

A third normal reflex that a newborn baby will have is a grasp reflex. When something (like your finger) is put in your baby's hand, he should hold on to it. It may not be a strong grip, but it should happen.

Shaking or Jitteriness

"Every so often, Alex will shake or twitch his arms or legs," said his mom. "Is this normal? It happens when he's awake and he seems fine otherwise."

The nervous system of a baby is very immature and is still developing at birth. Because of this, your baby may have a lot of shaking or jittery movements. These should be very brief—a few seconds—and then stop. This is normal.

Your baby should otherwise be acting well, feeding well, and sleeping normally. If he has prolonged periods of shaking, or appears to not be acting normally, then you should call your child's doctor for further advice.

CHAPTER 28

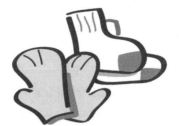

Arms and Legs

Funny Shapes of Hands, Feet, Fingers, and Toes

Rick asked, "Hallie's legs look funny. They looked really bowlegged. Will she have trouble walking?"

When a baby is developing in the uterus, the space is limited by the size of the uterus, the amount of amniotic fluid present, and the size of your baby. Based on this, she can be squished in there, and all the extremities (arms, legs, feet, and hands) have to curve to fit in this area. When your baby is first born, you may see the result of this.

All babies are a little bowlegged, and their feet curve inward a little. Sometimes, the toes and fingers may overlap slightly. Most of this will straighten out in the first few months of life now that there is space to stretch out. However, there are a few conditions that are not just the result of uterine space and may need to be treated. These are usually apparent on exam in the first few days of life, and your child's doctor should be able to tell you about them.

Nails—How to cut these nails?

Since your newborn does not really know how to control his arms, he may scratch his face by accident. To prevent this, keep the fingernails short if possible. Newborn nails are very soft. You may notice that they peel easily. Therefore, if you are uncomfortable clipping such small fingernails, it is very easy to trim the nails by using an emery board to just file the nails down. If you do this when your baby is sleeping, it might be easier.

Cold or Purple Hands and Feet

"Kevin's hands and feet always feel cold. I keep wrapping him up, but his feet even look blue sometimes!" said his concerned mom.

A newborn's circulation is pretty sensitive to the outside environment. If your baby is cold, his body will naturally try to warm up by bringing most of the blood to the center of the body. As a result, the hands and feet will often feel cold or even look a little purple.

As long as the purple color does not involve the face or the rest of the body, then this color is probably normal. Just try to warm your baby up or put on little mittens or socks. If the color and coolness improve, then this is a normal function of the body.

Sometimes feet or hands can look purplish if you are holding your baby in a position that compresses her arms or legs. If you reposition her, then the circulation to the extremities should improve and the color should return to normal.

If warming and repositioning do not help, you may want to mention it to your doctor to see if there is another explanation.

Clicks and Pops

The joints and ligaments of a baby are much looser than an adult's. As a result, you may feel little clicks and pops in your baby's joints, especially the knees, when you move him around. These are normal. It is just like when your knuckles crack.

It is not a sign of a problem—with one notable exception. If you feel significant clicking or popping in your baby's hips, then it can be a sign of a hip problem.

Some babies are born with a very shallow or malformed hip socket. If this happens, then the upper leg bone does not sit in the socket appropriately. This is called congenital hip dysplasia. With early treatment, the outcome is usually quite good. Generally, your doctor should be checking your baby's hips routinely to look for abnormalities.

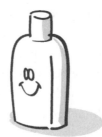

CHAPTER 29

Skin

Spots and Rashes

"I think he has a rash," said David's mother. "He's got all these little red spots on his body and on his face, too. I think they're spreading, but I'm not sure. I do not think this one was here when he was born," she said, pointing to a small, red, pimple-like spot.

When your baby is born, there may be some red spots on the body that look almost like little pimples with a little redness around them. This is a normal newborn rash called erythema toxicum. Despite the scary sounding name, it is a normal rash, which will usually disappear within a few weeks.

If you see any spots that appear to be clear bubbles or blisters, then let your child's doctor know, especially if mom has any history of sexually transmitted diseases, such as herpes.

You may also see some very tiny white bumps on your baby's face (usually on the nose) that also appear like little pimples. These are called milia and are also normal. These will generally disappear in the first few months.

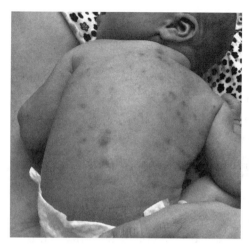

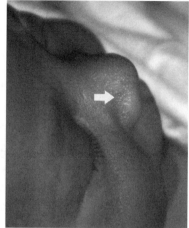

Normal newborn rash—small red spots

Normal newborn rash—tiny white bumps on nose (milia)

Jaundice: Yellow Color to the Skin

In the first week of life, many babies get a little yellow or jaundiced. Most babies do not need treatment, but they should be monitored closely by a doctor. The yellow color comes from a chemical called bilirubin, which is a byproduct of red blood cells.

Normally bilirubin is broken down by the liver so that we do not all turn yellow. However, a newborn's liver takes about a week to mature to the point where it can start to process bilirubin. As a result, the bilirubin builds up in the system and turns the skin and eyes yellow.

When the level of bilirubin is low, it does not affect your baby. However, if it gets high, it can damage the brain. Therefore, this needs to be followed closely by your doctor during the first week of life.

Your baby gets rid of bilirubin by peeing and pooping, so the more that your baby eats, the more bilirubin he excretes. For this reason, your doctor may recommend that you supplement your baby's diet with additional formula, especially if you are breastfeeding.

If treatment is needed, it involves exposing your baby's skin to ultraviolet (UV) light. The UV light works through the skin to break the bilirubin down to a harmless form. This can be done using a special UV light blanket

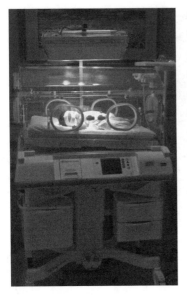

Phototherapy treatment for jaundice

or putting your baby in a special incubator with a UV light panel over it.

Sunlight could help, but there is a risk of your baby getting sunburned or dehydrated. It works only if the skin is exposed to the sunlight. Many people believe that putting the baby near a window helps. This does to some extent, but since most of the UV light is filtered by the window glass, it will not be very effective. Also, your baby may get overheated in the sunlight.

The yellow color of jaundice tends to start in the face and then travel down to include the chest, the belly, and the legs as the level of bilirubin gets higher. Therefore, if your baby's legs start to look yellow, then it is likely that the bilirubin level is pretty high. Your doctor can do a skin or blood test to determine the level of jaundice.

Some conditions increase the risk of developing significant jaundice. These issues include prematurity, blood type cross reactions, Asian or darker-skinned descent, or the presence of a collection of blood under the scalp from a vacuum or forceps delivery.

Treatment depends on the level of jaundice as your baby goes through the first week of life. A particular level of bilirubin is allowed for each hour of your baby's life before treatment is needed.

Diaper Rashes

Your baby's skin is very sensitive at birth. For the first nine months of development, her skin was bathed in a soothing balm of amniotic fluid. Then, suddenly, after birth, she is exposed to the elements and foreign materials like diapers, wipes, urine, poop, and clothes. When this happens, the skin gets red, and a rash may develop.

Commonly, it is the diaper area that gets red and irritated, and can sometimes even bleed. To help prevent this, make sure that you change your baby's diaper as soon as possible after he poops or pees. If the bottom is already red, apply a thick diaper rash cream (can be found in most stores that carry baby products). Put the cream on with every diaper change until the skin has healed.

Baby powders are also used commonly for diaper rashes. Be careful with baby powder since lung disease can occur if your baby accidentally inhales the powder. Also, powder may not be as effective for protection once the powder has absorbed a lot of liquid.

Exposing the skin to air and keeping it dry will help the skin to heal. This can be done by laying your baby out on a blanket or towel. Then, put an open diaper under your baby's bottom and another one on top of her genitals to help to catch any urine or stool that is produced. Letting air get to the skin will dry out the irritated area and help it to heal faster. Monitor your baby if you do this to make sure that the loose diapers do not migrate and cover her face!

True infections of the skin in the diaper area are not very common in the newborn period. However, if the redness does not improve in a day or so, spreads quickly, or has pus or bubbles, see your doctor.

Peeling Skin and Dryness

"He's really dry… should I put lotion on him?" asked Michael's mom.

Your baby's skin has been in a liquid environment for nine months in the uterus. Now that your baby is out, the top layer of skin will peel. This is a normal process. The skin will peel everywhere and appear dry. This includes the lips. There nothing that you need to do about this.

If the ankles or wrists are so dry that the skin begins to crack, you may apply a small amount of baby oil or lotion to those areas. Otherwise, just leave it alone and your baby's skin will appear more normal in two to three weeks.

Lotions and Oils

As mentioned before, a newborn's skin is very sensitive. Therefore, it is best not to apply too many chemicals to the skin during the first few weeks, or a rash may develop. If his skin is very dry and is getting cracked, then

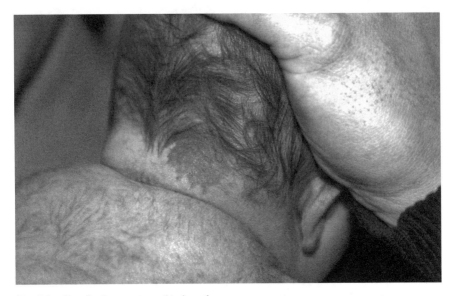

"Stork bite" or flat hemangioma birthmark

a small amount of lotion or oil could be applied. Generally, it is a good idea to wait until after your baby is two weeks of age to start applying any types of oils or lotions. When you do, apply only a small amount first to make sure that it does not cause a rash before you cover his body with it!

Many cultures use oils for massaging babies. Again, this is fine to do, but you may want to wait until your baby is at least two weeks old so that the risk of developing a rash is less. Avoid oils and lotions that contain nut products (such as almond oil) to decrease the risk of your baby developing nut allergies. While early exposure to nut products has not been proven to trigger allergies, limited to minimal exposure early on is still recommended.

Birthmarks

Red Ones—Strawberry Hemangiomas or "Stork Bites"

A common birthmark is called a strawberry hemangioma, which can be either raised or flat.

The flat ones are usually located near the middle of the forehead between the eyes or on the back of the neck. This type of birthmark is commonly referred to as a stork bite since it is where the stork was holding your baby for delivery! These generally fade by four years of age. The ones on the back of the scalp tend not to fade as much but will be covered by hair as your child grows.

Another common place for this flat, red birthmark is on the eyelids. Again, these will fade over time. When your baby is straining (such as when crying or stooling) or when your baby is warm (such as after a bath), these red marks may appear more prominent as the blood vessels underneath expand.

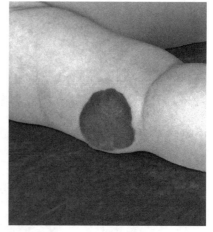

Raised "strawberry" hemangioma birthmark

Raised hemangiomas can be anywhere on the body and tend to rise up into a reddish bump over the first year of life. The hemangiomas can look rather dramatic when they get larger. These are often called strawberry hemangiomas due to their resemblance to strawberries. After about a year, these bumps gradually flatten out and then eventually either disappear or turn faint pink by the time your child is four years of age. Nothing needs to be done about either of these unless they are very large or are located in a place that may cause problems later, such as near the eye or around the mouth. The red color comes from the fact that they are made up of little blood vessels.

If your baby has a lot of hemangiomas, your doctor may refer you to a dermatologist or evaluate your baby further for conditions that may need treatment.

Blue Ones—Eyelids and Between the Eyes

This is not really a birthmark, but many parents ask about this. There are little veins on the upper part of the bridge of the nose than can extend into the upper eyelids. In a newborn, the skin in this area is pretty thin, and you can see these veins very easily. This gives your baby a slightly bluish

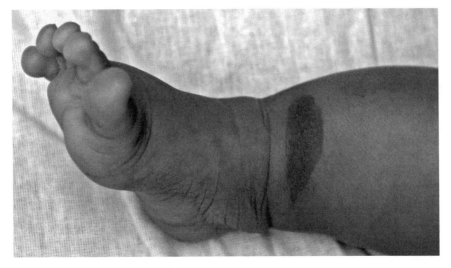

Mongolian spot birthmark

tint to the skin between the eyes. As the child grows, the skin will thicken and these vessels generally cannot be seen anymore. We all have them. You just cannot see them on yourself because of the thickness of the skin.

Grey-blue Ones—Mongolian Spots

Especially if your baby has darker pigmented skin (such as in Asian or African descent), he may have some dark grey-blue marks on the skin that appear almost like bruises. These are most common on the buttocks and can be rather large. These are normal and will usually fade by four to six years of age.

Because they can be mistaken for bruises, it is a good idea for your doctor to document their existence so that no one will question you about them later.

Brown Ones—Café au Lait Spots

A common birthmark is light brown in color and is called a café au lait spot. It is flat and is a coffee-colored brown (think coffee with cream). This birthmark should grow only as your baby grows. If your child has more than five birthmarks, visit your doctor to see if your child may have other

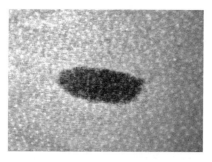

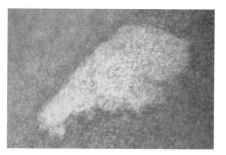

Café au lait spots   Ash leaf spot

findings that may indicate a disorder. If your child has only one to four of these birthmarks, then this is a normal variant.

Moles

Usually we develop moles as we get older, due to sun exposure. But some babies are born with moles. These range in size and can be anywhere on the body. Some may have hair growing out of them. Brown moles that are really big (more than 7 inches or 20 cm) are called giant nevi and are at higher risk for developing melanoma, or skin cancer. These need to be evaluated by a dermatologist. Moles that are medium-sized (.5 inches to 7 inches or 1.5cm to 19 cm) may be evaluated and followed. Hairy moles should be checked by a dermatologist as well.

White Ones—Ash Leaf Spots

Some babies have white colored birthmarks. If there is only one, then this can be a normal variation. The birthmark should grow only as your baby grows. If your child has many of these, has neurological problems, or has a spot growing faster than he is growing, see his doctor to rule out more significant medical conditions.

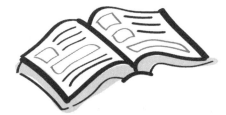

Finding a Doctor— Interview Questions

Practice/Doctor
Name:_____

Recommended
By:_____

Are all the doctors board-certified?   YES   NO

How many years has the practice been in business? _____

What are your hours? Do you have weekend or evening hours?

_____

Do you have same day appointments for sick visits? YES   NO

Will I see different doctors each time, or do I have an assigned doctor?
DIFFERENT   ASSIGNED

Are there multiple locations? Am I required to go to a particular office?

_____

Do you have advice nurses available for parents?   YES   NO

Do you use electronic medical records? YES   NO

Do you offer online access for patients? YES   NO

Are lactation consultant services available?   YES   NO

What do I do if I have an emergency? Who do I call?

_____

What's your policy on vaccines?

_____

Do you support breastfeeding? (if you are planning on breastfeeding)
YES   NO

Do you do circumcisions? (If not, then your obstetrician is usually who
performs the procedure.)   YES   NO

How much time do you allow for appointments?

_____

What's the average wait time to be seen?   _____

Does the office have a laboratory on-site?   YES   NO

And here are some factors you'll want to observe about the practice:

Is the location convenient?   YES   NO

Is the waiting room divided to separate sick children from well children?
YES   NO

Are there enough toys and books around to occupy children while they
are waiting to be seen? YES   NO

Is the office child-friendly?   YES   NO

Does the staff seem helpful and accommodating?   YES   NO

Other notes:

_____

_____

_____

_____

_____

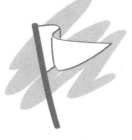

"Red Flag" List

Call the Doctor if any of the Following Occur!

1. Rectal temperature less than 97.0 ºF (36 ºC), or greater than 100.4 ºF (38 ºC).
2. Difficulty breathing, flaring nostrils, or persistent cough. Call 911 if there is blueness of the face or body.
3. Difficulty with feeding for several feeds.
4. Less than three or four wet diapers in 24 hours.
5. Lethargic, difficult to wake up, or sleeping more than six hours straight despite your best efforts to wake your baby.
6. Inconsolable fussiness or crankiness lasting more than two hours.
7. Projectile vomiting after most or all feeds.
8. Blood in stools, or frequent watery stools (more than five).
9. Bulging soft spot on the top of the head and fussy.
10. White-colored stools.
11. No stools during the first three days of life.
12. Yellow-colored skin (jaundice) of the entire body including the legs.

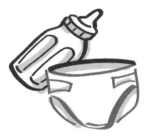

Baby's Input
and Output Chart

DATE	TIME	FEED (TYPE/AMT)	URINE	STOOL	SPIT UP

DATE	TIME	FEED (TYPE/AMT)	URINE	STOOL	SPIT UP

Checklist for Childcare/Daycare Interview

- What is the staff-to-child ratio?
- Are there different rooms for infants and toddlers?
- What are the policies on illness? What are the criteria for not allowing a sick child to come in?
- What are the facility's hours and holiday schedule?
- What happens if you are late picking up your child?
- What is their certification status?
- What kind of background check do they conduct on employees?
- What would disqualify someone from employment?
- How are their employees trained? Is infant and child CPR included?
- Does the same caregiver take care of your child every day?
- What is their employee turnover rate? How long have the teachers (especially the infant teachers) been there?
- Have they ever been the subject of an investigation? If so, what was the outcome?

- What are their hours? Do they provide care on holidays, weekends, or during early morning or evening hours?
- What is included in the fees? What must you supply?
- What types of meals and/or snacks do they provide? What is the feeding schedule?
- How often do they change diapers?
- How do they communicate back to you about the day? Do they give you a daily report?
- Do they currently have openings, or how long is the wait?
- Are parents encouraged to drop in to check on their children at any time?
- Do they provide closed-circuit monitoring via the web for parents?
- How do they verify the identity of the person picking up the child?
- What are their policies for handling accidents?
- How do they handle administering medications (prescription or over-the-counter)?
- Does the center have a policy of releasing children only to people whom the parents have authorized, in writing, to pick them up?

Observations to make while you are there:

- Does the staff seem flustered at being observed, or do they seem comfortable?
- Is the facility clean and neat? Are there age-appropriate toys and activities in each area?
- Is it easy for a person to enter the daycare center, or is there some barrier to prevent unauthorized entry?
- Do the children seem engaged with the caregivers? Or are the babies all sitting in swings and left to entertain themselves?
- How do the caregivers respond to unhappy children?
- How do you feel when you interact with the staff?
- Do children at the center appear to be secure and comfortable there?
- Is the facility well-ventilated, well-lit, and kept at a comfortable temperature?

- Is the childcare environment (both indoors and outdoors) safe and well-maintained?
- Are they organized?
- Is there enough open space to allow children to move around and explore their surroundings?
- Do the parents seem happy with the care that their children are receiving?

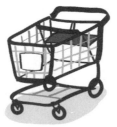

Newborn Shopping List

Equipment:

- Crib
- Bassinet (if desired)
- Portable crib (like Pack n' Play) (if desired)
- Stroller
- Car Seat
- Changing Table/Pad with Cover
- Rocker
- Diaper Bag

Layette:

- Onesies (5-10)
- Sleepers (4-5)
- Gowns (4-5, if desired)
- Thin receiving blankets

- Sleeper with swaddling attachment (if desired)
- Hats
- Socks
- Mittens (if desired)
- Bibs
- Burp cloths
- Outerwear/Bunting

Breastfeeding supplies:

- Nursing pillow
- Breast pads and nipple cream (lanolin)
- Breast pump and bottles to store pumped milk
- Nursing bras
- Nipple shield (if needed)

Bottle-feeding supplies:

- Bottles
- Nipples
- Bottlebrush
- Drying rack
- Sterilizer (optional)
- Formula

Sleeping and Relaxation:

- Nightlights
- Soothing sounds machine or CDs (optional)
- Baby monitor
- Pacifiers

Bath and Hygiene:

- Bathtub
- Washcloths

- Bath Towel
- Baby soap
- Baby shampoo
- Baby lotions/oil
- Diapers
- Diaper wipes
- Diaper disposal system
- Nail file and nail clippers

Medical Supplies:

- Digital Thermometer
- Vaseline (for thermometer and for circumcision, if applicable)
- Nasal saline
- Gas relief drops
- Vitamin D drops (if your baby is mostly breastfed)
- Infant's Tylenol (to use after two-month well check when your baby will get immunizations)

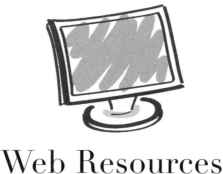

Web Resources

www.drsandysguide.com: Dr. Sandy provides online baby information, videos, photographs, and more!

www.cpsc.gov: Consumer Product Safety Commission—search for recalls on baby and child products.

www.nhtsa.gov/cps/cpsfitting/index.cfm: National Highway Traffic Safety Administration car seat inspection sites—enter your zip code to find local car seat installation inspection sites.

www.jpma.com: Juvenile Products Manufacturers Association—certifies that baby and child products meet ASTM (The American Society for Testing & Materials) International safety standards.

www.cdc.gov: Centers for Disease Control and Prevention—find information about traveling abroad and precautions against getting sick.

www.healthychildren.org: General pediatric information, sponsored by the American Academy of Pediatrics.

INDEX

ABOUT THE AUTHOR

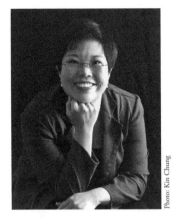

Photo: Kin Chung

SANDY L. CHUNG, M.D. is a noted pediatrician who has been named one of America's Top Doctors by the Consumer's Research Council of America and bestdoctors.com. After receiving her bachelor's degree and doctorate from the University of Virginia, Dr. Sandy completed her residency in pediatrics at the Inova Fairfax Hospital for Children and the University of Virginia. She has now been a practicing pediatrician for a large municipal community for more than eleven years.

Dr. Sandy has long been a leader in the pediatric community. She is President of Fairfax Pediatric Associates, PC, and serves on multiple boards and committees on a local, state and national level. With faculty appointments at multiple major universities, including Georgetown University and Virginia Commonwealth University, she has many years of experience training medical students, pediatric residents, and nurse practitioners in pediatrics. She has taught pediatric advance life support courses for the last ten years at Inova HealthSource for physicians, nurses, and emergency medical personnel.

Dr. Sandy has also made appearances at preschools and elementary schools, giving talks to parents on issues ranging from the H1N1 flu to nutrition and a healthy body mass index. She is a mother of four and thus knows firsthand the joy and stress of parenting. She aims to give new parents the skills and confidence to become great parents. Her website is www.drsandysguide.com, and you can read her blog at drsandychung.blogspot.com.

Sentient Publications, LLC publishes books on cultural creativity, experimental education, transformative spirituality, holistic health, new science, ecology, and other topics, approached from an integral viewpoint. Our authors are intensely interested in exploring the nature of life from fresh perspectives, addressing life's great questions, and fostering the full expression of the human potential. Sentient Publications' books arise from the spirit of inquiry and the richness of the inherent dialogue between writer and reader.

Our Culture Tools series is designed to give social catalyzers and cultural entrepreneurs the essential information, technology, and inspiration to forge a sustainable, creative, and compassionate world.

We are very interested in hearing from our readers. To direct suggestions or comments to us, or to be added to our mailing list, please contact:

SENTIENT PUBLICATIONS, LLC
1113 Spruce Street
Boulder, CO 80302
303-443-2188
contact@sentientpublications.com
www.sentientpublications.com

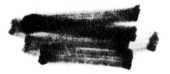

PATIENT PAVILION
HEALTH SCIENCES
FROST STREET
SAN DIEGO, CA 92123

CONTRADICTIONS

CONTRADICTIONS

poems by

BRIAN GLASER

Shanti Arts Publishing
Brunswick, Maine

CONTRADICTIONS

Copyright © 2020 Brian Glaser

All rights reserved. No part of this book may be
used or reproduced in any manner whatsoever
without the written permission of the publisher.

Published by Shanti Arts Publishing

Cover and interior design
by Shanti Arts Designs

Image on cover by
Wolfgang Hasselmann / unsplash.com

Shanti Arts LLC
Brunswick, Maine
www.shantiarts.com

Printed in the United States of America

ISBN: 978-1-951651-54-1 (softcover)

Library of Congress Control Number: 2020946940

For Andoe and John

Contents

ACKNOWLEDGMENTS

Grateful acknowledgment is made to the editors of the following publications where these poems first appeared:

Charge Magazine: "Essay on Tu Fu"

Diode Poetry Journal: "Trying Darkness"

The Magnolia Review: "Wake-Resilience"

Plum Tree Tavern: "Meditations in the Garden, March 22"

Tuck Magazine: "Sundown in Orange" and "Mendez v. Westminster"

SUNDOWN IN ORANGE

1.
There is no beginning—
the roads are still talking to you, asking
you the way.

So what is yours?—

your skin is made of glass;
it burns sometimes—

You are climbing the face
of and yet—

leave your quickdraws,

the cloud at the summit—
breath of the water, waiting—

where do you see this from, if not the midst
of your own life?

2.
First, do no harm—
harm to whom?

What if you were innocent
of the damage wrought by your politics—

if what mattered were your intentions alone
and the force that you were?

The American middle class
is terrified
of financial disaster—

and traitors, radicals:
though history moves like the plates of the earth.

3.
When you wake in the winter cold,
you doubt that goodness—

when the nurse calls us in—

we talk to the portrait
of the one

who does good by accident.

So—for reparations—we don't have
the expertise we need

in which children stole how much from whom,
in why

life is too brief for the whole arc
of morality on earth.

4.
Justice is volcanic,
poetry erodes.

One creates heights, one creates depths.

Looking deeply into someone's eyes—
a more vertiginous sight,

we should all have someone with whom
to share
that human vista.

*Note: Orange, California, was a sundown town through the 1950s.
This meant Black people were unwelcome at night. Chapman
University in those years shared with the Orange police
photos of its students so they wouldn't be harassed.*

MENDEZ V. WESTMINSTER

Lies—
some writers are openly proud
of their ability to tell them—

may a strong wind blow them away,
ashes on the Mediterranean Sea.

Students go to school
to escape from ubiquitous lies—

some say to use language is to lie;
each green leaf is as different from every other
as a star from a galaxy.

And the imagination,
the source of all our dreams,
may be amoral.

With all these forces arrayed against it, perhaps
it is a wonder
that the truth survives.

The truth is a relative concept,
it seems to me upon reflection—

we need enough of it
to keep goodness and beauty nearby.

It is when they go missing
that it is time for a trial—

time for a jury of school-aged children,
some of them wishing

with a passion to testify,

a passion
like earthrise in the Arctic—

the necessity of learning
from what has never been said.

*Note: Gonzalo Mendez in the 1940s sued an Orange County school
district that segregated students because of the color of their
skin. The rationale for the segregation was that it would help
students to learn English.*

Fairhaven Cemetery

One important thing about a work of art
is that it ends.

It is unclear to me
if the human mind can comprehend the infinite:

though I think
the imagination can be satisfied.

There is a monument in my cemetery
to the Confederate dead.

It is a squat obelisk covered with names
and a pyramid at the crown.

I have asked the county
to have it removed.

Those who fought for a lie—
those who killed for an indefensible cause—

their memorial art is the only art
that means whatever you say.

MEDITATIONS IN THE GARDEN

March 22—

The bee disappears
      into the trumpet-vine:
   forgetfulness.

March 23—

Grass pushing through the bricks—
      even in the garden
   of a gentle man.

WAKE-RESILIENCE

Rising

At my mother's beach house, we closed the metal blinds before
    bed, we were cautious,

and the children fell asleep before I did, as I lay listening to the
    seething rocks in the hints of moonlight,

and then in the middle of the night a thundering reverberation
    startled me awake,

though only I woke of all of us, and unlike the forgotten dreams on
    either side of it, I remembered the shock

in the morning, and walking out to the porch I found the glass of
    one patio pane shattered,

as my son and daughter said I would, and I thought—this is an
    early visitation of climate change—

the sea is angry, the sea is burning with anger, you can be good and
    still rouse the anger of nature,

you learn the right way long after you have begun to play, to play
    this instrument that gives you not music but life.

Casa Arcoiris, Tijuana

The superego is shaped by fear and, I think, the conscience is
    shaped by kindness,

though they are both less like the sound of the ocean—present,
    constant—than they are like an Aeolian harp,

the Romantic invention that made music in window frames as the
    wind passed over strings

connected to a resounding wood-chamber, making an effort at
    beauty out of the energy of chance;

we find our way towards goodness like a little globe of water
    wandering down a pane of glass,

like refugees, allowed to pass into goodness by grace, and seeking
    shelter under worn tarps

in the storms that constitute our failures, and the schools for our
    children that are like the sublime,

the sublime we have survived, that has changed us, that has saved
    us, that has told us we are always arriving,

even when we know, too, that we are always waiting, that time is a
    grace note, that time is a storm.

Coda

My daughter wrote a song on her ukulele about walking in the
    almost wholly concrete bed

of the creek that runs through our neighborhood, Santiago Creek,
    and she shared it on Instagram,

though now she has forbidden us, her family, a year later, to make
    reference to that song in any way,

embarrassed as she is by its innocence, and it seems to me that in a
    literal sense we have no innocence,

we have been like picadors to nature, but that music can create a
    sphere in which we are innocent,

in which, even, we can be surprised by the overwhelming evidence
    of our innocence—

a secret finally shared, a letter from a friend devoured with our
    eyes while the envelope burns.

21

THE MICHIGAN SONNETS

—for Justine Van Meter

1.

I don't know the names of the trees that hid me—
though the maples
were to that landscape
as the live oak is to the coast
I have come to love
and call my home.

One signature from the heavens
and a forest of them
a measurement of time
that broke its way
through the ground—

the roots work dawning.

Would the summer
of my childhood woods
be less filled with longing
if I could tell just how
those trees are called?

For they are not called by words
but by a feeling,
a feeling like a child sent out
to gather flowers—

as I have been—
and I found them, I who belonged.

2.
My favorite neighbors, the Klimeshes,
went to a Lutheran church
on Sundays.
They brought me
and my sister with them once.

I remember nothing of it
but the excitement of going
and the having gone.

Is that quite true?
I remember too the lustrous green of trees,
their crowns
high above me as I walked,
to or from, or after days had passed.

So the green of spring
and the gray of winter
in Michigan
become unforgettable,

the way that can be named—

a path between two places,
two childhood friends
who may never age.

3.
We drove across the state to the lake
and stayed in a cabin
built behind the dunes.

Pentwater:
it was a week,
enough time for creation.

Years later, when I went to the beaches
at Newport with friends,
the cresting
and crashing of the waves would feel something like
the advent of sexuality.

The rhythm of the waves of Lake Michigan
in no way prepared me
for the Pacific.

Lao Tzu, who said that water does not contend—
did he ever see an ocean shore?

Lake Michigan had one criterion
to be more real
to me
than any power revealed by abstraction:

it didn't wish to move me at all.

4.
My first memory is of waking on a blanket
in the warmth of sunlight
to the sound of a vacuum in another room.

I think it was the sudden knowledge of a pattern
that made it memorable,
though for years I thought it was the soothing sound
that impressed me,

and now, at the end of these poems,
I think it was my knowledge
that my mother was the creator of the sound—

it was my natural understanding
of the cause of the sound that made the moment
a good kind of shock.

My knowledge that my mother
could be many things,

that she could be awake while I slept,
that she could bear for me
to be apart.

State your name—
an island like a pilgrim,—

the right of a woman,
the first memory of the state.

THE LAND

The land will teach you to be nonviolent—
But you need to find the land.

1.

My father was a moral theologian;
He taught theology at the University of Detroit
For a few years before I was born
And a few more after my birth.
He didn't talk much about those days,
Though my mother has told me
That he was often called upon to teach
Theology to uninterested undergraduates—
Probably the general ed requirement
At a Jesuit school—and that he disliked
That part of the work. One story
He did relate to me was about the time
One of his undergraduates told him
He knew he had received a failing grade
And that if he didn't pass the course
He would lose his draft exemption and be sent
To Vietnam. He needed a fraudulent pass.
What did you do? I asked. He said,
I don't remember—and I believed him.

2.
There was one other story from those days.
My dad received a request from a stranger
Who said he knew him from his articles,
Which were often about conscience,
And needed some money because he was in a scrape
Of one kind or another. My father remembered
He sent him the cash. I would say of him
That he was by his nature a kind, curious man.

3.
To do violence to someone or to something
Is to treat him, or her, or them, in a way
That is contrary to their nature.
So not all force is violence. But what of the
Self-deputized customs officials
On the border of the Washington Territory
And Canada in the middle of the eighteen-eighties,
Enforcing immigration restrictions against
Chinese men seeking what was calling them here,
Those vigilantes and minute men?

Limitless freedom is transgressive too.
So some violence is inevitable. But I think we should
Always ask—whom does this violence serve?
The answer today, everywhere in the world, is:
Those with capital. How did this happen?
How did we get a system of allocation of wealth
And resources that treats so many people
In a way that is contrary to their nature?

Today I took my children to Laguna
To look at the tide pools in the rocky outcrops
At the north end of Main Beach.
There were barnacles on the rocks
And seaweed and seagrass everywhere
In reeking clumps, and I was moved
When we found two small translucent fish,
Fry really, in a pool of seawater gathered
In a wide pit out of the wet sand behind
A beaten face of rock where the waves
Resounded and crashed and sent up spray.

4.
I am reading a dissertation about American Daoism
That documents with unerring certainty
The pattern Edward Said called Orientalism
In the US absorption of that ancient system of belief.
The inclination of every empire is to find in its others
A kernel kept inert by superstitious tradition—

Then to stage itself rescuing that lost origin
And bringing it home as righteous wealth to the West.

So when I say that some phenomena are more natural
Than others, it seems to me that I am disparaging
A binary opposition where a spectrum is more apposite
But at the same time that I have no other way
Than the Orientalist error of imperial erasure
To ground to that judgment—

Still the future of the study culture lies in showing how
It contributes to health.

And I have been going this path
For decades already: in my early years teaching,
One of my first seminars in Duesseldorf,
I was standing in the center of a rectangle of tables
Holding forth on how Sylvia Plath's late poems
Were the record of a struggle towards maturity and peace.
An older student of Polish descent, one who had
Celebrated the collection of works of ancient art
In the vaults of a Berlin museum, said simply:
I object to the idea that art must be sane.

5.

Trade is as old as humanity, the libertarians say—
And capitalism is just the technical perfection
Of transtribal trade. I asked my wife yesterday
If she thinks capitalism is a more natural
Form of social organization than most others.
Yes, she said, because it is about freedom
And the rule of law. Up to a point, I have to say,
I can respect the idealism of anybody, especially
Those I love—and targets of idealism in a
Guatemalan adolescence couldn't have been
More plentiful than my own.

I remember talking with a classmate
In math during the end of the school year
Thirty years ago about the Tiananmen protests.
I was a socialist, like my dad—he was a Republican.
Aren't you inspired by these idealistic students?
He asked me. He explained to me his idea of
What was at stake. I didn't want to hear it,
Perhaps in the way that Zizek doesn't want to hear
About the tyranny of communists when he argues
That we are all complicit in the violence of capitalism
And so revolution is the ethical horizon.

As for me, now,
I am moved by the change in a once-Marxist friend
From graduate school who has found healing
In devotion to Jesus
On account of his self-sacrificing love.

6.
So, as a Westerner: am I trapped in the logic
Of the religions of my culture?
I read in a study of Daoism just today
That sacrifices of animals are a part of Daoist rituals,
Alongside food and goods and teas.

Recently moved back from Germany
Where I had chased work and fled from fascism,
Teaching the burdensome surveys of world lit
At my new college,
Near the end of the Bush administration
And the occupation of Iraq,
I observed my unfolding syllabus in despair
As the divinely decreed truce at the end of *The Odyssey*,
Accomplished after the father of Odysseus
Has killed the father of one of his victims who'd sworn revenge—
As this fragile vision of peace as an ending
Gives way to the vengeful decision of Aeneas
In the closing lines of *The Aeneid* to kill Turnus in the name
Of his dead friend Pallas
Because Turnus displays proudly the trophies of his kill.

He plunges his sword into him at the vulnerable throat.
My civilization learned nothing from the conclusion of *The Odyssey*,
It seemed to me, and so how could my students—
How could I?

7.

It is true and customary to say
That people with physical impairments—
Constructed as disabilities—
Are threatening because they remind everyone
Of the fragility of health and ability.
So most of the well stigmatize and look away.
In the same way, it seems to me,
Crazy people are unsettling in part
Because they sometimes don't act as if they have internalized
The legitimacy of consensual ideas
Of where bodies should and shouldn't be—
Which is to say, in essence,
That they have ceased to internalize
The legitimacy of the violence of the state.

My Romanticism teacher
Presented herself for arrest during the Occupy Movement
And was dragged by the hair
Across a public lawn on campus.
In discussing her decision to skeptical peers,
She wrote that a legitimate state
Would provide an adequate education
To its citizens.
Ad eaquus—towards equal.
This I know I believe: always only towards.

But it does seem to me that when Medea Benjamin
Interrupted a Trump official
Who was preparing the ground for war with Iran
And then went dead weight as they
Were carrying her off his stage,

She had crossed the threshold of madness
In the midst of a profound sanity—
Questioning the legitimacy of the millions
Of unspoken rules
That tell us how not to be moved by the state.

8.

At a conference on the environment and literature
Almost ten years ago
I was part of a panel which included
A religious studies scholar
Who proposed that we need artful rituals for mourning
Nature in the Anthropocene.

Hannes Bergthaller, an eco-critic I have come to admire,
Asked politely in the question period:
So, where should we begin our sense of what is to be mourned—
What is, so to say, our baseline idea of nature?
For it's been, he said, pretty rough going
For the megafauna
Since our species migrated out of Africa.
Nobody had an answer, as I recall.

Yesterday after an afternoon of thinking
I came to the end of a line of thought
That showed me for the first time mine:
August 6, 1945,
Around the beginning of the universalization of terror
And of leaving radioactive traces
In the geologic record of our polymathic ways.

9.
As I expected she would,
My wife today commented on the beauty of the canyon
Where we walked and watched for migratory birds,
And, as I expected, she said—
It's not Guatemala, but it's beautiful.

10.
I asked my son as he was protesting having to leave the house
For our walk in the canyon
What he thinks of when he thinks of nature.
Trees, he said.
What kind of trees? I said.
You know—Idyllwild—Yosemite, he said.
I felt a sense of accomplishment, of relief perhaps, of escape.

I accept the radicals' idea that capitalism has been, in part,
A mistake,
That it is unnatural in part.
But I do not accept their implicit idea of human nature,
That more materials are what we really want.
What is nature, what is natural—what is our nature?
Ask nature—nature tells you your answer.

11.
Putiidhem, the sacred site of the Acjachemen,
Has been taken for a school
Named for Junipero Serra in San Juan Capistrano,
And in the legal settlement some money was set aside
For off-site mitigation—
Meaning that my culture has given up on preserving the land
For its indigenous heirs.

Though it is hard not to think in a way
That the whole impulse of human history here
And our inspiring longing for cultural memory
Has been bought off,
The image that comes in a rush to mind
Is of the guardsmen with automatic weapons
Present at every hour
To guard the radioactive waste
At San Onofre Nuclear Generating Station,
Also known, with a terrorized absence of irony,
As SONGS.

12.
What will come to an end first—
Our masses of radioactive waste
Or our Western religious ideal of sacrifice?
Nuclear waste is dangerous to us because it emits particles
That destroy our DNA,
That alter its nature so that cancerous cells develop,
Unable to stop replicating,
Unable to cease.

Western culture is dead to me—
It died in 1945,
Though I have just realized that I have survived its end.
This is what happened to Eliot
When he was a younger man than me—
Then he chose denial, to return to the comfort of forms,
To be satisfied living with a ghost.

So what do I have left?

As you approach Tijuana from the north on the freeway
You can see a set of high ridges wholly covered in architecture,
Crowding out every organic form on that easel,
Contrasting with the brown hills
Of southern San Diego,
And it can seem, as you move towards it,
Like a tsunami may appear
To a novice of science in the worship of nature.

OC PRIDE

1.
Hope is what I have instead of pride
in my ancestors.

2.

I have given my statement on hope in another poem:
Hope is a question.

Sometimes a desperate, aggressive question—

spoken with the self-involvement with which my elder son
shows words to me he's learned to sign,

a language I have no intention of understanding well.

3.
My eldest is transgender—
I am still working on what he calls my pronoun game.

When we went to Orange County Pride last summer,
sitting together at an intersection in downtown Santa Ana—

all of us feeling caught up in the passionate energy
of goodwill and progress, growth—

I had to walk up the street to look for a bottle of water,
and I heard protesters on a side street,
chanting with a bullhorn:

"No Justice—No Pride!"

By the time I got back out to the street they were leaving;
I followed them
and over the music I rasp-spoke my questions at them,

to ask what precisely they wanted,
but they didn't hear me—though I was right behind them—

or—it dawned on me—
they knew I wasn't worth talking to.

4.
Somewhere close to me on my maternal family tree
is a man named Andrew Jackson Brodhead.

My branch of the Brodheads includes as a great uncle
a general in the Revolutionary War
who led the massacre of Seneca villages,

and others, to me unnamed,
who were holders of slaves.

More recent Brodhead uncles include a Congressman—
a lawyer, a landscaper, a dishwasher—
a loveable salesman who died by suicide.

5.
My former student works for Downtown, Inc.—
an organization of developers in Santa Ana.

She has organized literary festivals, art-walks, legislative efforts,
including what she calls a sunshine ordinance.

Last weekend, she gave a talk to the Orange County Greens titled:
Is Redevelopment Without Gentrification Possible?

She seemed to be suggesting, reluctantly,
that it isn't,
when she was interrupted by two women from Chicanos Unidos.

It is hurtful to me,
said one of the women,
that you as Greens would invite a gentrifier to address this subject.

We don't need our communities to be developed,
she said.

We need a moratorium on development in Santa Ana.

We already have—
and here I can't remember precisely the word she used—
working communities of our own.

6.
After more had been said,
a woman in the back of the room said:

I like how the two of you could complement each other;
Madeleine brings an academic perspective
and you, Gabby, bring the essential energy of an activist.

Gabby began to speak and the woman said,
I'm not finished yet.

It would be wonderful, she said,
for you two to work together instead of against one another.
There is clearly a great deal of common ground.

Gabby raised her chin slightly and said,
That's something I would expect from a white woman.

You don't know anything about me,
the woman replied.

7.

In his speech at my rehearsal dinner
sixteen years ago,

my father quoted Vaclav Havel,
who said that hope is not optimism—

it is the belief that there is meaning in however things turn out.

I quoted this in my eulogy at his funeral.
My undergraduate mentor,

who attended the wedding, who attended the funeral,
said as I left her at the airport:

you are like family,
you can call me for anything—
even when you don't know why you're calling,

when you don't want to make sense.

8.
I want from art what I want from life—
inventive solutions to intractable questions.

The protesters who staged an anti-gentrification action against
the Orange County Center for Contemporary Art
in downtown Santa Ana

have something to teach me:

art should not be a backyard garden.

Art is a way of looking at the human imagination
from a somewhat cold premise:

to begin to make an artwork carries the seeds of the irrational,
since you start from nothing each time.

Then comes meaning, like wild mustard—
everywhere in April, brittle tinder in July.

9.
If I were to contemplate
a world in which there were no differences

between art and life,
as Wallace Stevens does in "Ordinary Evening in New Haven"—

I think of the faintly audible window taps from the detention center
by which the inmates acknowledged

our protests below—

10.
Why do I feel the need
to endlessly educate the working class?

My uncle's suicide.
I identify with him.

A chilling reversal of values,
a bullet ripped through what we're told to think of as good.

And so perhaps I envy the sane ones:

I know better than they do
what they are capable of.

11.
It's okay to have killed yourself.
I had to tell someone once I knew.

My uncle, my grandmother's mother—
they were not sinners,
they were not failures.

This is not to say,
as I understand Sartre to have been saying,
that you probably should kill yourself.

Just to say that those voices
that tell you
that there is something cursed about those

who do the ultimate violence to themselves,
that their joy was less real,

that they are on the wrong side
of morality's inaugural prison—

to tell them
that they will forget their secret word someday

or find that it has changed.

Eleven Prayers to a Creek

1.
I don't
want to pray—my first step is away from you.
Why have you hidden

yourself across this distance, where the dust is an angel?
I have seen the hidden:
the disks of fungi together on the tree-limbs

in the green-decked creek.
Look at how those roots find the hidden water—
the signal of their success

is that the crown grows away from the hidden water,
heavenward.
It is easier to grow than to heal.

2.
The ugliness of God—
like vomit,
like the time my son was sick with fever for days

and threw up standing in a doorframe in the afternoon
and was suddenly well.
On my daily walk to the creek last week, I passed a grocery cart

burdened with trash,
or what seemed to me like trash—paper, bottles, wires.
And a sodden mattress under the bridge.

Like God's vomit—
some days that's the only thing a believer can do,
accept his disgust.

3.
There are two kinds of bridges
over Santiago Creek.
There's the freeway thirty feet above the path,

from which you can't see the creek at all—
and then the railroad,
a lower bridge, from which you can see the creek

if you look out the window
at the right time.
Descartes' evidence for the existence of God—

that we can conceive of him, and—therefore, he must exist—
makes an argument of thirst.
I prefer the realism of the seasons: no water, no life.

4.
And what of the evening
my daughter ran into the house from the side-yard pool
to tell me

she had just saved her brother's life?
If I believe that water
is God, I should perhaps keep that conviction private

in the way
that I wish to keep that memory of my negligence private—
or only make art from it

like our scenic painting of a lake,
not like the handwriting on the walls above the bed
of the public creek.

5.
Eliot called the river a strong brown god:
since water is amoral,
the human project of morality would be incomplete forever.

My son learned in school
that the Tongva believe humans keep separate the realms
of good and evil

which reside above and below our earthly home.
So some who found
this creek-cut to be a boundary a thousand years ago

believed, as I do,
that morality is a purely human accomplishment—
    like language, mortal;
like language, a vow to a child.

6.
I saw a heron and a rabbit on my walk today
and an orange dragonfly,
not once but twice, though it wasn't the same dragonfly,

I know,
which raises the question—of the two roots in
our protolanguage

for water, one which names water as a substance
and another,
they say, named water as a spirit—

what do we mean when we say they name the same being,
except to say
we don't believe them anymore: their stone has worn away.

7.
In the dream I was a lawyer for enlisted men,
helping them desert.
Of the smells along the creek-side walk—

rosemary, dried grass, eucalyptus, damp earth—
the haunting one
is the marijuana smoke, sometimes coming from

under the oaks,
sometimes, often, from the guys at the picnic table
under the bridge.

The faithful for generations had mortal arguments about
the ritual of incense,
the legitimacy of the baptism of the young.

8.
I was raised a Catholic.
Ritual, community, sacrament, tradition, display—they are what
I believed in, too.

So I sometimes miss their authority as I worship water.
The overwhelming
comfort of the tribe. The proof one is not insane.

Today on the walk
white and bright yellow moths were everywhere,
and I know

that most moths are nocturnal—so these were day's pilgrims,
illustrating the air,
protected by heaven from the lure of electric light.

9.
In the dream she became a river
as we made love.
Today along the creek I paused in the oak's shade

to watch an archer at the range.
He studied
the distance for more than long enough

to wrestle with a doubt.
The arrow was black, was fine—I couldn't see it reach the target
once it flew.

My music was from the cloud: Shostakovich.
The clouds are for silence:
every song to them has long been said, and yet they stay.

10.
The thinker who turned me against Hegel described why
he prefers James
with a phrase spoken like a banishment: no absolute.

His eyes were mad with conviction.
Now that I have
found a way to worship water, retrospective irony

allows me to ask: what is lethal about the absolute—
is it pollution?
For, at least to me, they seem to be opposites.

To be taken out of the solvent, to be absolved—
I can't give it up, entirely—
may the disgraced solution save one who has been burned by the sun.

11.
Water is not a jealous god.
The Greek deities, who rape and punish mortals
for their sexuality,

the brooding God of Adam
who made a woman to tempt him out of paradise—
the God of the killers

who blow up the unbelievers in the controlling passion
of their jealousy—
water was the same cold clarity to me

when my son and I went fishing on the jetty in Dana Point
as she is at the creek—
as I strayed, as I cast a line from the rocks for pleasure.

Taoist Daybook

August 4

Today at the Palm Springs Air Museum with my family, the sheen of the polished planes made their violence seem of our moment again, as if it had just happened. In the European theater hangar, I thought for as long as I could bear of the children killed by the bombs dropped from those planes. Melanie and Andoe and John had disappeared into the center of a bomber on their tour, and I watched the only other visitors there—a mother in a hijab with a father and three children too young for school, and two mothers speaking to their children in Japanese as the kids climbed in and out of a cockpit. This I remembered as I was sitting on the balcony late tonight in the warm, dry air at the resort, in a wicker chair on a balcony overlooking the pool, looking up through the water vapor in the air at the few stars and marveling at how much care it has taken for each of the bodies that were there at the pool in the afternoon, now all disappeared too, to get the fresh water that makes up more than half of their mass, every one of us.

August 11

Reading of the beginning of the thousands of years of continuous
civilization in China, held together by writing and war, the first
dynasty troubled by rumors of an unfaithful wife, a scandal
debated by historians for millennia—out of the vast culture that
gives us the harmonious dynamic of yin and yang

Father nature: my feminism must involve reimagining male
sexuality—I write this as my younger son reads Greek myths
on the couch across from me in the living room, on the night
before school begins—I cannot tread any further yet than these
words, father nature—here I feel I have invited into my innocence,
contemptuous laughter—

August 12

I burnt myself with steam tonight preparing dinner—invisible
labor, my friend calls it, the work done by migrants from the south
in restaurants all over this part of the world, kept deliberately
behind walls, unseen men, open secrets—my father's father died
when my father was sixteen—it was a heart attack. I never asked
my father how he felt about the loss of his dad so early in life—I
knew the question was taboo; I knew so deeply it was knowledge
hidden from me until today—

Today watching the line of first graders leave my son's
elementary after their first day of the year—they looked
a little stunned, utterly alert—they will learn to read this
year—I wished I could do something great for them, their dark,
intelligent spirits—as for my colleagues who sent out a death
notice of their writer friend yesterday—I am glad they made
me uneasy by speaking of the dead——who else could be as
essential to talk about as this person who has made me feel
deeply, this absent, shadowing light?

August 17

Meditating in the backyard at night after reading about the Tao in a book of the sixties—my posture on the black disk of a cushion was my habitual Zen posture, which the book says is foreign to Taoist meditation—the Taoist is to sit with his bent knees in front of him, with his buttocks resting on his ankles—and not to count his breaths, as the Zen novice does—

Outside in the warm evening of late summer—the book tells me that Taoist awareness involves a non-rational state of dissolution between self and world—how can I allow to arise the non-rational—for my dragon: I cannot see him in the dark—my dark dragon, my life's composition in the minor key—of all my errors and mistakes—it is not fear of the dragon—sitting in this darkness makes quite evident what I had not yet seen, the brevity of the dark dragon's life—

TRYING DARKNESS

—for Livia Kohn

1.

The valley spirit never dies:
so says Lao Tzu.
The purpose of the valley is to express
a monument of survival.

As you walk the boulevards of Tijuana it is not unheard of
to see prostitutes in doorframes.
You can find this image in public films as well—
some women avert their gaze

as the camera passes—
the river shapes the valley with the energy of shame.
This will be my first poem like a sex-worker—

not at work in bed, but on the street—
and the camera must cut like a channel of water,
as moral as a cat.

2.

My first reading in a Tijuana newspaper is about
an abducted child—

his mother is an addict who must have fled with him to the capital,
his father says hopefully.

And the second is an article about a presentation
at the university
of the work of a poet on the hundredth anniversary of his birth.

The dark enigma of which Lao Tzu speaks—

we said in the liturgy of my youth, too:
let us proclaim the mystery of faith.

An unbearable mystery:
in every imaginable film he would be found.

What have we made of the unbearable—
God's will, monarchs, genres of the night.

3.
Sadness, post-coital melancholia—
the experience
of the hollows of *eros*;

I don't think you can imagine your way to them,
nor can I,
in such a way, know the fear and contempt that are the trials
of the prostitute this afternoon in Tijuana,

and to try is a test of the health of my sense of humanity
in a strange game—
looking for a moment across the fence—my culture calls literature.

Scripture may have something to temper the act of risk
at play in empathy.

Buddha says to desire is to suffer;
Taoism says to find out *li*, the sandy erotic pattern in the grain.

4.
Someone who might know
because he has been a therapist for thirty years
says sex is initially transgressive
in adolescence, and remains vitalizing to the extent

that it is still a transgression
in adult life.
A book about prostitutes in Tijuana says

that they are at as much risk of disease from romantic partners
as from their johns.
All this only seems to confirm my sense that there

is something especially pathological about straight male sexuality.
And just today I read for the first time
that Freud called happiness the fulfillment of a prehistoric wish—
sex without gender: the exit in desire.

5.
Taoism is without the idea of fallen sexuality
and carnal sin.

It has its versions of the Kama Sutra and recommendations
for sexual yoga,

and for a child of Catholicism in a Puritanical culture
it gives room for hope
that the body could be loved as the body is.

And yet the focus of those texts seems often to be
on stealing or retaining
one's *qi*, the vital energy and life force that produces longevity,

than which there is no higher good in Taoism.
So there is too a coercive element
to Taoist teachings on sex—
corrupt silence on the subject of pure pleasure there too.

6.

The discourse of pleasure reminds me of college
where everyone the age I am now
seemed to be despondent about Reagan and to be getting a divorce,

sleeping with students, too.
The aspiration to pleasure brought the peaceful defeat of the good,
hardly anything more.

And that dark place reminds me of
returning as a ten-year-old
from a family trip to a cabin at Lake Michigan
to find that a group of teenagers had broken into our home

and stolen my thousands of pennies from my room—
I remember the police, their forensic white dust
on revealed fingerprints,
some of them the transgressors' and some of them mine.

Essay on Tu Fu

1.

If I begin in sadness again
it is because I hope to write towards sadness leavened by joy.

A bombing at a mosque in Afghanistan:
the killers made the roof collapse, crushing sixty worshipers.

It is necessary for me, necessary to do properly:
absence-thinking.

If I had loved one of those worshipers
this poem would be obscene.

Perhaps that is what freedom means, at its darkest depth—
to love yourself for no good reason.

2.
One philosopher writing on John Dewey
says to believe in democracy requires a sense of the tragic.

I wasn't able to ask the naturalist at our walk
how evolution explains poison fruit.

Not to know—
Lao Tzu says he who speaks does not know.

And he who knows does not speak;
so the poet speaks—to become unknowing, to dream for another.

3.
If there is a primordial void
there must be a first vessel, a dwelling for emptiness.

Thus, absence cannot be before all things—
the meaning of the Tao may be understood without difference.

Keep the fish, says Chuang Tzu,
and let the net that caught them be forgotten.

If you have been touched by presence in this way,
absence is a mortal danger.

All poetry is translation, says a friend—
words die without translation.

4.
Reading Tu Fu's early poem
written across a distance to his little boy:

the poem—like many others in this section of the book—
acknowledges the presence of grief at its end.

An insect—it is unusual, I don't know its name—
climbs up the page and turns around and descends.

Among the gifts of fatherhood,
light and unexpected was the innocence of poems.

5.
As I was explaining the Tao to my younger son, he said—
so, basically, it's just like the force.

Yes, I said, sort of—the force without all the magic.
Oh, he said.

Spring rain, wine in a garden with a friend, the waning moon—
it is as if Tu Fu discovered

someone would still listen after he said that—oh—to mortality.
His poems of war and refuge are another matter.

I do not find them to offer any consolation for suffering.
This is their eloquent case against life.

6.
Tu Fu rejected Taoism, I think,
for more or less the reason I can't be a Christian.

The doctrine of the omnipresence of the culture's consecrated spirit
is out of our range.

One timeless way of absence:
so David Hinton translates Tu Fu's late verdict on existence.

When there is joy to be found here,
it belongs to neither silence nor to words.

ELEGY

1.

Getting a haircut today
the stylist told me the story of the homeless sex offender
who loiters by her door and pulls his pants down in the bushes,
and another story

about a client's boyfriend
who raped her three young children, two little girls and boy.
What is the name of that country where they just kill people
for doing things like that?—

she asked—it's a European country.
They don't have these kinds of problems over there anymore.

2.

The president of the Black Student Union at my school asked if she
could take my course

on human rights.

She's writing on disparities in incarceration for black and brown
    inmates—
the essay ends asking how older judges will ever unlearn
their racism.

It's mostly talk,
the human rights movement—nation-states have all the money,
nations and corporations. In this, it's like the elegy, which, according
to Peter Sacks,

is really about sex.

3.
As I was raising my young children in Santa Ana, in my thirties,
working in sustained fright about keeping my job at the college,
a Vietnamese poet

named Nguyen Chi Thien
spent his final years in the same city, the city where I kept the embers
of the sacred flame of poetry alive in my own life as well.
He died in 2012,

leaving behind prose memoirs
of his years as a prisoner at the Hanoi Hilton, and a book of poems
which he went back to prison for smuggling into the British embassy,
published in English

by Yale, the CIA hotbed.
I am reading these poems slowly, learning from how conflicted he was,
not like the serene dissidents I know in Santa Ana who risk their
        private peace
to protest injustice

in America and the west,
but someone who could not rest until he had defeated dictatorship
        personally,
who didn't really understand the source of his passion,
who learned he was sad

because he wept.
Lao Tzu says a victory should be celebrated like a funeral.
Does it follow that a funeral should be like a victorious rite?

4.
Elizabeth Bishop

shocked me in a letter
when she said that she believes *The Waste Land* is about impotence—
not symbolic impotence, that is, but, as she put it, the thing itself.
How can

one disagree decorously?
Sacks says the elegy rewards desire with symbolic triumphs—
thunder becomes the syllable of Sanskrit, which becomes scripture,
which is the climax.

There are a thousand
volumes in the Taoist canon, more than a layperson could ever read.
The peace of celibacy: as symbol, as the thing—there is no
        distress of the erotic
in the poems of Nguyen,

it is as if
he may have never felt that tear that transforms a lover into a father,
what Cather called, speaking of a professor, his nature modified
        by sex.

5.
The defeated prisons—

Nguyen misunderstands,
to me, the bond across generations, a link fragile as a daisy-chain.
He imagines someday summer will burn autumn on its pyre,
that joyously the young

will celebrate
the defeat of the devils he calls the Communist thugs and liars.
Some have, some would—but as a teacher I find most young minds
are fascinated

mostly by themselves,
their futures, their fates, their ironic survivals of the burdens
of their fallible parents' love, which most of them are fortunate
        enough
to know.

Poetry is a
brown-skinned woman, long lustrous black hair
and warm, piercing brown eyes, eyes that look up from the page
        of life
and find me,

ashamed,
to be so old and not have solved for anyone the problem of desire.

6.
What is victory?
At the cemetery on Memorial Day the jets fly over us, all of us
sitting on the grass, me half-listening to the artful rhetoric and
    music while
the young ones

play tag
and run in circles at the edges of the strange organic shape we make
by gathering to listen on the earth that keeps the dead hidden forever.
What if the west

is wrong
about heaven—that our forebears are not there, safely, waiting,
but that they need us still, they need not only our worship, the custom
of the Vietnamese,

but they need us
the way our lovers need us—not with the indecency of desire, no,
but with its same indefatigable recitation, like words it has chosen
to memorize,

to condemn
the dreary unlovable prison, to give us the taste of morning?

CLOSE HELD ELEMENTS

Wood

A face cord,
steadfast
and split
underneath

the father,
oak bark,
bought for winter
and stacked

by his son
who survives
somehow here—
wood teaches

you beauty,
the memory of
a woodpile
stacked like earth—

we all need
a copse of
living brothers of
the oak—

each oak
quarters after
its heart,

the grain,
if you run your hand
along the broken
splinter-surface

as it calls
you to,
you feel the
yielding strength

only slowly,
this is the way
one grain
teaches

Fire

A campfire
smoldering the night
through and you,
chaos,

never,
a companion
in the morning,
cold like a cut

in the tent—
Chaos as darkness, too,
the darkness
of smoke—

what is burning?—
the good
dead-wood
of autumn, living—

The forest
you need
like an ancestor
is cut, too,

cut to ash,
though the forest
can grow
when its guardian

is gone—
it is
the guardian
who lingers

like smoke,
the one who wakes
you:
don't fear

the chaos,
they took me—
the smoke
remembers

Water

This frozen
pith of life
should not float—
find the ice

on the sea floor
and you have
the claret-world
of theory:

crossing water
to grow
more innocent—

but because
its danger
is the
time thaw

to time
at the door—
dark calving:

they are already
there,
the stateless,
their hidden bid,

the visible
disappears,
reality
torments the boat,

this danger,
it can't be
thought away—
the rupture

of water
makes nothing's roof
and floor—

the pattern doesn't
always end—

Metal

The way
of the world
in Gaza,

again,
for the first time,
again,
a silence

is not the silence
of children—
of course—
we will never

extricate our eyes
from the blood;
can you bear
the hate-garden,

the matted
hair of love,
soaked purple
like an eggplant

with blood—
The iron there
is the element
of munition—

you have tasted
what killed them,
and if you say
their names

the hate-garden
grows
like blood
in your saliva—

so say them,
you who would spit,
this poison
comes from heaven—

Air

Music is impossible
without you—

we know,
we two—

ABOUT THE AUTHOR

Brian Glaser was born in Detroit, Michigan,
the eldest of two children of Jack Glaser, a
theologian, and Mary Ellen Glaser, an educator
and social worker. He was educated at the
University of California, Berkeley. In 2003, he
married dancer and choreographer Melanie Ríos,
with whom he has two children, Andoe and
John. In 2005, he joined the faculty at Chapman
University, where he currently teaches in the
department of English. His previous poetry
collection, *All the Hills*, was published by Shanti
Arts Publishing in 2019.

Shanti Arts

Nature · Art · Spirit

Please visit us online
to browse our entire book
catalog, including poetry
collections and fiction, books
on travel, nature, healing, art,
photography, and more.

Also take a look at our highly
regarded art and literary journal,
Still Point Arts Quarterly, which
may be downloaded for free.

WWW.SHANTIARTS.COM

Wrong Highway

*To R.E.S. who paved the way
and to "The Indignants" who helped us along it*

Wrong Highway

The Misadventures of a
Misplaced Society Girl

STELLA T. JENKINS

Edited by Mark E. Smith

hancock
house

ISBN 978-0-88839-708-9
Copyright © 2011 Stella T. Jenkins
Second printing 2012

Library and Archives Canada Cataloguing in Publication

Jenkins, Stella T.
Wrong highway : the misadventures of a misplaced society girl / Stella T.
Jenkins ; edited by Mark E. Smith.

Includes index.
Also issued in electronic format.
ISBN 978-0-88839-708-9

1. Jenkins, Stella T. 2. Jenkins, Stella T.—Family. 3. British Columbia,
Northern—Biography. 4. Yukon—Biography. I. Smith, Mark E., 1950– II. Title.

FC3826.1.J45A3 2011   971.1'8   C2011-903404-2

All rights reserved. No part of this publication may be reproduced, stored in a
retrieval system or transmitted, in any form or by any means, electronic, mechanical,
photocopying, recording, or otherwise, without the prior written permission of
Hancock House Publishers.

Printed in South Korea — PACOM
Editor: Theresa Laviolette
Production: Ingrid Luters
Cover Design: Ingrid Luters

HEADIN' DOWN THE WRONG HIGHWAY
By TED DAFFAN
© 1945 (Renewed) UNICHAPPELL MUSIC INC.
All Rights Reserved   Used by Permission

All photos by author except: P. 190-192 by Mark Smith
Map by Eric Leinberger, UBC

*We acknowledge the financial support of the Government of Canada through the
Canada Book Fund for our publishing activities.*

Published simultaneously in Canada and the United States by
HANCOCK HOUSE PUBLISHERS LTD.
19313 Zero Avenue, Surrey, BC Canada V3S 9R9
1431 Harrison Avenue, Blaine, WA, USA 98230-5005
(604) 538-1114 Fax (604) 538-2262

www.hancockhouse.com | sales@hancockhouse.com

Contents

Preface

This is the story of a young couple escaping the strictures of the 1940s city life by "going north" into the British Columbia and Yukon bush of those days, against family disapproval. In doing so we experienced many inappropriate domestic issues, extant even today, but especially when joined by my children from a previous marriage.

This story is much more than a family saga, dealing, as it does, with adventures encountered and the lives of a lot of very old people scattered through the pines and spruce, whose influence on us was inevitable. The story is built in part from my own notes taken at the time, from 1948 to 1958. The title of the book is taken from an old record, *Headin' Down The Wrong Highway*, and refers not only to the Alaska Highway but also to the supposedly wrong road we took in life.

Initially, I changed the names of people to avoid disturbing the living. The names of most towns and settlements had also been altered, with a few backgrounds in a generous haze. This enabled me to write frankly. Once the story had been written, however, two of my sons prevailed upon me to reveal real names and places, using the argument that this is, indeed, a valid snapshot of days gone by and that truth is more fascinating than fiction, so now the names are real and the names of places stand as such. All the elders have gone on, as well as most of our contemporaries, but I crave the indulgence of any survivors who should not be too incensed when they recognize kinfolk by what took place so long ago. I hope they will feel, as I do, that those were great days and we were all human.

One or two liberties have been taken with the truth to help things along, but they are based on absolutely true facts strung together as a composite, as with Charlie Lindquist's deeds, and with Mrs. Boyd who represents several women. In some cases, too, the names have had to be fictitious because I had either forgotten or never known them.

Charlie Lindquist did rescue Effie at a different time and she was indeed inspected by a social worker. Mrs. Travers lived a little further down the road but her home was as described inside and she and Hattie did look exactly as delineated, as do all the other characters. The two women really were friends but I'm not too sure about the golden eggs. Hattie's true ending did not include winching a boy out of the well but she was terribly worried about my boy falling in. This ending does portray what she was doing and of what she was capable. They did have to break in to find her.

Originally intended as a tale of those balky elders met in the bush (whom I dubbed the Indignants because of a lovely malapropism used by Tatty), with stories of them like beads strung together, it became evident that our story was the thread binding us, and carried more beads. The account gradually turned into a narrative of our flight and the flak raised by relatives. We met the Indignants while having our own indignations.

In addition, I did crib shamelessly from a trapper, Mr. John Tetsoe. Bob knew all the trapping methods, but I could not remember them, and most of Mr. Tetsoe's sounded familiar. His were the yarns about tapping the ice around a beaver lodge to find an entrance, shooting at a mountain wall to force the moose closer, and seeing a bird's feet touching the fish. Otherwise most credits (I would say ALL) belong to Bob Smith.

Finally, since the themes come up so often, I hope readers will be interested in how we handled the hurdle of remarriage, extended family, and interference sixty years ago.

— STELLA JENKINS
Victoria, BC, 2008

10

Headin' Down the Wrong Highway

Too many sweethearts and none of them true
Done too many things that I shouldn't do
I made lots of money all spent the wrong way
Headin' down the wrong highway

I made lots of friends but now they're all gone
Too many mem'ries that still linger on
I had too many drinks both night and day
Headin' down the wrong highway

Too many heartaches and too many tears
Crowded too much in just a few years
I want to go right but I've lost my way
Headin' down the wrong highway

I've lost everything lost all my friends
God only knows how all this will end
Drinking and gambling each night and day
Headin' down the wrong highway

—THERON EUGENE "TED" DAFFAN (1912–1996)

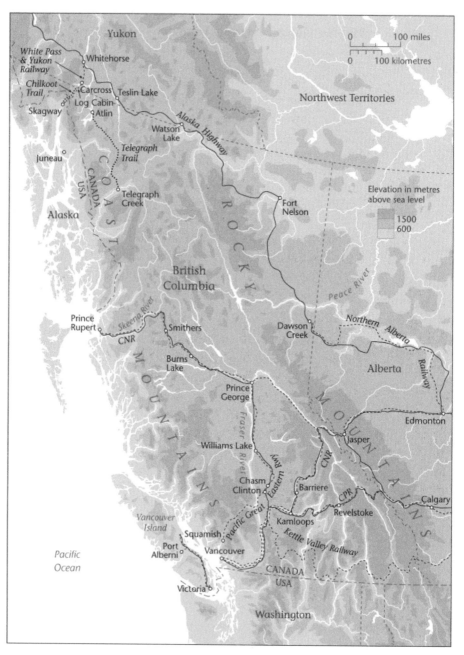

British Columbia in the 1950s.

CHAPTER · I

Traps

"This country is so boggy you can step on one end of a field and the other end goes up." So went Bob Smith's journal, written in pencil most nights by the light of his fire. "Been skirting bogs all day. I got this Indian guide, Shorty Johnson, to take me down to the end of Teslin in his canoe. When he put me down, Shorty said I was nuts."

Robert Edward Smith had set off with his pack to walk from Teslin Lake to the British Columbia coast over the Trail of '98 to come out at Telegraph Creek. At the same time, unknown to my adventurer and me, the BC writer and explorer, R.M. Patterson, (*Trail to the Interior*, MacMillan of Canada, 1966) was heading up the Trail of '98 while Bob was walking down it. Mr. Patterson headed for the Dease Lake branch and so the two men did not meet.

It was July 1948, and while everyone was engrossed down south with the Fraser Valley flood, my thoughts were up north because the only light of my life at that time was in danger of going out altogether. And he needed company.

A detailed map of British Columbia covered a wall in my office. As a government clerk, every morning on arrival, I stole up to it and studied the terrain between Teslin and Telegraph. Each day I looked at the map and tried to estimate how far Bob had gone. I could not know then if he had survived or if the grizzlies had got him, but in due course a great fat envelope would arrive which contained his pencilled journal. I read it, dying a little death at each entry, for, apart from fields tilting when he stepped on one end, he had crossed rivers by unreliable cable, undergone all dangers and was without food for three days until rescued by a trapper with pack horses, an Indian wife and small children, all seemingly living off the wild rhubarb stuffed into the panniers. As I was taking this in, Bob was calmly making his way from Wrangell, an Alaskan town on an island off the mouth of the Stikine River, back into the interior of BC, looking for work.

Bob Smith, as a wanderer, was a direct result of the unsettled state of veterans after the Second World War. He was adrift on the country. In 1948 he was like other returned men, fidgety and picking up jobs only to put them down again. Now he was looking for work near the Babine country. Footloose, though not entirely fancy-free, he had finished that walk from the end of Teslin Lake to the settlement of Telegraph Creek on the Stikine River and felt fulfilled. For the time being.

I was a newly divorced woman, aged thirty-two, dark-haired with blue-grey eyes, standing five foot eight and a half at one hundred thirty-eight pounds, which "wouldn't make decent broth," according to my father, and was in my first job ever, having been taken into the Parliament Buildings literally off the street. With a background of very English parents, teachers, and beliefs in all things British, I was still fresh from the domineering presence of a sea-going spouse, who, although he loved me dearly, used to say, "Catch 'em young and treat 'em rough." He had received me straight from the schoolroom and the arms of a dominant mother in 1933. I believed everything they said. And World War II had everything to do with everything.

Were it not for the war, there would have not been those anxious days listening to reports of the battle on the Atlantic; the heady excitement of brief reunions; a sailor's infidelities; love stoked up by the sight of a uniform, then disillusioned by its wearer; keeping the home fires burning and wondering what for. Real trouble had begun when my husband trapped himself with a part-time mistress he was sorry for, who began being proprietary. He actually compared our letters, hiding nothing. Absolutely nothing made any sense to him unless he could tell me about each achievement, like a cat laying its catch on your doorstep. I finally grew up and said, "Sauce for the gander is sauce for the goose," meaning, "Just you see how it feels!" I plotted revenge successfully, going on a couple of outings with other men, but such a stance didn't suit me; it made my skin crawl. Of course, when he realized my intention was to have revenge, everything hit the fan. Still, a divorce would never have been necessary but for the totally unrepentant attitude of this restless vet who flatly refused to give up his habit of rescuing wallflowers who needed "serving." My sister reflected, "He thought he was doing them a favour." His stated belief was "every bull needs a harem," and he continued his philandering. Then he began to hit me, and it was over.

The sad part was that otherwise he was a very fine man. Passionate about the sea, he was a good seaman and navigator, and a dutiful workaholic. For instance, he had single-handedly rewired his ship, a passenger and freight vessel plying up and down the west coast of Vancouver Island which he operated with his partner, another naval veteran. They were well known for their cheerful assistance and generosity towards coastal settlements that could use their aid.

A friend who worked for them said, "I know nothing about their domestic lives, but they are great guys to work for." During the war, when my ex was transferred from command of his minesweeper, some sailors leaning out of a port as he went down the plank, were heard to say, "There goes the best damn skipper we ever had."

George McCandless and Esson Young formed the Barkley Sound Transportation Co. Ltd. in 1946, replacing an existing shipping service started in the 1930s. The small ship referred to was MV *Uchuck I.* An interesting history of the ship and its successors is online at www.mvuchuck.com/mv-uchuck-3.php (as at January 2011).

Looking back, our break-up was so sad and senseless. Bitter recriminations slid the whole thing to its inevitable, stupid end.

Arrangements were made. In those days one simply did not get a divorce as easily as today; adultery and beating were the only grounds, so men faked "grounds" in order to have the break become legal. With our families having been so close for almost twenty years, I simply could not bring myself to even tell my mother, let alone say publicly, that he had beaten me. In those days it would have shamed the entire family, and the rest were fine people. I kept it to myself and my parents went to their graves never knowing.

During our divorce proceedings, the judge said that our "arrangements" amounted almost to collusion because we appeared to be so amicable, and he nearly threw the case out of court. Our fifteen years of marriage came to an end in 1948. While in those times divorce was something to be avoided at all costs, after the war my elders would have their heads together, saying, "It's in every family."

For the first time, I was flying solo, apart from the two youngest children I'd had to bring with me to Victoria, leaving the two big boys, thirteen and twelve, with their father—which seemed best, as they needed a father. They were to work after school on his ship. But I'd had to keep my daughter with me, and the youngest boy had to have a mum.

I was full of a desire to show everyone what I could do to survive, without an ounce of confidence in my ability to do so. My insides had been full of black chaos before I met Bob while on my way to volunteer at the *HMCS Naden* canteen. Chicken behaviour vanished in a hurry. He had the pluck to ask for my phone number and, to my own total surprise, I found myself giving it. When he called and suggested things like coffee or walks on the beach I accepted and found myself with a happy, solid companion. He was also quite "proper" as the divorce proceedings went on, saying, "You won't ever drag *me* into this; your marriage was busted a long time before *we* ever met!"

Bob took me at face value and expected only practical optimism.

He looked like a short, stocky kid of five foot two and a half, with a wrestler's build carried on slim, almost delicate, legs.

He had red wavy hair, mud-brown eyes and freckles blended into a smear, and his classical, almost pretty, features made him look about sixteen. He was, in fact, almost twenty-six.

He had demobbed from the war as a navy commando dressed in round rig, which would be transformed into a tweed jacket, slacks and brogues, holdovers from his university and golfing days when in civvies, but it was the bush life that showed his real image. There he wore his commando gabardine "blouse" with the insignia torn off, over a red plaid jack shirt. These went with green whipcord pants, hiking boots, and, on top of the red curls, an everlasting ski cap—before ski caps were so popular. He would shade his eyes with its peak, defensively sometimes, and never wore it in any position but dead straight ahead. His cockiness was combined with modesty and did not run to being a smart aleck; the truth is that, like me, he was the product of Anglo-Saxon parents and, like me, could not completely shake off his traditional origins for all his bush poses.

What got to me was not any of these facts, endearing though they were. It was that he understood me completely and seemed to like what he found. And if he didn't like what I did he would soon tell me, one to one, without being critical. It was a new feeling, because up until then I'd had to live inside a suit of armour.

Now I didn't know if I was in love with him, exactly, but I was hooked.

While Bob wandered, my own life down in Victoria was in a state of flux. After packing up and leaving, the two kids and I had gone straight to my parents. They understood my misery, but my mother, not knowing all the details, felt I should have stuck it out. They had known my ex-husband, George, since his childhood and thought he was a fine man. My father was very unhappy with the situation but kept quiet about it. A divorce in those days was a shocking scandal to be avoided at all costs. At the same time I was going through this, my sister Faith was having difficulty with her second husband's alcohol abuse. It was only many years later she and I found out Mom was far more sympathetic to our plights than she let on. She thought both of us had "deserved another go."

With regard to my budding relationship with Bob, Mom told me, surprisingly, that she thought every woman should have a romance, but should know when to cut the cord and end it.

Having three of us there soon became too much for my mother, who was over seventy, and she had to ask me to find some other way out. She kept Robert, who was five, while Joan, who was ten, moved with me into a hotel.

In the hotel, Joan and I were treated to the sounds of mating coming through a wall and I knew I had to get her out of there fast. A walk-up in a seedy district near town was our first home on our own, all stairs and linoleum, and a cooler hanging out the window. The next step was retrieving Robert, who happily discovered that his first school ever was one block away.

On his first-ever day at school, Robert, not quite six, admitted himself, all alone, without a whimper. I had to be at work at eight. He and watchdog Joan separated at the gate, as she proceeded to her own elementary further on. Now an eleven-year-old, she was a honey-coloured kid as to hair and suntan, with hair parted in the middle and two long braids, while Robby was a skinny puppy with large hands and feet and an observant mind. He had been observant enough as a toddler to listen to Red Skelton from his high chair and bring forth, "If I do it, I get a licking—I *dood* it," dropping his porridge bowl on the floor.

My humble pay packet was ninety-eight dollars and my workmates every type imaginable, but I was befriended by a partially recovered polio victim who dragged one foot while she showed off by heaving around great mail sacks. "You let your emotions rule you," she accused, meaning that I was wavering between grief at the divorce and eager anticipation of the anecdotes that dropped regularly through our mail slot. Bob was literary-minded, with no other willing recipient of his sometimes utopian prose; his letters, though carefully noncommittal, kept me going.

On the Line

Bob had been pumping a bartender in Burns Lake for news of work available when he met Harry Larsen, a trapper he failed to describe; eventually I was to meet him. He had a long, distinctly Norwegian visage above the usual mackinaw, with a dirty ski cap pulled down over his nose to hide shrewd blue eyes. He had a huge family hidden in the woods and a trap line. When he met Bob, the trap line was for sale. Harry had seen Bob with his packboard at his feet and had eavesdropped, as was customary in those parts. So was his intrusion.

"What kind of job d'you want?"

Bob always took things like nosiness in his stride. "Mostly logging. I can run a green chain and I can cook," he said. "After the war, me and my brother ran a hunting lodge in the Kootenays and I did the cooking. Until," he added lamely, "his wife left him and we sold out."

"Ever think of trapping?"

"Yeah. There was a Yankee in Whitehorse wanted me to go trapping with him around Atlin. And I hunted a lot as a kid."

Harry got an idea. "You look as if you could do with a meal. Come on home with me and meet the wife."

Effie Larsen liked Bob at once because he was respectfully cheeky. "Anything for a free meal," he'd said, laughing and blushing.

It turned out that Harry and Effie had ten children in their home in the bush, mostly girls. Effie really was something of a hillbilly mother, with a lot of wisdom and capable of a loud voice when needed, which was frequently. She had a heart like mush and took in all strays. Harry was much older, already in his fifties. Effie, tall and gaunt, was in her late thirties. She had been having children since she was twenty.

After Effie assessed Bob, she introduced him to an old man sitting in an armchair over by a window, Charlie "Gunnar" Lindquist, a greying blonde Swede and retired trapper. They were all in the big kitchen that served for eating and general living purposes. Effie said her usual, "sit in," to the visitor, indicating the end of the table for the men, as far away as possible, I gathered, from the little ones and the baby. Gunnar would have come out of his corner to step into his ordained place beside Harry at the far end, facing Bob.

The picture presented to me in Bob's letters was of this male threesome as a fixture at meals when Bob visited, with the two oldest girls trying to chip in while their big brother corrected them. Yarning went on unhindered during the family clamour and fidgets. The younger girls served the meals and took turns spooning food into the baby.

Effie's hospitality that night was the beginning of Larsen's long friendship with Bob. Before the night was over, the sale of Harry's trap line to Bob took place in Gunnar's cabin, a stone's throw from Larsen's, across the CNR tracks and beside a big lake. Decker Lake. Gunnar's cabin was a ten-by-ten affair with a lino floor, a bunk, stove, table and chairs, and you took your boots off on entry. Gunnar's door faced onto the lake and ducks swam along the shore. That night a case of beer disappeared while the three men argued, bartered, and spun tales. The evening wound up with Gunnar saying they'd better have some java and Bob had better get busy setting up the cot that was under Gunnar's bunk. Before Harry went home, the two older men got up and stood over Bob, saying they'd see what he was made of. The tall elders smiled down with evil patronage on the short young one, who sat, as was his wont, with one knee crossed over the other. He used to wriggle back into his chair without uncrossing his legs.

"Yeah?" he cried. "First I got to see this place. Don't take me for granted." Then he added, in his account to me, that they needn't think he was the kind of transient they were used to or that he was a complete fool. He told them that he had five hundred in the bank down in Burns Lake and that was all. The rest had to come out of the sale of skins. Satisfied, as he was desperate for money, Harry arranged to go up the trail to the trap line first thing in the morning.

Bob took possession and an immediate rapport began. Besides enjoying Harry's company, Bob liked Effie's tart remarks when he got her going. He did not have much use for children, but as children were always around he endured them for the sake of the company. This was evident in his letters and gave me pause for thought.

He did think enough of the three oldest children to mention them in his first report to me: the eldest son and the two oldest girls. The youth was a long-faced, silent "yard of pump water" [tall and skinny] with a scholastic nature, who was very accurate with a gun. His closest sisters were at puberty and tried to appear as teenage knockouts in innocent and hoydenish ways, always difficult with an earthy mother watching every move.

"I took them some grouse the other day," wrote Bob. "Effie said, 'What kind of a man is it who fills a bird with buckshot and breaks our teeth?'" At such times, he would retort with something like, "That's gratitude!" But Effie was hard to match.

Gunnar intrigued Bob too, as a "dear old guy" who acted as grandfather to the Larsen brood. When Harry was away working, Gunnar would cut wood, fix things, run errands in town and listen for hours to Effie's tales. Her brothers and others brought deer and moose meat, and many consumed her meals, but few bothered to help her.

Bob collected old men like nuggets. It did not matter to a young man like him that Gunnar no longer hunted but just sat about. Old men loved Bob for his avid interest in their yarns and for his respectful yet brassy manner; he got their stories by teasing them. These tales were disclosed to me in batches, sometimes in letters, but later on, often over mugs of coffee beside some tin stove. Bob was a great mimic and past conversations came out verbatim.

From then on, I received a letter for every trip Bob made into Burns Lake with furs. Sometimes a letter would turn out to be no more than a journal. It made me long to see the situation for myself, but of course I wouldn't have dreamed of suggesting it. My role was that of friend and confidante with just enough romance to keep me wondering. Having just created a different life for myself as a single mother, I was in no rush to pull up stakes and create another. His descriptions were of the sort that said, "You would love this and that," rather than, "I wish you could get away and see it." I don't think anything crossed his mind other than joy in what he was doing.

I felt that trapping might be just a stage and that one day he might move closer to the coast.

It was six miles of trail from Harry's kitchen door to the nearest cabin on the trap line. It must be realized that using traps and wearing furs was not considered deplorable in those days. Trapping was a legitimate occupation, and still is, if you can go against the outcry.

The light was golden in September, right after Labour Day, the legal time for hunting. In the deciduous forests, the poplars and alders scattered their gold coins everywhere and their trunks gleamed white. In Bob's area, the trees gave way to jack pine but the woods were fairly thin, and shafts of sunlight bathed the cranberry leaf tops. Some of the bushes were waist-high and waves of delicate green rippled under the breezes.

In the days when I came to know the Interior, I found such woods full of little rendezvous spaces where parties of nature-lovers would want to linger rather than keep to the trail. But nature-lovers in those days were anathema to the natives. Government surveyors, ranchers, and prospectors could get by them with good will; construction workers got by them with a good push; otherwise the locals tolerated no dilettantes in short leather pants.

During his first night on the line, Bob sat down to record his emotions after he had got a fire going and had eaten supper. He described thick layers of moss and kinnikinnick (a bearberry ground cover), and then forest where game shelter looked better.

"We went several more miles," the saga of his hike with Larsen continued, "until the forest broke out into the clearing by a little lake. Hidden under the trees I saw a small cabin, weathered black, but it seemed in good shape. No moss or signs of a caving roof. Small outhouse by it. There is a little dock at the lake made by one big plank with stakes in the mud and there's a raft among the reeds. I figured I could live on ducks if nothing else.

"When we got to the door, Harry stopped me from going in. He banged on it, kicked the door open, and jumped back. 'Pack rats,' he said. 'Never go into an abandoned cabin straight away. In this country they nest and breed in there. Big as cats or small dogs. You daren't corner 'em, but they're afraid if you make a big noise.'

"Nothing came out. There was no smell of rats either. The place had everything. Good bunk, long cooking counter under the window with enough crockery and cutlery, a good little airtight heater, a table and captain's chair."

Since my soul was as romantic as his, if not worse, I sighed with envy as I read. He didn't have anything to do at night, once his lamp was lit, other than scrape skins and listen to his radio, and write. Each fur delivery gave him a chance to mail a graphic report on working the line.

Meanwhile, down in Victoria, life went on. I was busy shaping up in that first job and proving certain points of a new lifestyle to family and friends. I was easily and apprehensively influenced by family opinion then, but was trying to get out from under it. The government had put me to work doing humble clerical recording because my credentials were nil. Then a kindly supervisor lent me his own typewriter to take home and I learned from a manual how to type at forty words per minute. The required speed was eighty.

Also, I attempted a course in speedwriting, though not successfully. Sometime later my mother said, "You have surprised me!" It had been taken for granted by all that I was an unemployable wimp because, loving harmony and wanting to keep the peace, I had hardly ever fought back.

In retrospect, long before this, before my marital fiasco became final, I had thought to get me a job to keep from brooding. "You do," my spouse had exclaimed, "and I'll go down to see the people and get you fired. This is your job. Running the home." (His other idea was that bull seals always kept a harem.) Later, when I had pulled out and "gone home to mother," she had not been unsympathetic toward my misery. However, she had been a merchant woman of some standing, accustomed to giving orders, so that when she finally came to the conclusion that she should have packed me back to my husband on the first train, it never crossed her innocent mind that she did not have that power.

They were a pair, my spouse and my mother; duty and appearances were everything, so that, in the course of time, they got along together well enough because they were both active movers and shakers. They had both tried to bundle my feelings back and forth between them and were amazed that I'd had the gall to slip through their fingers. My parents, of course, never, then nor ever, had any idea of what actually went on and thought everything was talk and bluster. I still cared enough about my tormentor not to sell him down the river or destroy their illusions completely, both for his sake and the children's; he was really a fine man when he wasn't a complete fool.

Now I was free of all that and had to prove up, and Bob's letters were heavy anodyne. They nearly always ended in the same way: "Time to make shavings and turn in." Shavings, I learned, were the starters made by whittling a piece of kindling into a fan of long wooden curls that were not quite cut off. There was no newsprint in the bush and all these needed was a match.

There were breakfasts of bacon and bannock; a billy can and tea bags on the trail; his frying pan, sleeping bag and brush shelters at night; logs to be pushed end on into the red core of his all-night fire, for the cold tends to induce stoking. This would be in the freezing part of fall, but not in sub-zero temperatures.

Before Bob, my idea of the bush had been an excursion into farm country where patches of forest smelled all piney, or you could push through salal and come out on a beach. There was an Alpine Club trekking round about Victoria outskirts, but I wasn't in that league.

Before freeze-up, Bob wrote, "The lake is so quiet here. When a fish jumps you can hear it far off. They say the Indian kids are so used to quiet that when a fish jumps, it makes them jump too. Of course I've got my loon family here. Ever hear the cry of a loon?"

No, I had not.

"I find I average twelve miles a day with my pack, tending the line. Just heard mice are good bait for marten."

Bob had many tales of Gunnar.

"Up where he was trapping, the fish were coming into shore and ducks everywhere. In fact, the ducks' feet would touch the fish, which would take off. I'd never have believed him if I hadn't seen the fish in creeks near Atlin. You could almost kick 'em out."

By October he was snowed in and the lake was frozen thickly. He cut a water hole and noted regretfully that his near-by beaver lodges were mounded over.

"I can skin a beaver in half an hour but they tell me a good Indian trapper can do it in eight minutes. It takes a good light and a very sharp knife."

Then he went off the deep end of credibility with tales of the wolverine. "The Carcajou. Effie laughs at me and says I read too much when I call it that."

Eve in Eden

Just before Thanksgiving, Bob had had enough of his own company and the Larsens had had enough of hearing about me.

"Why don't you get her up here? She can stay with us if she wants. Get her to take a long weekend."

It was a small matter to send both children by train to join their brothers up-island over the Thanksgiving weekend while I was supposedly going to Vancouver to see friends. Of course, I would have to pass through Vancouver to see those friends. It all felt like cloak and dagger plotting.

The Larsen home was up the railway line a little from Burns Lake and Bob met me with their truck. The place was set back in the bush not far from Gunnar's foreshore on Decker Lake, which the CNR followed. The house itself was slightly distant from the railway line, except for Effie's snow-mounded vegetable patch, and completely surrounded by deciduous forest. It was a one-level conglomerate of additions, with a bit of porch here and little tarpaper there.

What I saw when I first came into their kitchen was what Bob had seen on his first night: a very big room with a long table down the middle covered with an oilcloth and set with condiments. Children were running in and out and the very youngest were playing with the baby on the floor. The old man in the armchair by the window was our fair Swede, hair grey with blonde streaks, whose seamed face bore a long nose meeting his chin. A thick grey bush shirt was open, revealing long underwear with the top button done up. The rest of his attire was the usual bush uniform of rough black bush pants and heavy grey wool socks, his boots being laid by the door. Gunnar Lindquist looked scrubbed clean.

This man was Bob's first "nugget," the old paragon so often described. To me, he was what my parents would have described as a "rough diamond," or most damning of all, "one of nature's gentlemen." It took me some time to stop seeing people that way, but Bob's outlook was infectious and pretty soon his friends did a good job on my city standards.

Effie made short work of me with a "take us as we are" statement. It is true that, primed as I was with Bob's descriptions, I was still not prepared for reality. My experience of country folk had been limited to a few Gulf Islanders who are quite a different breed, friendly enough but not as rough and ready as these Interior people.

Effie said she had been likened to Ma Kettle, the prime hillbilly mother of 1940s fiction, but I could see she was not that scatty or messy, and I settled that quickly. She was fair and faded with straight short hair and seemed to be dressed in layers of cloth, likely a cotton dress and covering apron. There was cloth all around the room that made me think of calico. It was at the windows and covering an old settee along the wall, and served as dishcloths, mop-up cloths, and everything boilable by the look of it. In those days, much use was made of bleached cotton flour sacks, sturdy and white.

At any rate, I had arrived with no parka but wore a Cowichan Indian sweater with knife-pleated wool gabardine slacks, folded at the calf into heavy socks and gumboots. The gumboots wouldn't do, "as they'd fill up in a minute and anyway you have to let your pants hang down outside, and, besides, your socks are too short," all this from a ring of little girls around me. One of them lent me her boots.

Harry and the eldest boy, Helge, were not there this day, just Gunnar, Effie and the girls. At table they had fun baiting Bob for a rookie when he tried to impress me with his skills.

"Dis guy," squeaked Gunnar, "you ought to seen him. We was sittin' in my cabin wid de door open and grouse starts walkin' up and down outside. He's got his .22 beside him and I sez, 'you get him,' and he takes aim and misses! Holy yumpin' Yesus, how could he miss? It weren't five feet away."

"Easy," shouted Gerda, the second oldest girl, rocking from side to side with laughter.

"You want to hang on a hook again?" growled Bob. His eyes got bigger and bigger, a habit he had when he wanted to transfix. As I wanted to know what that was all about, Gunnar took over.

"Well," he began paternally, regarding Thora, the first-born girl, and Gerda, "dese girls got wind of Bob's brudder paying him a visit and nuttin' must do but dey must come snookin' around my place when dey hear de boys are dere."

The young men had said hello to the girls but paid them no more attention. "But dat didn't do, did it?"

Thora tossed her head. Apparently the girls kept showing themselves and interrupting conversation, but when they were ignored, they started calling out insults. Spoiled by Gunnar, and often humoured by Bob as it turned out, they couldn't take no for an answer. They had retreated to a distance and plotted attack.

Effie did nothing to interfere with this recital but sat calmly.

"So who trew rocks?" Gunnar looked heavily at Gerda who had stopped swaying and now sat hunching her shoulders up and down.

"And dis one," he indicated Thora, "got so mad that she used her tongue too much and de boys had to cool her off in the lake. Den Gerda starts trowin' rocks right at de boys. Dat did it. Bob's brudder hung her up on my washtub hook by her belt. Laff! Never did see so much kicking and hollerin'."

Then Bob began telling Gunnar how he shot a beaver, which sank and he wasn't going into ice water after it; now it was frozen over. He was getting a stream of advice about rescuing such a catch when Effie cut in.

"You better can the chatter and get goin'," she remarked, looking at us, "or you'll never get back by nightfall." She winked at Bob over my head.

Trial Run

There was a scurry to get me kitted out; they lent me a muffler and toque, and I had mitts. We were seen off with cheers and jeers. It seemed we were to travel on snowshoes, which I had never seen before outside of museum Indian relics. Bob buckled me into them and went ahead, illustrating how to proceed.

"Just lift a foot and put it down. Swing your leg forward from the hip. That's right. You'll get used to it."

I did. I had never known such agony, but somewhere halfway along the six miles I got my second wind. Swing. Swing. They were large strides, though. This was the test; deliberate, to see if I had the stuff to be a fit mate. In his pack were supplies for two, I found out, and a few frills for me, like eggs.

Bare white expanses twinkled in the sun and were crossed with animal tracks everywhere. Snow crunched under our weight but produced powder sprays off the arcing snowshoes. The air was mild but drew a tingle in the cheek. At about half-past three, the sun went in for good and we entered the forest. All was as it should be. Loaded fir branches hung close to snow hummocks and more interesting game trails appeared. Peace prevailed.

"Do you know what that is?" Bob pointed to a set of little footprints. "That'll be marten. If you weren't here I'd do something about him, but I've got to get you to the cabin." He studied my face. "You gotta keep going. Swear if you want to. It helps a lot."

The pain in my hips and thighs allowed no energy for swearing and I decided not to give him the satisfaction of seeing me crack. I did not know why it seemed such hard work and didn't know when we reached the cabin or how long it had taken. The pain had long since enveloped me in a sort of red stupor.

What I saw was something like a postcard from Banff or Jasper: a little cabin with a good foot of snow on its roof despite overhanging snow-laden firs and a flat white expanse that was the lake, a clearing that was three or four feet deep in snowdrifts piled against the cabin walls, and a path dug to the door, with another branching from it to the water hole.

Inside the dwelling would be my fate, or something I could expect to see more of if all went well. What was I doing here? My usual motto, "All for love and the world well lost," was only slightly hampered by common sense. With very mixed feelings I went into the cabin, followed by Bob's anxious, defensive self. The place smelled of pine needles and pelts and, in fact, there was a skin on a stretcher.

It was more comfortable than he had described. A bear rug half covered the bunk, the window was clean and free from cobwebs, and white oilcloth gleamed on the long counter. His mugs and plates were stacked neatly at one end: two thick mugs, tin plates, cutlery enough, also a wire toast rack to extend over the heater's open lid. Behind the stove hung the everlasting frying pan. He had padded the captain's chair with skins. Harry would probably have toted up one of Effie's old cushions, but Bob just had to stick to his theme.

With no coaxing at all, he made me rest on the bunk while he picked up ready shavings and started a fire in the heater. The lower part of my body was aflame with pain; I couldn't move. Pretty soon the kettle was singing and he brought out a bottle of rum. That cheered me in spite of its implications. He had one thought in mind, however, at that time, and that was to make up for the ordeal of my snowshoeing, all done on his behalf.

After a couple of rums, I was soon normal but one thing was clear: there was no way I could snowshoe another six miles back to Larsen's with night coming on. I was quite sure Effie had known it but I didn't enjoy the feeling: one sees where one's life is heading and puts on blinkers.

"What on earth will Effie think if I stay?" I objected. "It will be dark soon."

"She won't think a thing. Didn't you see her wink at me?"

I stayed. Eventually I was to find that it was quite easy to walk to the cabin and back in one day, and be back in time for supper. But that first journey had been uphill, we had started late, and in the snow each mile had seemed like ten. Still, I would not hide behind the fact that I had to stay, and that was another milestone, declaring my private life before strangers.

We did not talk of future plans. He lived for the present and assumed he'd keep on trapping, while I was afraid there'd be no future plans if I pushed ahead with suggestions, especially since I had a couple of young, two-legged reasons to be cautious; but my kids had to be pushed outside all of this while I got my bearings.

The moments in the cabin stayed complete. Radio news broke the silence, which Bob said was the bush man's delight. "You know, an old guy up here knows more of what is going on in the world than some people that do have a newspaper every day. There's no distraction. He has all the time in the world to listen to the news of the world."

Our socks were extended towards the glowing stove with our feet resting on the shared chopping block. The rums were scalding and buttery. Bob began to brag about his take. The only thing that jarred me was the row of steel traps hanging on the back wall with their jaws and springs. I tried to be practical and not notice them.

"What kind of game we got here? Everything. Though mostly small stuff except for the moose. No mountain goats or sheep like we had in the Monashees. I like to get marten. It's richer looking than mink, I think. It's fluffier. But we go for everything: mink, ermine—that's just a white weasel with a black tail tip, the Bonaparte weasel. We're pretty close to Babine country and get some of their game. We could get lynx, badger, beaver, river otter, muskrat, but only the last three sell well. Plenty of deer. The trails get messed up with jumping mice and snowshoe hares but they're great for bait or the pot—rabbits, I mean. It's wolves that get me and I still have to meet my first wolverine. Brrr."

He was good at shivering dramatically.

The place was heaven. Not a sound except the soft plop of snow. Once during the night we heard a wolf howl. I wished I could have stayed forever. I envied Effie.

The outhouse was a step outside and I came back puzzled. "Why is that board on the front of the pit all broken away at the bottom?"

He laughed. "That's porcupines. They're after the salt." Porcupines were his constant friends and he told me that one day he had found one in his sleeping bag.

At breakfast he cut bacon from a slab while I, as ordered, started a fire. While the bacon fried in the pan on the heater, he cut more shavings for the next fire and then said, "Here, you try," handing me the knife. I thought this training looked promising and picked up some kindling, but my wooden curls were much thicker than his and only went halfway down the stick. A beautiful fan was beyond me. I did take the water bucket down to the lake and dipped it through the water hole, which I had bashed clear of ice first. I felt like an old hand.

Then, too soon, there was a train to catch and the resumption of a life I did not want to think about yet. There was no hanging about after we'd eaten and the snowshoe return to Larsen's took half as long and was twice as easy; my painful hamstrings seemed to welcome being loosened up.

Effie searched my face carefully, with motherly interest. If she had been any other woman, I would have been furious.

"And now what do you think of a man that makes his living so cruelly?"

"I told you," Bob began, giving me no time to reply. "A trapper has no grocery store in the bush and he has to get his grub from it. You eat moose and deer meat, don't you? If you get something for the skins, what's the difference? A man has to get by. Getting meat from the bush is no different than…"

Effie was laughing at us. "You better get them snowshoes off and some coffee down you. And you better get her to the station pretty quick. Gunnar's in the house. He wants to say goodbye."

As I paid my thanks to the Larsens, Effie pulled me aside.

"Make him marry you!" she hissed. I flushed scarlet.

Trapping by Mail

Sometimes Harry's struggle to find work further afield was mentioned in Bob's letter, or he relayed Effie's description of her latest calamity, but mostly he had some new tale of Gunnar's trapping advice.

"Today he taught me how to call a moose," or, "Now I know a better way to set beaver traps."

He learned to fire at a mountain wall behind a group of moose to make them move nearer and how to make one stand up out of the long grass by rapping a set of antlers with a stick. Or by rubbing a big bone against a tree, which sounds like antlers being rubbed; sometimes a moose would reply by rubbing his.

All he thought about was his trap line.

He wrote, "I know how to get beaver under ice. You look for a food pile nearby. You can see the airway into the nest because it's full of frozen air bubbles. Beavers are so smart that if they hear a trap go off underwater they don't go near a trap again.

"Well I've got to get my kit ready for morning," he would write, "so I'll knock off. They say that to waterproof a pack you should rub melted candle wax over the canvas but I hate the idea of a mess. Mine's pretty waterproof but if I want to cover anything I just turn my old bearskin rug inside out on top of everything."

Nobody had a packboard like Bob's. During the long winter evenings, he had constructed it of two polished pine poles with three flat bands of pine carved and curved between them, the whole covered with a stretched black bear skin laced taut from behind with leather thongs. It weighed scarcely over a pound, and wherever he went it was his hallmark.

It was obvious from his letters that he was going to hibernate and I'd have to make my winter plans alone. What they would be I did not know. Beyond the routine of work and bed and taking the two kids, Joan and Robby, to Sunday dinner with my parents, I did not want any plans and was just in limbo. Apart from some old friends who took us out for drives, and little homilies from my work colleague with the dragging

foot who kept jerking me into reality, life just went on. I discussed Bob with no one.

Winter in the Interior proceeded and everything was shut down around Decker Lake. The local sawmill was shut down and everything was still and quiet except for the snow crunch. Jokes at Larsen's made sport of such tracks as went into teepees and didn't come out again.

By the first of November, Bob was getting depressed and restless. He went on as ever about fur runs into Williams Lake and visits with his friends.

"The kids are getting to me but at least they are happy kids. Running all over in front of me and making angels in the snow. They're a nuisance when you're trying to talk. But you should see how Gunnar handles them. Harry's away job-hunting again. Gunnar bought the kids skis.

"Something tells me this can't last. It was a good idea to start with and I don't regret it but the take is low. If I can't make enough of a stake I'll have to push further north…"

I tried to read between the lines. My own life was untenable and having a far distant boyfriend was not helping matters. It was only untenable because I didn't have a goal beyond being with Bob if possible, and we were so hard up. The kids were good, but it was no life for them in a dingy walk-up in a down-at-heels district. Eventually I would be forced to plan something, but it needed time.

On about Bob's second visit to Victoria, before going trapping, he had met my children, whose reactions were not as he expected. Robert had curled into a pretzel on his bed and said nothing, and Joan had been shy but curious. Bob was to remark later, "I expected to get along with the girl well enough but thought the boy would bring trouble." It would turn out to be exactly the opposite.

When Bob had first written about the Larsen children, I had tried to fathom whether he was amused by their company or truly irritated. I needed to know. I had also tried to decide whether he was sincerely smitten by the bush or whether it was just a phase. Gunnar complicated the issue by piling on bush-style enticements.

We did not know it then, but our star was rising as Gunnar's was setting. In retrospect, his importance to us was that he was the first in a chain of very old and very stubborn bush people (whom I was to dub "The Indignants") who lived alone and wanted it that way. Our admiration of him and his fellows would be immense, especially when they encouraged us with quips and jeers into emulating their past achievements.

We were both, for different reasons, smarting from others' attitudes towards our styles of living. "Like a cat in a packing case," was my portion, while Bob's people expected him to raise his sights a lot higher.

For us, before justification, there had to be a beginning. One day, added to one of Bob's journal-like reports, was a rash statement that settled everything. "I am dying to marry you," it said.

Stinkers, BC

Outcasts

The town was Smithers, but more often than not we were to call it Stinkers. Not that "Stinkers" is a good description of anything sanitized by winter; it is just what we felt the place deserved from late spring to fall. When we arrived in early December—with me were Joan and Robert, completely trusting— the snow was a foot deep and piling up, while the temperature was fifteen below and going down. Our train pulled into a sort of Christmas movie set, complete with main street and false front, all sandwiched in between two mountain ranges. Main Street was blocked off solidly at each end by gloomy sentinels with sharp white peaks cleft by glaciers. Below them, two man-made barriers—the railroad station and the courthouse—were planted more or less facing each other at either end of the road, as though to discourage any wandering off among forbidden slopes. Those two buildings proved to be the chief hubs of local existence. On that night, as on many nights, their lights spilled out on the snow in wakefulness. But down on the deserted main road there was only a pall of white, while one lone neon sign shed a ruddy glow.

Bob's trap line life had lasted only until mid-November

due to lack of money and restlessness. He was after higher goals. The time he had put in on the line had seemed much longer to us than it really was, and he had abandoned it back into Harry's care, to be leased to any worthy applicant or else sold. His agreement with Harry had been paid off because Bob couldn't stand debts. Working "ever northwards," he had taken a job near Smithers and had begun to wish for company.

For me, this was a jobless, houseless plunge into refrigeration. "City girl goes north" was now my motto. No more crazy rents, loaded buses or frustrations of the nine-to-five civic life. There is always an incentive for such impulsiveness, and in this case it was a man who had been fool enough to commit himself on paper. I had said nothing to my mother about the letter, for by this point I think she'd pretty much given up on me.

Up to this point, my emotional and domestic lives had been things apart; one didn't know what the other was doing. Also, living with children in that old walk-up on those low wages, under the accusing eyes of well-meaning relatives, was not to be borne when we could do our starving in private amid healthier surroundings. I'd had a lot of help by mail in judging what was healthier. But it was a lonely waif who had come under the gaze of Effie Larsen that fall and I knew Effie would be rooting for me.

My private theory was that the north was like any other place if you tackled it the right way, but from the first it settled in to tackle me. I was supposed to forget everything I'd ever read about its opening up and development. The results were not the "true north," locals were to tell me, but the abhorred approach of civilization. The next thing to forget was time, because here time was no object. After that I was to forget any preconceived ideas about the correct winter garb.

Huddled on the Smithers railway platform, two kids with bare knees and one determined mother, we tried hard to look optimistic as the station grew emptier and emptier. Voices faded and truck doors slammed. There was no sound and nothing moved save diamonds winking in the snow.

I surveyed the ground with my chin tucked into my fur collar, and wondered what to do. After a few moments I became aware of a pair of odd but familiar feet right beside me, which had approached noiselessly. The feet were clad not in flapping overshoes or ski boots or any such predictable footwear, but in thick grey socks thrust into rubbers. These were called "moccasins," a travesty of the Indian ones. They were built up to cover the instep like old men's slippers but were in fact plain-old fashioned galoshes like those worn long ago. Felt insoles were inserted against the cold when leaving a warm house to go out into the snow.

My footgear beside these was a pair of high-heeled black velvet overshoes, fur-trimmed. Atop these was a black cloth coat with a generous black fox collar, no hat, and underneath the coat, my only suit, of smooth grey flannel, with a pink pullover. My companion looked as he had before: green drill bags, red plaid shirt under his commando jacket with the everlasting ski cap upon his copper curls.

"Oops," he snickered nervously. "Guess I'm a bit late."

And so it was that, taking only what the kids and I needed and leaving a trunk to be dealt with later, our ill-matched feet fell into step for the few hundred yards into town while my two excited youngsters ran on ahead.

No arrangements appeared to have been made for us, which alarmed me. That is, there were hotels, but nothing was mentioned beyond that.

Smithers then had three hotels: one good, one medium, and one quite bad, depending on the points of view held by Interior travellers on what was good or bad in a hostelry. The best from my point of view had comfortable beds, storm windows, and running water in the rooms, the last running water we were to have for nearly three years.

The beds had candlewick spreads over very heavy quilts; the heat came from a big oil heater on the landing, flowing down a long corridor laid with linoleum and in through a transom over the door. One left the door ajar when the corridor was empty, in order to warm up.

Having seen us registered, Bob left me to get the children into bed and join him later. Since they had eaten at the last train stop and were too dazed and tired to think, they fell asleep almost at once.

The Dog Kennel

In Smithers, music filled the night. By day, in summer and winter, it came from a little shop, a focal point on the main street that featured candy, toys, records and radios. By night, during the winter, music rose from a big, black pile of an arena, from the top of which a crater of light fanned its image upwards. The sky was high and the stars were bright as the *Skaters' Waltz* blared up to meet them.

On that first night, finding my way past the black shadow of the arena as instructed, I saw two big log houses in the dark beside it. Across the street from them, under the purity of an arc light, stood a little church. It was the kind of church children draw, with a little cross sticking up on top. And there beside the church was a very little cabin, rather like a dog kennel, so small it was.

Music also came from the kennel on that first night and smoke curled up from its rakish chimney. Light shone through two small curtains covering a glass pane in the door. Being expected, I knocked and opened the door in a proprietary manner and saw not one, but two, young men in a scene that remains with me forever.

There was a bunk and a table, a chair and a black leather rocker, a washstand with a basin on it, a chest of drawers and a hot little cook stove. The walls were panelled with red linoleum and on the grey battleship lino that covered the floor was a small, familiar black bear rug. Protruding from under the bunk, which was fairly high, were boxes, snowshoes, skis and guns.

Bob and a young male, a stranger to me, were waiting for me. The stranger, full of voyeuristic curiosity, occupied the rocker. My young male was seated on the bunk, staring at the door, his feet not quite touching the ground. As I came in, the music changed and he reached overhead suddenly to turn up the volume of a radio on a shelf above him.

"East is east and west is west and the wrong one I have chose."

Noise filled the shack. I started to say something but the wide-open, limpid brown eyes I knew so well defied me. I was to learn that when he got what I called his "wall-eyed" look, he was about to either challenge me or to tell the most bald-faced lie imaginable.

Don't bury me in this prairie, take me where the cee-ment
    grows…
I'll love you in buckskin, or skirts that I've homespun—

The heedless stranger was now on his feet and jitterbugging violently.

But I'll love you longer, stronger where yer friends don't
    tote a gun.

Up went the volume another notch. The walls shook.

It was the first time I had heard the song Buttons and Bows, and it was the first popular ballad we heard together in the northwest. I was challenged; anyway we both loved our drama.

This was the guy who had written about longing to marry, but things seem different in a lonely little cabin than they do when reality walks through the door.

The subject of marriage had come up before in a roundabout way. On one of his rare visits to the coast, in fact after he had met my two children for the first time, he was sitting in a restaurant booth with me, having tea and hot buttered toast, when he said quite out of the blue with a nervous little laugh, "Well there's one thing. If your kids ever come to me, their old man will have to go overboard." The breath had gone out of me as I saw our entire romance dissolve, knowing what I had to do. Where my children were concerned, he had crossed a boundary.

"You go to hell," I said.

"Oops!" he laughed. "Guess I went too far that time."

And that was that, crisis over. Justice meant more to me than anything in life, and being fair meant everything to Bob. He'd been trying things for size.

The happy-go-lucky stranger was soon turfed out; I never did catch his name. There was coffee with rum in it. After a while, responsibility returned and I wended my way back to see if the children were warm enough.

Everything connected with this romance going smoothly depended on my being able to handle domestic and work affairs as efficiently as possible. On the other hand I was not going to allow romance to overrule family.

Of School Masters and Post Masters

My priority the next morning was to get the children back into school. It had not been possible to wait until term end because I had to get a job settled before Christmas. And of course I had not been able to wait to get out of Victoria. What I had done in order not to burn bridges was to wangle a six-month leave of absence from the British Columbia government, without pay but without loss of seniority, to see if I could find an opening in an Interior government office. Merle Campbell of the personnel department made this possible for me; she turned out to be my government lifebuoy for the next twenty years.

The grade school was very big compared with other buildings around town. The principal was very young and embittered and his manner towards his charges was more of the bulldozer than the patriarch. He led us upstairs to his office and the classrooms, after charging a path through the noisy rabble that seemed unimpressed by his passage. His commands were more rough than righteous.

My chatter and optimism about the school and the town were received in a dour, friendly way, typical of the Smithers native. I happened to mention water problems in general and thought it would be rather muddy when snow went.

"Wait until summer," he replied lugubriously. "The whole place is built on muskeg."

Part of his dim view of life was explained later when we

heard that, on a previous Halloween, the big men in grade eight had beaten him up. A couple of years after we left the place there was something in the paper about Smithers that involved a policeman's son, a gas ring in a school lab, and the principal's hand.

Meanwhile, braziers of coal burned outside but most of the children were inside, where they attempted volleyball and the like in huge playrooms. They were a tough bunch and rugged, especially in language, but they took over my novices tenderly when I left. The children reported on that second night that the local kids had helped them up and down snow banks as if they had never seen snow before, adding, "We were the only kids in town with bare knees."

The next step in our survival was to get something between the elements and us.

The town contained a lone dress shop—useless to us—some meat and grocery stores, the usual amenities like a bank, hospital, Canadian Legion Hall, post office and one real estate office. The entire field of commerce was up and down Main Street behind false fronts. The place still needed a big general store, or some such pioneer establishment, which was conspicuous by its absence.

Over the street from our hotel was a large clothes emporium with bush jackets, sleeping bags and plain shirts in one window, and ladies' and babies' things in the other. Upon entering we found these goods segregated by a large pot-bellied heater, in the vicinity of which wandered a couple of old men who were presiding over the merchandise and, one felt, over all souls in town.

They pondered our family needs carefully, being full of helpful suggestions and questions. I bought dark green ski pants, fleece lined, a brick-coloured parka, overshoes and muffs for myself. Mitts and earmuffs were all that Joan needed and a cap with ear flaps for Robert, who suddenly became a rosy-cheeked cherub in a bonnet. Warm wool slacks for both kids completed the job. They had Indian sweaters that had been passed down from their two older brothers who were even then working after high school for their father. The older boys had a stepmother already and these children just had me. This was our status quo.

The next expedition took me back to the station to see about our large trunk. I could not imagine placing it in a temporary hotel room or in Bob's "kennel." We were making fairly good use of the cabin though mostly while its occupant was at work.

The station agent said we might leave the trunk where it was until we were settled. Since he was chatty I expanded into discourse, asking about vital matters in a guileless manner. It turned out he was one of the town's chief grapevine tenders; although I had not asked directly about work available, whatever I had let slip paid off.

It was the most fruitful grapevine really, seldom a bitter one. They minded their own business in Smithers—after finding out first what was going on—then expected you to mind yours.

That first morning's gossip brought the mountain to Mahomet.

That afternoon we were all three in our hotel room while I sat on the big bed counting change. I was force-feeding myself with studied optimism, because in those days I had developed my own pipeline to God, but in fact I was absolutely terrified by the future. We were quite on our own, unsubsidized and not dependent on Bob in any way. My purse was upside down and remaining assets were parcelled into heaps, when there came heavy footsteps down the passage, followed by a knock on the door.

Sweeping up the monetary mess, I jumped up and found standing in the hall a six-foot male with a long-nosed gloomy Irish visage, half framed by a red-lined, fur-trimmed parka hood, which covered a golf cap added for good measure. Mr. Kilpatrick, the postmaster of Smithers.

One would guess work was in the offing. It was. But in truth my eye was on the provincial government agency at the end of the street. Flattering though it was to have the Feds at my feet instead of the agency people, I decided to risk toying with both. I managed to ask him all the job requirements, to demur and defer decisions. I must have been crazy.

If I took part time work I would lose out on a chance to get back into clerical work. The only alternative, judging by a quick take of the town's business section, was to sell things on my feet all day or wash dishes. I was to find out later that the town was not anxious for me to do either. It had me in its sights.

My austere benefactor left. He would await my verdict at the end of the week. He was short-handed for the Christmas rush, now beginning, and hoped to take on a permanent clerk afterwards, as someone was leaving. He spoke of sorting mail. The hours of work would be hard on a working mother, from 8:00 a.m. to 6:00 p.m., but all other businesses kept the same hours. In addition, the ancient custom of keeping stores and the post office open until 9:00 p.m. on Saturday was very much in force. Smithers was a market town and, small as it was, a hub.

In retrospect, with a six-month leeway for getting into the agency, or any agency, I could have walked straight into the post office, but I panicked and didn't think of it. I was too afraid of being locked out of the B.C. civil service.

With heavy hours as an excuse to project me into finding easier ones, I attacked the citadel. The only person I was allowed to see was the government agent, K.D. McCrae, and I knew that after his verdict there would be no appeal. He looked at my flimsy credentials and after listening to my palaver he got rid of me by promising to attack Victoria, the capital, for permission to hire an unwanted clerk, but held out no hope. He suggested that if I had no temporary work at the end of the week I should come back and ask again in case he had been successful. He knew I was not fooled but did his best.

Bob was off in the bush during the day working for a lumber company. Trapping and old trappers were a thing of the past for now. Apart from using his little house for meals, the children and I were completely on our own and that is how he wanted it. It was his idea of a training programme; if we could not make it in the world of northern jobs and schools we'd better go home. It would show we didn't belong. He did not say as much, but it was only too evident.

His attitude made me smart so much I was determined to get the kind of job that would put him in his place. Although his letters right up to train time had been ever-loving, since our arrival the magic word had not reappeared. In any case it was impossible to backtrack.

We went on like this through the first week, with teasings at night about the day's progress. He seemed quite interested in seeing if my kids could handle the local kids—or measure up to Effie's, I had no doubt.

One day I was proud to tell him that my six-year old Robert, who had never seen skates before, had hired some, tied them on, had stood up in them and, taking a deep breath, had lashed out across the rink ice with flashing feet, finally sitting on them when he felt himself falling, to keep sliding on the impetus until he hit the end board of the arena. That had been one up.

Search for Shelter

In all fairness, Bob could not possibly have been expected to find work for me, but unknown to me he had been doing a thorough filtering of accommodation rumours among his pals. House hunting in bush country is not a matter of constant searching but of good connections. Usually there are no real estate offices. To gain connections one must live in the area for several years or know somebody who has and we didn't. Since Bob was of the roving kind, or had been, his connections were pretty queer. Most of them were to be found in the three licensed hotels, but the best leads were found in the worst one.

The bad hotel was fascinating. It had the same oil heating as the best one but it didn't go in much for lighting, which may have been a good thing. Over each door was a square gap in place of a transom, to let the heat from the hall into the rooms and the noise from the rooms into the hall.

The sounds in Smithers' three hotels could be graded like the hotels themselves: decorous, nondescript, and awful. In other words: civilized, somewhat noisy, and blueing the air. Strangely enough the noise and bad language in the bad hotel

44

did not penetrate the licensed parlour downstairs, where the clock ticked quietly on the wall, as grizzled old Gus thoughtfully wiped off his bar and the old men sat and sat. One of them, who always sat under the clock, was to become my landlord.

I had walked up and down past every house in Stinkers for several days until the choice was narrowed down to three places furnished by the sole agent: a nine-room barn that would have made a fine boarding house and would cost a fortune to heat; a big log structure with noble rustic aspect but with peeling plaster inside and an unlikely twisted, topply brick chimney, unsupported as it rose through the second storey where wiring lay all over the floor; a furnished shack that out-shacked many, with tar paper flapping in the wind and miles from anywhere down the highway leading out of town. Although in town the temperature seldom fell lower than minus thirty, it got to be almost forty below along that road. Nothing was habitable without expense, and our money was almost gone.

We were due to leave the hotel at the end of the week. I wondered why I didn't throw in the towel, wire for help and go home. Yet I did know why: pride and cussedness. The children were game. As long as they didn't have to suffer too much for too long, I didn't care. To return was unthinkable.

"Well, it takes me to get action," said Bob, very full of himself. "You've got a house."

Of course my response was, "Where? When? What like?" His answers were evasive and very fancy.

"It's just got two rooms. Easy on the heat. Furnished! Good stove, a bed, table and chairs, light and water, a block or two from town, and ten dollars a month! Takes me!"

My great relief was mixed with chagrin. It would have been nice to have found it ourselves and to have proved our independence. I didn't fall for his line; having gone over the area with a fine-toothed comb I was very sceptical, but held my peace. I made a mental note we would take the place no matter how it looked until I could show him what we could dig up later. Our relationship was jockeying on both sides.

Pride burned in showing Bob what I was made of and what my children could do.

He was not especially hard on the kids; more amused. I had forgotten that he'd once been in their shoes when his banker father had been moved up country and he'd taken his well-pressed little britches into the northern bush, and that after his squirrel hunts he'd been able to go back to a comfortable over-stuffed home and his mommy's pies. He had been a city child and was still his mommy's boy, having always been her favourite, even now. He did his best to poke our pride with constant little cracks to see if we could take such hardships. My aim was to show that not only could we take conditions as they came, but could improve on them without the least sign of effort. Thus we furthered his training programme without knowing it. If he was going to be stuck with us he wanted us shaped to be worthy. The little blister was a challenge.

This first Saturday I was to apply for that government job, since it was a working day locally, and in the afternoon I was to go with Bob to see my new home. On the following Monday the children and I were to check out of the hotel and move, job or no job.

Somebody Up There

Sometimes a reckless person is motivated by a force that does not appear on the surface. I had my Higher Power.

For a year there had been secreted under my pillow a little booklet called *The Golden Key*, given to me buy a woman minister whom I had consulted during previous troubles. It was pulled out frantically as soon as the kids were asleep so that I could get to sleep myself. Its theme was that if you keep your eyes off the negative and concentrate on the positive, or on what you are asking for, you'll get the latter. This is dynamite when it works, as you often get more than you bargained for. Eventually I was to find one is supposed to keep an open mind over what one will get, compared with what one wants, but in those days I could not afford such licence. I was a freak under cover. Nobody then had heard of the Age of Aquarius and its possibilities. If any sceptic sniffed out my religious game I was prepared to quote, as an example, Second World War air aces and the terse prayers said with their backs against the sky.

With a case of sublime faith I walked up the road to the agency. This was the "come back at the end of the week" suggested by the agent in his put-off. While I walked I held myself deliberately in a sort of vacuum of faith, carefully not thinking, passing the post office with a speculative eye, as if to say what will be will be. My attitude may have been over-dramatization of an ordinary job hunt, but in reality it was Russian roulette: if I did not get back into the government it meant I was "throwing up a career for a man."

The agent McCrae seemed reluctant to attend me. I suspected he'd made no attempt to contact Victoria and had no intention of taking on staff. He had not heard anything from Victoria, he said, and had I been able to locate work of a sort for myself? On being told not, he suggested that I try one of the little district offices upstairs as one of the supervisors was purportedly looking for an extra stenographer, the hiring of whom was outside the agent's jurisdiction. He gave me a name.

Armed with the name, I sucked in my frightened stomach and, muttering something like "God is Love and God is with me," I floated up the long wooden staircase to a region where there was a long room—the courtroom—and two or three small offices representing various departments of the government. One of these was the district engineer's office and in it was a rather big woman, who seemed both smart and capable in a menacing sort of way. I decided to keep my affairs for the right pair of ears and asked for the engineer personally.

A short heavy man with a bald head and a trace of military bearing turned from the window, where he had been looking at papers on top of a nearby filing cabinet, and walked towards the counter. "Yes," he said, leaning amiably, William E. Bottomley, bedight.

Looking neither to right nor left but directly at him, I smiled as though we were alone in a drawing room and remarked that the agent downstairs had said that this office might need a steno, in which case I'd like to apply.

"Well," he demurred. He seemed at a loss and a sudden silence made the room oppressive. Without allowing him time to think further I began a light-hearted spiel about what I could do and had done (as a junior clerk with that typing speed of forty words a minute) and for once made no mention of what I couldn't do. I repeated that I was on six months' leave of absence without loss of seniority in hopes of reinstating myself in this agency and town and then, as there was nothing more to say I waited, airily detached and fatalistic. There was no way I could know that incumbents of government agencies in small towns are as kooky as the people in the streets of their towns and that nothing surprises them.

"We don't exactly need a steno," he began. "Don't know who told you that. Winnie here is our stenographer and my secretary. But we need someone to type up payrolls and take memos, as it's too much for her. You have shorthand?"

I said no and he should have said no too.

"Come back after the first of January and we'll give it a week's try anyway."

"Thanks very much," I said, scarcely breathing.

He turned from the counter without looking at the other woman, although my entrance had seemingly interrupted a discussion, and oiled through a door into his own office.

As I hurried along the street, such a warm wave of humility and relief overtook me I thought I would burst. For I knew without being told that the week would stretch into months or for as long as needed; I also knew the soft-hearted engineer should hire a proper clerk-steno and that was why he had slunk back into his office. He was going to catch it from Winifred.

I should have been salaaming in the streets and raising my arms to the sky. The next few years would teach me. All I did was to accelerate along the road, mumbling "Thanks. Thanks a lot," accompanied by goose bumps all over.

I passed the post office and remembered Kilpatrick who had offered me a job and was still waiting for a reply. I'd have to tell him. I couldn't see why he'd have trouble keeping a permanent clerk or why I should feel guilty about it. Besides, the post office was a federal institution and would not transfer seniority of service from a provincial government. Eventually we did find out why clerical material did not linger in Smithers, especially in an office right on the main street in hot weather.

His response was dour and aimed at my departing back.

"There goes another one." Then, "Hey!" he called, as I reached the door. "You say you don't start at the agency until after New Year's. What do you think you are going to do between now and then?" He had me. Both of us had forgotten the Christmas rush. Now all my family needs were met.

That afternoon I met Charlie.

CHAPTER · III

The Pennsylvania Dutchman

The Watchbird

In appearance Charlie van Alstine seemed of a benign brooding blackness.

"I've got his house key," said Bob, "but you'll have to meet him first. Naturally he will want to look you over."

In the licensed parlour of the third hotel, right beneath the ponderous wall clock with its pendulum, sat a big man in black clothes: black suit, black shirt, black elastic-sided boots and a black Stetson. No hats came off in this place, neither did Bob's ski cap.

Charlie was about seventy-five and should have looked like an old gangster in those clothes; instead he looked more like some old bird. His bulk hunched down in his chair, his face was full and long, his nose large and hooked, and his eyes were dark, inscrutable and hooded. The charm of Charlie, the absolutely delightful surprise of Charlie, was that true to his ancestry this Dutchman from Pennsylvania was smoking a long white clay pipe. Near him on the floor was a polished brass spittoon and I was to learn that when the pipe was not in his mouth he chewed snoose and his aim of the resultant

50

stream was perfect. He never seemed to move from his position under the clock except for meals and closing time. The spittoon stayed where it was.

He didn't rise as I approached his table. No man in that country got to his feet for a woman except for a few officials and bank clerks; rather was I led to the throne.

"This is Stella," began Bob proudly.

Under the black brim the eyes became more hooded, as he surveyed me.

"With the man of the hour," was Charlie's acknowledgment.

His voice was low and rumbling as he took in my grey suit, pink pullover and the pearl earrings I had thought to put on to meet a landlord. His insult swept me with ice until I realized he was just being dry. Later I learned that nearly all his remarks were philosophical and dispensed at local humanity from his vantage point.

"I hear you have nowhere to live and you have a couple of children with you. Well we can't have that. I won't be using my cabin or leaving the hotel before break-up so you are welcome to use it until then. But I must ask you for enough to cover the light and water bills. You'll find plenty of wood outside but you'll have to get young bucko here to split it for you."

Light and water. God knows what I had expected when living in a town. I thanked him enthusiastically. Although I was itching to inspect the place, we had to sit for a couple of rounds while I got acquainted. Time was no object.

Charlie did not pump us. Nosiness was not his line. It was obvious what he thought of our relationship and that he said, "Well, well" to himself and kept his peace. I could not say to him "It's not what you think" because we did not have anything to go on and were feeling our way.

In fact we had suffered in another way from passing glances at as unlikely a pair as anyone ever saw. After the war, when we first met, we had both been sitting down, on a streetcar. Then Bob, full of daring, asked me to go off and have a cup of coffee with him, stalling my rebuff by adding "but you wouldn't, would you?" When I looked at his cute wistful face

I agreed (the bit being between my teeth at that time.) As I got up to leave with him he gasped in dismay.

"I was afraid of that." He came up to my chin. Worse, he looked like a cherub. God knows what made me accept the coffee that got the whole thing rolling; probably his fetching, gloomy self-negation. "I appealed to the mother in you, that's what it was," he'd tease me.

At another time that winter, in a Smithers cafe, somebody passing our table was heard to murmur "Sonny and mommy having a nice outing?" Bob's fists on the table showed white knuckles, but he sat there and took it for my sake. "I told you there'd be days like this," he said.

The way to Charlie's cabin was down a lane just off Main Street and near the railway tracks. A little path led off the lane and down beside Charlie's outhouse, which backed onto the lane. There was a reason in Smithers, which became apparent later, for having outhouses placed on the alleys. From Charlie's outhouse a slatted boardwalk led to the cabin's only door.

It was a neat shack, looking like something on a railway siding, sheathed in tarpaper with a roof sloping down in one direction from front to back. Out of this slope stuck the usual tin chimney, while the electric wire from the lane led to a white porcelain fixture beside the door. Inside were two rooms. The manner of partition was a wall that did not quite meet the end wall so that you passed around the divider to get into the other room. By the door in the main room was a tap with a bucket of water beneath it, frozen over. Against the dividing wall were a table and a couple of chairs, while opposite them sat the cook stove.

Such stoves are worth describing, as they cannot be found anymore unless a wood stove craze is reviving them. Made of cast iron with a stove top measuring three feet by two and standing up about three feet from the floor, each had a nice little oven and firebox that would take an eighteen-inch length of wood. One could bake loaves in the little oven, or a pie or a roast. As long as one had such a stove one had comfort, no matter what the surroundings. It could cook a person right out of his dwelling when stoked up.

The outhouse system is best understood by describing what happened to Joan one day. Like every other convenience in town, ours did not contain the usual pit but had a bucket under the seat. These were known as "honey buckets" and the honey-bucket man drove down the lane with his truck, picking up the full ones and replacing them with disinfected empty ones. On this occasion Joan was caught and flattened herself against the wall as a hand reached in.

The children, in their permitted and unpermitted explorations while I was tied to a job, found out later where the honey buckets went. Joan's bike had been sent up by her father. Taking a ride over the tracks and out of town, they went to the dump and sure enough on the edge of the fill were rows and rows of peaked piles. In summer they reported the place as a wild drone of flies with rats running everywhere; and even a sunny day in mid-winter was not exempt.

On the morning of the move I kept the children out of school to help with lugging cases down the street. After we had dumped everything into Charlie's cabin and spread a few things around, they went back to school and I reported to the postmaster. It was now nearly term end and close to Christmas.

The station agent sent our trunk down and we placed it under the bedroom window. In it was all our bedding and all our household possessions. By dint of making a pad on top of the trunk we created a second 'bed' for Robert, the younger and shorter. He cried all night. His sister, at the age of eleven and an old woman already, wearily got out of the small bed she was sharing with me and traded places. With my first week's pay from the post office I bought a cot.

My daughter became the mummy after that. At her tender age Joan's idea of doing potatoes for supper was to put a pot of ice water on the stove with tiny pieces of potato cut up in it and wait forever for it to boil. In spite of that, in their own self-interest, both kids became good at making a fire very quickly. I had no recourse but to trust them to be responsible and they were. They had their share of advice, lectures and threats, but were naturally sensible.

Charlie's place was only a few blocks from Bob's, and Bob and I managed to meet at night for a while, but it was awkward. He worked full daylight hours and after he'd cleaned up and made his own supper in the kennel he would sometimes feel like going for a beer. Or he'd mend equipment and with mugs of cocoa at the ready, wait for me to join him. After the next move, we were closer still.

Working in the post office was quite exciting, as I never minded doing dog work that bored other people, and all the populace came in and out. It was a top-flight observation post. It also gave me a quick knowledge of the layout of the town and surrounding farms and settlements, which came in handy later. My job was to share the mail sorting with another girl and to hand out general delivery parcels for Christmas.

One day I had been sorting in the rear when a voice called through the wicket "It's Stella, isn't it?" There of all the dirty luck was one of my old classmates, untrammelled in her thinking of course, as though straight from St. Margaret's, the private school we attended in Victoria. This woman had a husband who was posted here and probably thought Smithers a lark. She was obviously lonely because she insisted I visit them. It was the last thing on earth I wanted to do. She was always full of questions and her little pointed tongue flicked in and out while she waited for your answer. I ran into her thirty years later at a reunion and the first thing she asked me in front of a lot of people was, "Did you marry that man?"

The children made our Christmas while I worked to the last hour. Over the tracks again they went at ten below, bundled up and with the earflaps of Robert's cap framing his rosy cheeks, to look for a suitable tree. Going along a ridge of willows they saw only bear tracks and very few conifers. Finally they found a young one, bent it over and chopped off its top with their hatchet. This they somehow set up on top of the liberated steamer trunk.

Meanwhile, Bob had split us a great supply of firewood, working out in the sun of a Sunday at thirty below with his shirt off and fully conscious of the effect. The children stared and stared at his pads of muscle. In my own family men were thin and spare and too much muscle was considered obscene. Bob soon had us running around carrying wood. We all survived.

Later a dampening note was struck when Joan received a big soft brown blanket from her paternal home, through the mails for Christmas, which was meant to make a point. And *of course* we needed it. She also got admonitions by mail from her paternal grandmother about the two kids "braving the storm" by hanging together and looking after each other. In those days my temperature was boiling with outrage. Afterwards I could not even recall being cold.

Christmas Day was not memorable. I suppose I put a chicken into the little oven but don't remember which of us supplied it. There was always rum. It was one of those times when Bob did eat with us otherwise he was pretty mobile.

As it happened, the children and I enjoyed the brief week between Christmas and the New Year. It was the first fun we had had together since leaving the coast, the first time we had dared to feel light-hearted. We went up into the bush looking for animal tracks. Sometimes Bob went with us, and his knowledge made it better. We explored as far as our feet would take us and went down to the frozen river. This I told the children they were to keep off, on pain of death, if I was not with them. Later, much later, they confided cheerfully that they had built a bonfire on the ice in order to roast wieners. But they were a good deal older, and handy with their hands in defense against a flailing mother on the warpath, when they told me.

We did get another house, one of those beside the arena and, as it happened, directly across from Bob's place. On Christmas Eve I had been paid off, and with nothing to do between then and New Year's, I found the new home just before the first of the year, so that another simultaneous move and job switch was entailed. The house was just a shack beside two bigger houses, but it was quite new and commodious in its two rooms. By now I had started to buy bits of furniture, the first of which had been the cot. The new place also had a double bed.

Brünhilde

The main thing on the agenda now was for me to sell myself to the district engineer and his militant girl Friday. On the second day of January I climbed those stairs with the usual knot in my middle because of my amateur typing.

They gave me a good desk with a great big machine and a window at my back to cast light on the copy. In the middle of the outer office, between the public counter and the wall opposite it, and at right angles to both, was an enormous double desk with a divider on top, which was full of pigeonholes that stored mail, memos and correspondence. The wall beside the double desk was shelved and held file boxes from floor to ceiling.

Winifred's side of the desk faced the engineer's door, which she could see through the divider; facing her on the other side was the chief clerk whom she could not help seeing. This individual was a thin, balding youngish man whose main sport in life was baiting Winnie in an unsmiling and self-amused manner for all the traffic would bear. When he got a rise out of her he would cackle like a hen. His presence was a pleasant surprise as they had not bothered to mention him; he made an ally when Winnie got too rough, which did not occur until after I had got my bearings and had begun to show some personality.

The payrolls involved road crews and machine operators, there being many machines in the big district. Each paylist needed fifteen copies for the main district office and headquarters, and fifteen copies with accompanying carbons were what I rolled into that brute of a typewriter. I set to work in a pall of fear against making a mistake. Winnie listened grimly while I struck each key with love and care, but she said nothing.

Instead she scolded the clerk. "Either smoke that cigarette or put it out. If there's anything I can't stand it's a butt left in an ashtray. Pyew!" He would put it out sullenly each time she said this, saying there was no pleasing her.

When she became aware of my stealthy erasures of fifteen pages, one at a time, she became vocal.

"Chuck those away and start again. You can't have carbon

smears. Take your time. If it takes all day don't make a mistake. But you'll have to buck up pretty fast. You'll soon have other typing to do."

I was a clerk, not a typist, but there would be no clerking for me here. Their volume of work was pretty high for such a small office and Winnie's day was spent taking inquiries at the counter and writing the boss's letters, from dictation. It kept her more than busy and she had no time for memos, but I did.

With knees knocking I took down my first dictation in a scrabbling type of longhand while the engineer averted his eyes. It was time for all my strength and will power to do a job beyond my experience and make them keep me. The correspondence course on typing had helped considerably and I remembered enough speed writing to resurrect a few short cuts. These questionable skills had never been tried out on a government before. Therefore I ground out memos as fast as I dared, trying not to have false starts in my wastebasket or to go back to the engineer for clarification. Such trials passed.

It transpired that Winnie was a widow, but she had been married three times. She was very droll about this and was currently dating the game warden. Rather like Bob, he was short, stocky and outdoorsy, whereas Winnie was comfortably built, very tall and used to coastal niceties. It would be more explicit to say that she had run with the Victoria "Four Hundred" who made the society pages, and had "seen better days." The fact that she was so tall and that the game warden was so short (and nobody's fool) heartened me no end.

Gradually I became expert with the payrolls, but attending at the counter was out of bounds. Almost all the office business was handled by the chief clerk, or by Winnie when he was out of the room, and by both of them at once at times. Curious glances used to come my way from men on the other side of the counter and finally Winnie had enough of intercepting the direction of these. As soon as the room was empty after one such stare and she was back in her chair, she swivelled around and gave me a level look.

"I'll have you know that I'm the queen bee in here and that's the way things are going to stay. Is that clear?"

Bob laughed heartily at me that night and had no sympathy.

"Serves you right for letting her get the best of you. If she can get the best of you she deserves to."

There was more, which affected me. A year later, my sister, after hearing a very brief version of the Smithers experience, smiled small smiles at me as she told me that she had known Winifred socially some years before as one of the Victoria "Four Hundred" social set and was familiar with her humour.

However the office began accepting me and we had fun. One day the clerk was telling us a yarn while leaning back against the counter. Suddenly he was overtaken by a big sneeze and his teeth flew out and scuttled under the main desk. We women laughed ourselves silly while, red-faced, he retrieved the plate with a long ruler. He was livid with us, which made us laugh the harder.

Winnie also had a way, after or during an especially hard day, of leaning back in her chair with her arms hooked back over it and dangling behind pathetically.

"I want my mother," she'd say to the ceiling.

Not only did I find this hilarious but also rather fetching. As a transplant Winnie wasn't such a big success either.

The clerk was friendly in a grudging sort of way. He tried strenuously to stay hard-boiled in a female atmosphere. He was no match for Winnie and when she was out of the room would try to get even with dour suppositions about her love life. I gave him no encouragement on that subject but kept steadily typing or remarking, "You don't say." Funnily enough she was not above a few conjectures about *his* domestic felicity when stung. Although Winnie was often a plague to me I felt she would be a loyal friend as long as I did not step on her toes, and so it proved.

There were few monotonous days at work. Once, a moose came calmly down Main Street and into the front door of the agency before beating a retreat. At another time Winnie was standing at the counter when I noticed a blue mark on her leg, showing through her stocking. When I asked her what had happened, she kept turning ledger pages and replied, "One of my husbands bit me."

And so it went. We seldom saw the engineer. He would check in first thing in the morning, do a raft of dictating and then disappear. He seemed to be all over the district. He was a quiet man and uncomplaining. Once when I was taking a memo he thought to ask how the children and I were getting on. I gave him a graphic description or two because I thought he would understand, then got around to honey buckets. Bill Bottomley raised his eyes to look at me.

"You can get used to anything," he said. "Anything."

For years afterwards during our struggles up and down the land I'd think, "You can get used to anything," and for the rest of my life I would remember the engineer and how he looked when he said that. It was one of the aphorisms of the north, summing up how civilized people could abandon all they knew to pig into some pretty awful situations, becoming like the locals in looks and language and loving it.

Such a one was a woman in Smithers who wandered up and down the streets with a goat pulling a little cart, collecting things. She also owned an old horse that pulled a bigger cart and sometimes the goat was tied to the horse as they went along. I supposed the woman was completely nutty but never spoke to her to find out. Everyone knew her and called her Crazy Daisy. One night I mentioned her to Charlie. He seemed to think she was a former educator who had written many textbooks, but she was completely unknown to us.

"Poor woman. People are so unkind to her," he said.

We used to see her going in and out of beer parlours alone and heard some of the jeers. At one time I saw her come out of one with all her skirts awry and half way up her back, smiling away, after using the parlour's facilities no doubt.

I thought Daisy must have tried to convince locals of matters too esoteric for them, and beer had not helped. Daisy was unaware and uncaring and made me heartsick. But she seemed happy, always with a smile on her face.

Daisy was born in 1892 in Buxton, England, christened as Kathleen Daisy O'Connell, and is listed in Burke's Peerage. Her passing in 1980 was the subject of a short tribute by Ponnie Wilmot of the *Smithers Interior News* (used by permission): "Another chapter in the story of Smithers came to an end with the death last week of Mrs. Kathleen Casler. How many youngsters have danced in a fairy ring under an ancient oak tree by the light of the moon? Kathleen did. Maybe that enchanting night is when she received her gift of fey imagination. Long before it became fashionable, Mrs. Casler began doing 'her own thing.' Her more conventional fellow citizens disapproved, but Mrs. Casler called on her inner resources and so became somewhat of a legend in her own time. She never forgot a kindness. She expressed her opinions regardless of the consequences, and allowed no one to pull any tricks on her.

In failing health the past several years, Mrs. Casler spent much of her time in hospital, the past two years or so in extended care. Here she brought great joy and a sense of fun to those who cared for her. Maybe right now the angels are chuckling at one of her rapier thrusts of wit. We'll miss you, Kathleen."

The Klootchman

Our evenings with Charlie continued. Various people joined our table at times, but usually we three sat alone. It was while we were in Smithers that the Indians obtained their franchise and were allowed into licensed parlours. They came in droves at first but couldn't handle their liquor. There began to be sundry local scenes.

One night found a real aboriginal at our table, by which delineation I mean that there were no traces of modern living about her; she had only a few words of English and got by with signs.

Bob had a thing about the Indians, much the same as he had for old pioneers and any old man worth knowing.

This night in the parlour Bob's regard for Indians was put to the test. He treated the woman who had joined us uninvited very courteously, even though she was stoned, and he kidded her a lot. He did not know what lay ahead.

"You know somebody's got to see her home," remarked

Charlie. "Oh yes. When she gets home her old man will beat her up. You just can't let her go home alone in that condition." She was really out of it by then. "And if you take her home by yourself," he said to Bob, "he'll think the worst and beat you up as well. And he's a big 'un. Your lady here will have to go with you." Charlie avoided using my Christian name out of old world manners and dodged any other title under the circumstances.

We found ourselves out in the dark with a woman, dead drunk, hanging between us whose feet got pulled along. There is no such thing as leaving a drunk to sleep it off up north in winter. A person would freeze to death in minutes. You can't even grab the handle of a train door on a passing freight, as many vagrants found, because your hand welds solidly to the metal.

She did not live far. We went down into an alley into the back of some building, pretty horrible in the dark, and on hearing our commotion a deep voice called "Whozzat?" It sounded terrifying. The Indian came out and for once Bob's knuckles went limp. Then the man saw me. He had been sleeping one off himself, and he could not equate me with what he thought his wife had been doing, so he gave the poor woman a push inside and closed the door.

One day after our little family had moved into the house opposite his, I commissioned an Indian to bring us a load of wood. This the man did, and as the sun was hot that day he asked for a drink of water. I gave him a tumbler full and stood waiting until he had finished it. As the man left Bob suddenly turned nasty.

"Now take the glass inside and boil it," he commanded. "Go on. Take it inside and boil it!" He was inferring that I, as a city girl, would never touch the glass again unless it was boiled because an Indian had touched it. His outburst was totally uncalled for as I had no thoughts at all about the glass.

"Do you know who he is?" persisted Bob, practically in high C. "He's the nephew of Simon Peter Gunanoot." Everyone in the valley except me knew the legend of the Indian outlaw who eluded the Mounties for years.

61

Simon Peter Gunanoot had been the subject of the largest manhunt in Canadian history, vanishing into the wilderness after being accused of a double homicide. Thirteen years passed, and then one day in 1919 he turned himself in with a lawyer at his side. He was acquitted of the charges.

Chuckout Time

By now Bob was fidgety again. Our going to a pub at night was only a token and something to do after the kids were in bed. This was no hazard, short of an earthquake, as the little stove would be banked down for the night and I'd see them settled. In any case Joan was very responsible and Robert did what the little mother told him to. If they had known of to-day's options for children I could not have moved a muscle. As it was, nobody in the office or in town seemed to question the situation.

Some evenings he would go off by himself to find friends and I would write letters or read while the kids did homework. Occasionally, Bob and I tried other places. One particular night out with Bob brought both of us near the brink of notoriety.

Two Mounties came into the parlour where we were, off the main street, at about closing time. At exactly three minutes to the hour they spoke to the bartender who called, "Time, gentlemen, please!" Everyone arose as bidden, intimidated by scarlet tunics and Stetson-shielded eyes, but not my man. Instead he rose majestically, the better to rebuke them, took a stance and slowly withdrew an old railway watch from his pocket, looked at it studiously, then looked into the face of the nearest Mountie who was coming towards us with "chuck out" written all over him. Bob was just starting a preamble about our having two and a half more minutes to go when I pulled his sleeve mightily and finally got him spluttering out into the air.

One does not work in a government agency without knowing what Mounties do and how they think. In those days they were intent on getting the newly enfranchised Indians home and generally policing everything. It was a new experience for us as well as for the Indians.

"If it hadn't been for you I'd have hit that guy!"

And he would have. He had peeled a great many potatoes in the Navy for impudence unbecoming a sailor, even if his officers had had to muffle their smiles. Mounties do not have that sense of humour.

"Yes, and you'd have landed both of us in jail." I knew full well that I'd have been rounded up too, as they did not stop for niceties and asked their questions afterwards.

For once next morning I had something interesting to report.

"I nearly didn't get into work this morning. You would have had to bail me out of the lockup downstairs."

They were more impressed with an encounter with the Mounties than with the comic situation; they knew about the RCMP too and considered we'd had a narrow escape.

Spring Fever

As the weather warmed most men got restless. One Monday morn the engineer came out of his office tearing his hair.

Over the weekend two bored heavy-machinery operators from our district had cooked up a wager that each could prove his machine superior to the others and they had staged a duel. Using their cranes and buckets, which made the machines look like long-necked dinosaurs with a lot of teeth, they set upon each other in the middle of the street and bashed away. The thought of these iron-jawed monsters snapping away defied description. Winnie and I were in hysterics, but also deeply sorry for our boss. Much of that and Victoria would select a new engineer.

By now the valley was veering into spring. Break-up in the river was due and I was to learn that when flights of Canada geese trailed overhead in wavering V formations Bob would start looking over his packsack and equipment. The cry of the geese was too much for him.

"The call of the North," he'd say, as if he had invented it, looking at me in innocent splendour and growing to twice his size. My heart would sink.

As the sun came out and less snow was on the ground I was taken for a "moose hunt." What he meant was that if we saw any moose tracks well and good, otherwise at least we would have an outing. Off we went with the packboard, getting a workout into the surrounding bush below the mountains.

After a while we found moose track holes as if made by poles thrust two to three feet into the snow, but the snow was settling and encrusted and the droppings were old, which meant it was warm enough for the moose to have gone back up towards the hills.

Somewhere along the trail I had my first experience of making tea with snow water and eating beans with bacon beside a fire started with twigs from trees. To make a fire in snow you scoop the snow out from under a fallen log. The fire in the hollow burns out part of the log and makes a protected place to do your cooking, away from wind.

I felt very capable and carefree, dressed in my bottle-green ski pants with T-shirt underneath my Black Watch viyella shirt and no parka. I was hardening up to the feel of things while my companion was getting very much disgusted with all this domesticity and no action. I liked to tease him. Once I went too far; I'd called him "my glorious northern Apollo." He turned on me furiously.

"Don't you ever, ever laugh at me again."

By the first of May he was fit to be tied. One Sunday I was told, "Come on. You're going to see what a real bush hike is like."

Down the highway and off under the mountains some two or three miles was a lake in its own natural park, which was where we were heading. The snow was all gone, it was warm—almost hot—and I peeled off layers while Bob stripped to his swim trunks. Silently aching with fatigue I helped spread out our blanket in the woods near the lake and we sat down to eat lunch.

"This is more like," he said. "There could be moose and deer around here." Whisky jacks inquired and red squirrels ran up and down headfirst among the pines. "Not a soul in sight. Now you begin to see what I mean." It was true. We had found no solitude since leaving his trapping cabin. We basked flat on the rug in the woodsy sunlight while he dreamed his dreams no doubt. There was no sound but for a little scurrying.

"Ah," he sighed. "This is the life."

Then on the warm air a familiar sound pricked me back into reality. A bicycle bell. Sitting up I beheld coming along the forest track my own children. Joan was riding her bike extremely slowly while reading a comic book and Robert was trotting along beside her. The packboard for the big hike lay beside Bob; my kids had trumped his ace.

Partings

When no further developments seemed to transpire, it never occurred to me to ditch him for breach of promise. He thought everything was as ever and I did not want anyone else; the mere thought sickened me. I did not know him very well then or the signs of restlessness would have been read for what they were rather than as signs of desertion. He was a lemming, a migratory animal, making his annual run like the geese.

It was true he had started to chafe at the chains wrought by a woman and kids around his bachelorhood. The peak of this had come one night when we'd had a load of coal delivered to my house because we could not keep a fire going all night using wood. The children had gone out that evening with a sled, muffled up, to begin the tedious task of getting the stuff off the street where it had been dumped, and naturally we thought we were putting on a good show until Bob would offer to help.

What we beheld, as we worked away that early evening after supper, was Bob emerging from his kennel yonder, dressed to the nines for a night on the town: Harris jacket, collar and tie, good slacks and Scottish brogues. He went down the road without glancing sideways at us, his head held very high and defiantly. When we saw there would be no help from him we threw coal after him for as long as we could reach him.

Before the second week in May he was gone. To be sure, there were jobs locally but they were mostly lumbering in the valley, mining and farming, the money poor and they did not offer him the future he wanted. Without a qualm he had joined the United States Forest Service in Alaska.

In mid-May, after he had gone, we found a decent house and moved into it. Before we moved, the lingering old snow mounds had gone altogether, and, with its pristine purity removed from hollows around the dog kennel, objects could be seen twinkling in the sun, a sea of tin cans that had been hidden under the snow. I thought he'd taken the freedom of the north too seriously and wished his friends could see them. One of them did. Gunnar.

Before we moved into our proper big house I had a letter from Effie Larsen saying Gunnar was going to be up our way and would like to pay us a visit. I was very dismayed about how to entertain him with Bob gone and there was no telephone at her place or time to notify her before he came. How he found us says something for Smithers' communications, but come he did. It was a Gunnar I didn't recognize. He had cancer of the throat and could hardly speak; he was making his last rounds of the country.

Gunnar had time between trains to have dinner with us and hear all our news but he could not reply except with a croak. I gave him the softest dinner I could manage, but his eyes were full of unshed tears while saliva ran down his chin as he ate. I felt kicked in the stomach and sent the children from the table early so that he could eat slowly and in peace, trying not to notice anything myself. Naturally he had come to say goodbye to Bob and I did the best I could to substitute.

Gunnar's final end was in the Burns Lake hospital the following summer, but of course we knew then that this was it. He would not let me see him to the train and, in the hour or so he was with us, was constantly overly grateful for everything, which made me feel worse than ever.

Dear old men were disappearing out of my life with Bob away. News had reached us earlier that my landlord Charlie van Alstine was in hospital. Bob had gone up to see him before he left and had commissioned me by mail to visit him, though with some misgivings.

"He won't like it," was the main thought, "but you'd better go anyway."

There was an excuse now for me to sit with Charlie because if I had sought him out personally in a beer parlour both of us would have been embarrassed, especially with "the man of the hour" now flown, as predicted or inferred at our first meeting, where Charlie had thought we wouldn't last. Bob and I got used to that sort of scepticism as our days together ebbed and flowed.

Charlie was in an old men's ward and, like Gunnar, on his way out. I crept towards his bed diffidently because I was such an intruder into his old man's world. His face was grey although his hair was still black, and he was uncomfortable about me standing there. The inevitable bottle hung below his bed and it was that as much as anything that made me turn and run after a few words, to leave him his privacy. He had not known what to say to me. I never did find out what his nemesis was, but his courtliness had deserted him.

Further visits to the hospital were out of the question. Charlie was one of the north's mystery men; he never said a word about his life or work, only that he was a Pennsylvania Dutchman, though it was likely that he had worked on the railway. His white pipe was always beside him. He had merely existed on an even keel doing nothing but observe the world around him. He may have been an invalid when we met him, but we were never to know.

CHAPTER · IV

||||||||||||||||||||||||||||||||||||||||||||||||||||||||||||||||||||||||||||||||||||||||||||||||||||||||||||||||||||||||||||||

Lambing Time

May Day

After Bob left I expected to feel lonely, but I was so numb that an ensuing string of community events, which kept the children and me occupied, became also my therapy. Perhaps I was more outraged than damaged, and perhaps I felt guilty about expecting him to remain in this hole.

Our newest home was a decent log house with a porch on the front and an actual piece of lawn beside it, or what passed for one. A green duroid roof sloped to cover the porch, which was glassed in at one end with old mismatching windows. There was a pump in the kitchen sink and the water smelled of sulphur. This house was also off the main street, at the end of a cul de sac. Beyond it were meadows.

On our walks we had found an Indian encampment on a grassy plain just outside town, with teepees and real live female aboriginals dressed in buckskin and beads, as opposed to the town's usual Indian women in cotton dresses with their heads bound in scarves. In those days the Smithers Indians still owned a lot of native regalia and used it for festive affairs, and many Indians of the area still lived in tents, or appeared to. As well as the tents, they possessed a few big wigwams and when celebrations took place in town they camped in these nearby. Some still dragged travois that they brought into town for processions, along with their deerhide drums.

Shortly after we moved into our new home, Smithers and its districts had its annual "May Day" parade on Victoria Day. The parade had the customary funny attempts at floats with six or seven Mounties on horseback, merchants' efforts, a band of Indians aforesaid beating a drum and dragging a travois, and Public Works heavy machinery.

At the head of the procession was Crazy Daisy. She stood up in her tumbril, taking the reins over its high front while her two children sat down behind her. Their dog ran beside the horse. I looked at lonely Daisy with her son and daughter and thought my wry thoughts.

Joan was also watching. Her gaze was upon the boy, who was her own age, and she was feeling very drawn towards him as he sat with his knees huddled to his chin to squeeze out embarrassment. Daisy was to repeat the performance on Klondike Day, this time alone in the cart while her son and daughter led the horse. Attached to the bridle of the horse on one side was her goat; on the other side ran their dog. She was very well known, evoking whistles and shouts.

Smithers itself was as well decorated for May Day as it would be for Klondike Day. On the latter day fake false fronts were put on anything that needed to be disguised and hitching rails were set up in front of them, especially in front of the Dirty Shame Saloon, which was really the Elks Hall. The town seemed so flat, sparse and semi-deserted in aspect during summer, with houses scattered about; yet dispersed through the valley were roughly 3,200 people who came in to trade, some of whom became a seeming populace in town to make the most of these events. Everyone lined the hitching rails to watch.

Running the length of Main Street and adding to the piquancy of the situation was a big open sewer. It was a good six or eight feet across and much too wide to jump over. The smell from this in summer and the dust clouds were our chief reasons for calling Smithers "Stinkers." That and honey buckets.

And we were not exempt from smells down in our dead end lane because one day the honey bucket man turned his truck around in front of our house too sharply and tipped a couple of buckets off. He did his best to clear the mess but we lived with the residue until sun and wind took over.

Bob's letters came regularly. He was making a lot of money cutting trails for the Americans, who thought much of his prowess. He was also learning how to build with logs. By early summer he came back on leave and we finally married on July 7, 1949.

Packin' In

The manner of our marriage is worth recording.

Bob was given a week's leave for the event and made short work of seeing the agent and civil registration. He also made short work of our lawn with a scythe. He refused to be married in the courtroom as he wasn't going to "stand up like a monkey and be looked at." Instead McCrae, as agent, married us privately in his office, while Winnie, the chief clerk, the engineer and his wife stood as witnesses.

When Bob came bounding up the stairs into my office that first time, Winnie took one startled look. She had never actually met him before. She used to throw dark hints at me like, "You may as well be married as live the way you are," which infuriated me. Or conversely, "If you have the slightest doubts run like hell." The clerk would then, when Winnie left the room, gossip with rich surmise about her marriages and about her right to give advice. She in her turn had surveyed him. Now she was looking at me.

Bob had bought a Stetson in Juneau to replace an old favourite that had flown down a canyon when he'd been doing that walk from Teslin Lake to Telegraph Creek the summer before. It seemed incredible that all these lifetimes had barely spanned one year.

The counter in the public works was a high one and came right up to his chest. The big hat seemed to put a lid on him, which in his hurry he did not think to remove.

Between the hat and the counter, his innocuous, boyish freckled face, showing splendid teeth, completed the picture. Winnie threw herself back in her chair again saying, as in any crisis, "I want my mother."

The clerk wanted to know, did this mean I would be quitting? Bob and I both said "No" at once and he explained that he was only on leave for now.

"So you are putting your wife to work?" asked Winnie ominously.

"Yep," replied the chosen one. "That's the kind of hairpin I am."

Before the ceremony the children were picked up by friends and taken away at my request. They had suffered already from the presentation by mail of the fact of their father's remarriage, which came in a large portrait of him and their new stepmother on the occasion of his "re-hitchment," sent by my successor to underline her position. He looked awful, which did not escape the kids. I saw no need to rub in further cruelties.

After the ceremony we all repaired to my house where we stood outside in the sun on the "lawn" and watched my boss uncork champagne that he had had the foresight to provide. They refused sandwiches and after a decent interval the office bunch moseyed off, knowing we had a lot of packsack loading to do and a train to catch.

They had all been very kind. After the wedding poor Mc-Crae's golf game was ruined for weeks because his friends would hail him loudly across the so-called golf course with "Hi padre!" Everyone had rallied around very understandingly once the wedding was in the wind. Winnie grudgingly took on my memos for a week and the parents of one of Joan's school friends devised a means for us to have a honeymoon. The children went to stay on a farm these people knew of, near Terrace and beside a creek that ran into the Skeena. In those days I thought that the parents of school children would be responsible and that these friends of Joan's, whom I had met, would be reliable. I had no qualms.

Our wedding journey took us half way down the CNR line

between Smithers and Burns Lake, where we got out at a tiny whistlestop called Forestdale. We stepped out onto a dirt road and organized our packs. This time I was to pack in for real. Bob's load weighed over seventy pounds and mine was about thirty-five.

Through the woods we went on a faint trail of about three miles, to Day Lake. We walked single file, my pace trying to match his, stepping over a lot of fallen jack pine. Though my legs were longer, his stride seemed bigger and was certainly faster; he was going at half his normal speed. It was hot and there were baby grouse everywhere, though it was a religion with him not to shoot out of season and spoil the crop. Eventually we came to the barely visible remains of a sawmill by the lake, which was our landmark. Working along the shore some distance from it we pitched our tent and made our first little camp, staying for two nights.

Mosquitoes were thick that evening, after sun-drop behind the hills, but in the hot morning sun with a constant breeze making the lake choppy they disappeared back among the trees. We had a tiny beach and flat grass for a campsite. Near us some scarlet-breasted flickers nested in a hole in an alder trunk. The birds paid no attention to us and went on feeding their young as we ate in peace and watched them, not ten feet from our cooking fire.

There was an old raft abandoned nearby and after breakfast we pushed around on that, sitting on a packing crate. Dragonflies followed us and all the birds and squirrels along the shore. Hawks and eagles soared and owls hooted at night. The lake was too rough for loons to settle easily so that their penetrating cry, the signature of the north for me, was a discovery of the future. A certain frog sat on a fallen tree that angled into the water and he seemed to orchestrate a froggy chorus.

Bob always had a fund of anecdotes, dreams and hopes to talk about. My use to him at these times seemed to lie in an empathetic understanding of what he was about, a willingness to learn, sincerity, a caustic wit to match his when crossed and, it seemed, the ability to please his eye. There had to be something in it for him; just as a dear friend wrote to me, "He must have something for you; otherwise you wouldn't be going along with it." The comment did not imply a physical attraction. Always, good-looking men had put me off, unless there was that "something." I did not need columbines and roses this time and imagined Bob didn't either, since he often called me "Chum." I was wrong. He needed romantic loving.

The short break was soon over. We had done nothing but laze and yet we seemed to be busy all the time: frying bacon, making bannock, washing up, scraping pots with sand, having another coffee and finding firewood.

On our return to Forestdale we took a better look at the little general store and post office among the jackpines and the old folk in it. We had bought matches and milk there on the way in. It was the only building for miles around that had survived the demise of the sawmill, as the bush had reclaimed everything. Not a soul within miles either but the store's owners.

They were very old, and standing side by side looked exactly like the figures in the painting *American Gothic*, where the dried-out old man in braces stands holding a pitchfork and his wife is all apron with sparse hair strained into a bun. This man was tall with baggy pants braced up to his rib cage. She was short, wispy and toothless in a faded old dress and cardigan. Over the dress was a big white apron that came down to her knees and they both wore boots.

They saw us young people off politely, standing on a stoop built of half round slabs. Bob had found out that the old man was so restless during the long nights of summer that he patrolled the store half the time and slept on a shelf; they never left the place as they had nowhere to go.

Too soon we were back at my house, which was now Bob's. He could not stay to claim it. The morning after our return a friend fetched him away in a truck and as it backed out Bob gave me a long, long look. It was a terrible look, as if he were memorizing my face for the last time. My blood ran cold. But the spoken plan was that he would continue working until the end of the summer season until he knew what we should do.

Strawberry Time

My life was now focused on the children. At the end of their allotted time on the farm they were returned in such a rush I could not tell if they had been ejected or had wanted to run away. They were delivered at the door of course, but the tales they burst with once we were alone made me thankful of my ignorance of their welfare.

Their hosts were the parents of Joan's playmate Lucille, an eleven-year old girl, prematurely pubescent, who didn't know what to do with her body. The mother was easygoing and normal, but the father, a Mr. Trueman, was puritanical with children. I had seen the strictness as safety and thought in terms of farms and cream from the cow. The children's recent adventures now became uppermost in my mind.

All had been well as long as the children were at Truemans. There were chickens and a goat. The two girls wandered through daisy meadows while Robert had chicks to watch. So far the only thing that put Joan off was that Lucille would sigh and fling herself about and flump into chairs in abandoned positions. Her preoccupation with the facts of life, in her conversation, escaped her father's notice. Privately Joan thought that what Lucille needed was a couple of brothers.

My kids were to stay at Trueman's for two weeks. Time hung heavily. Trueman made Joan write to me and stood over her reading every word. To kill time the girls parted in different directions. Joan, who had just turned twelve, accepted an offer from kindly workers to run a grader on a nearby road and Lucille, who thought this unfeminine, undertook to be all womanly and cook the road men a meal in their trailer. To Joan's disgust this meant opening cans of beans, quite forgetting that her own favourite offering to Robert was wieners and beans.

Then it was thought the girls might make some pocket money picking strawberries up the Skeena River. Consequently they found themselves in a commodious shack on another farm by the river and in the care of a forty-five-year-old good-looking man and his lean, listless wife who smoked a lot. Robby stayed behind with the Truemans, out of harm's way.

Again Joan was allowed to run machinery, this time on the strawberry farm. All went well until she fell off their little farm tractor onto its footplate and, unable to shut off the ignition switch, headed straight for the swirling river. Her boss legged across the field and cut the motor in time, but was more concerned about losing his tractor than her probable fate.

They picked berries all day on one day, which were packed into flats and ferried across the Skeena the next day, to be carried through a forest to the CNR line. The fun began when their boss took one of the girls with him each time, Lucille going first. She came back happy enough. When Joan's turn came a certain apprehension overtook her when her boss deliberately watched her as she went into the woods for nature's call. He kept frightening her into staying close to him with tales of wolves and bears. She had nothing tangible to disclose to anyone on their return but unsettling episodes began to happen.

As the days between trips were for farm chores, Joan found herself one day in the barn alone with her boss. He proceeded to milk the cow while she played with kittens. Laughing, he sprayed the mother cat's face with milk straight from the udder. Suddenly he walked over to where Joan was as she tried to put their big Newfoundland dog between herself and her employer.

My kids were taught to respect elders and not to hack shins; no preschool classes in those days on how to handle strangers. When she jumped up from behind the dog he put his hands on her shoulders then slid one down over her bottom, telling her that she had a "nice little posterior" and that she was a very nice little girl. The next scene found this man sitting on the edge of the big double bed the girls shared in the main room of the shack. He was going to tell them stories. Joan conceded that his stories were very good. While telling them he lay down beside them. Lucille in the middle fell asleep and the paternal raconteur then leaned right across her and gave Joan a great mouthing kiss. His wife, who sat there smoking listlessly as usual, paid them no attention.

Next day he commandeered Joan to help ferry berries again. She backed down, asking him to take Lucille instead, adding desperately as only a kid can, "She's more what you want." Just as he was telling her he didn't want Lucille, he wanted her, there was a great commotion and dust storm as the Truemans drove up and Robert burst across to his sister in tears. "He hasn't stopped crying since you left. We can't take any more of it." The wages Joan was supposed to be paid did not materialize either.

Somebody up there must have been watching over my children, as I seemed to be doing such a rotten job of it.

Reckonings

The summer went along happily with expeditions into more daisy meadows, where we gathered wild flowers and pressed them in toilet paper between the pages of *The Secret Garden*, one of Joan's few books. We had never seen such wildflowers before or so many of them. We walked and walked one Sunday to the foot of a glacier but knew we could not go on exploring because of having to walk back.

The Truemans were very kind and took us for a drive, going along the highway to Kitwanga to see the totem poles. Trueman said the village was called KitwanGA, not KitWANGa. When we passed a mountain that fascinated me in the Rocher de Boule range, he said it had a small locomotive still at the top of it, left there after being hauled up piecemeal for a mining tramway and not worth lowering down the mountain.

Then another milestone approached that could not be averted.

Enthusiastic letters were arriving from Juneau with talk of good pay and future possibilities that did not sound as if they included me too much. Because what about my kids? From the sound of things Bob simply could not handle them and do the things he wanted to do. Now I had to write and tell him I was pregnant and wait for the outcome. In addition, the news of our marriage had circulated down to the coast and an aura of worry and apprehension was wafting up towards me. No wedding presents wafted up either, except from my sister who surprised me with a great big Hudson's Bay blanket.

Bob moved swiftly. If it could be put into words he sometimes used, though not in this case as far as I'm aware, "I seen my duty and I done it." He was not his sterling father's son for nothing. My father-in-law, whom I had not yet met, appeared to be a kindly man, decent in all things, whose influence on his sons was very strong. Selfish little beggar though he seemed to me, Bob was trained in where to draw the line. In those days I couldn't see the forest for the trees, but now I know what I did to a man like him, in pulling the wings off Mercury's feet.

"I have formulated a plan," he replied, with another favourite expression, "and I have decided to move to the Yukon at the end of this season. We can join my brother in Edmonton and drive up the Alaska Highway to Whitehorse. But you'll have to make arrangements about the kids. We can't take them there on spec and there won't be room in the truck."

With a baby coming I had no choice. One could not stay pregnant on the job in those days for very long. I wrote in a panic to ask my ex to take the children until we were settled. He was absolutely delighted and his wife was livid. He replied that "they" felt the children's schooling should not be disrupted and the children should stay with them for one full school year, to give my marriage a chance he added facetiously. Later in August he would send my boys up for a holiday and they would take my other children back with them, as well as our dog. It was a handsome offer. As to the dog, in their loneliness the children had acquired a black lab pup that they christened Snoose, who slept on their beds and went everywhere they did.

It was time to give in and I knew it.

I had seen enough of my girl in working jeans and a coarse scarlet turtle neck with a gold locket hung around it—little knowing that jeans and heavy pullovers would be designer stuff thirty years on—with her hair hidden under a peasant turban thing. Dressed thusly she would emerge on hands and knees with her friends from culvert pipes as their idea of fun. When I got her back a year later they had chopped off her lovely honey-coloured mane and she descended from the train with a long scarf trailing from around her ears like a tarty tennis player's.

Meanwhile, I had not been all that bad as a mother. Once Joan did a painting of a deer's head on the back of a paper plate, with which she was going to cover a stove hole in the wall. It was a work of art. I sent her on the train once a week to take painting lessons in a nearby town. The child was really talented.

That summer of waiting went by pleasantly enough. Bob was finishing his stint in Alaska and salting away his money. My office was busy with its network of roads and men and I could do fifteen payroll copies without strikeovers. I knew the names of all the heavy machinery vehicles in the country, like "Bucyrus-Erie," the names of all the construction bosses who held government contracts, and I met most of the big cat operators.

I had no private life except by mail and did not seek to know the townsfolk. I knew instinctively they would do something to my marital life, as Bob was not explainable to anyone or amenable to civilization.

"You are turning your back on your own kind," remarked Winnie, my uninvited watchdog. She always said aloud what I tried not to think. At any rate the office antics kept me amused.

Coming events were now to turn us strangely back into Gunnar territory.

Gambolling

Sometime during the summer I received a news clipping that showed my oldest son, David, as winner of a prize that would send him to Ottawa. He was fifteen and the "best all-around cadet" in a sea cadet contest. The close-up photo looked like something on a Life magazine cover and revealed him in "round rig" bearing a rifle. He looked older than when I had last seen him, but no different otherwise.

One of the things I had avoided thinking about was the love I bore him and his nearest brother, which was the kind that wipes a mother out. I had been a kitten raising kittens. They were so close to me in age they were the breath of my life. When the break-up came I had to leave them where they were safe and settled. They would have bucked at coming with me anyway, it turned out. Of course I hung on to my only girl and had to keep the little boy with me. As stated before, splitting the children between us had caused a family furor, but I had wanted to teach my skirt-chasing spouse a lesson, not kill him by taking away his entire family. It had been hell.

David's trip to Ottawa coincided nicely with the plan to send the boys to me. I met the CNR train that connected with his returning one; my other boy, Henry, was to come up from the coast.

No child of mine got off that train. There was a six-foot sailor at the end of the platform who began walking in my direction with long arms extended to the bags he was carrying. This man said hello with a deep growl. I said, "David?" He bent down and embraced me.

"It can't be you!" Where was my lovely boy, my boy, my boy? I walked along stunned saying nothing but "I can't believe it!"

Suddenly he put his bags down in the road.

"Look," he said, in his usual pedantic way only two octaves lower. "If you don't stop saying that I'm going to turn around and go right back." That was David. Warmth flowed through my veins for the first time that year.

The sailor suit was stowed as he got into his favourite bush clothes. Then Henry joined us. Always my naughty monkey, he was not as tall as David but was beginning to be debonair.

We all went on foot to explore the country again and see it afresh through the boys' eyes. On one of our hikes Henry found a good shovel lying in the bush.

"Here you are," he proffered. "Just what you need."

I told him to put it back where he had found it; that everything in the bush is on trust and nobody touches anything. Sulkily he replaced it.

"You would. I knew you'd say that."

Nothing had changed after all. They were each of them as

they should be and the four of them ran on ahead of me with the dog chasing after them. For a while it was a little bit of heaven.

Nor were we forgotten. I had a week off from the office and Bob must have written to Larsens about my boys' visit and must have hinted that we'd need somewhere to have a holiday. Whether he contrived it or not, a letter from Effie invited us all to come at once and soon we were on the train heading back to Burns Lake.

The Trail Again

Larsens' welcome was an eye-opener for the children. Effie's kids took mine over in a sort of swarming action. We stayed almost a week, but afterwards I didn't remember much of what we did except that it was felt by all to be mandatory that my kids see Bob's trapping cabin.

The two six-footers, Helge and David, led the way accompanied by Henry and Thora, with Effie's immediate fry attending Joan and Robert. Almost immediately there started to be a bucolic romance. Thora had matured since my previous visit, when I had never really noticed that she was so blonde, firm and fully rounded, nor that my quiet David, who had so shaken me by looking like a bean pole, was now ready for this. A feeling of life escalating too rapidly took hold of me: the pregnancy, young men for sons, and now calf love. All three young men were carrying rifles while I had Bob's little .22. Gerda and Christie, the next Larsens in line, were soon flat on their bellies in the moss, with Joan and Robert, feeling for kinnikinnick (bear berries) with which they juiced their faces red.

Until this rest stop it had been blazing hot along the logging trails where nothing was recognizable from the previous winter. In winter you can have a logging road firmly packed with snow above stumps a foot high and not know they are there, while the summer trail can be a mess of stumps, small deadfalls, vines and high grass. It was a little hotter that August than when Bob first saw these woods the previous September.

Some of the jack pines had been logged so that there were open spaces. In the forest there were dense patches. In a blazing hot clearing stood an abandoned sawmill, one of the many dotted around the land. It was by a small round pond and the bunkhouse was beside it. The air was heavy with a sweetish smell. Helge sniffed it.

"Pack rats! Stand back everybody!"

Going up to the bunkhouse door he banged on it, wrenched it open and jumped aside, gun at the ready. A horde of fat, sleek rats poured out in a pack and streamed by us. They were bigger than cats with grey fur and I could not help noticing that their pelts were absolutely beautiful. If they had not been so loathsome and had not smelled so sickly they would have made good pets. This speculative reaction was not shared by my sons, especially Henry. He raised his rifle and shot one. The boys were not trigger happy but well trained at Sea Cadets' rifle butts and David had been hunting in his home hills. Vermin were vermin. Helge was facetious about Henry's "brutality" and made him feel silly. Helge had a great time and certainly had Effie's sense of gentle mockery.

The trail was ascending slowly and my legs were beginning to remember how they had felt on snowshoes, as Helge led us up a long rise of seven or eight hundred feet. In the winter I had not noticed it as a climb because I had been following blindly along that snow-packed way and everything had looked and felt the same.

We entered the proper forest and sat down for a rest in the shade. Helge said we were about half way. Harry's "high bush cranberries" swayed above our heads and the hush was beatific. Nobody spoke for awhile as we all sat surveying our shoes. Helge had a camera and took a picture of the boys and me, saying later that the picture was as dull as we looked "due to exercise on the mountain grade." He was very waggish, but we liked that.

This was a time when Helge showed us what he could do. On the trail the year before his father had bragged to Bob about the way Helge caught fool hens. We witnessed him reaching out and nabbing them with his hands, then he would swing each bird by the head in a swift arc to break its neck; he then split the breast skin with his thumbnail and peeled off the feathers in one movement, like taking off a glove; the next thing was to take out his knife and pierce the breast just below the rib cage, snap the bird wide open and remove the entrails with one hand and in the same manoeuvre chuck them on the trailside; the clean, featherless carcass was then folded up neatly and stuffed into his rucksack. This went on here and there until we had enough grouse on that particular walk to feed a family its supper.

"See," he said, showing us the naked little pink victims, "no buckshot."

At last we came to the cabin clearing, and how different it was from winter beauty. The cabin, jack pine and spruce were tinder dry and the lake, small, triangular and totally black, was surrounded by thirty-foot spruce bottle brushes reflecting their blackness in the water. Its dark depths concealed fat, pink-bellied rainbow trout, flashing in and out of sight, and soon Helge and David were poling offshore on the half submerged old raft. It measured about seven feet by five and had a crude bench on it. David had some fishing flies in his pocket and Helge had found some old fish line in the reeds. They had soon cut rods from the bush and, poling just beyond the reeds, began to haul in rainbow six inches wide.

It was David's idea of paradise, girls forgotten. It was also the start of a friendship with Helge and his sister that was to affect his life for some time. A born bush rat, David only needed a little contact with them to begin combating the standardized influences he was getting at home. (Here it should be explained that in my former life, and my son's current life, everything was supposed to be "pusser" (Royal Navy slang for a member giving 100 per cent service), line ahead and KR&AI (King's Regulations and Admiralty Instructions)—references to my ex's British roots and military background. I was accused of not caring how I lived, like a cat in a packing case. David inherited my rebellious outlook.) Henry was not bothered by any of these considerations and regarded this holiday as just one more experience to chalk up to the rich game of life.

It was blissful to be in the cabin, which was really Bob's No. 2 cabin, Helge explained. I had not known that, as it was the one he had lived in. The inside gave me pangs because all the dear smells of pine and fur were still there.

My loving nostalgia was soon shattered by a large poster over the door of a prone and naked woman with very rounded thighs, which had not been there before. Furious that my kids should see me shamed, I raised my .22 and let the pinup have it right through the butt. Unfortunately the thick log behind the target was not all that thick. We drifted outside and saw Henry approaching along the trail as our party had split into two groups. He came towards me wearing his calmest poker face and held out his hand. In his palm lay the spent .22 bullet.

"It landed at my feet," he said dryly.

Not being content with that heart-stopping lesson, there was to be one more occurrence where I would get stupid with a gun and inspire sheer horror at myself. Every hunter has something to be ashamed of no matter how well trained he is.

The trap line expedition took place on the day after our arrival at Effie's. We got back to the house at dusk, it taking half the time to return downhill. Again I stewed with chagrin over the time taken by that snowshoe trip and the dilemma about staying overnight. But then we had not started at the crack of dawn as I had with the boys. When we all came down into the fields with the big boys in the van, two huge owls winged silently over their heads.

In the matter of sleeping arrangements we were disposed of throughout the labyrinth. Effie insisted on giving pregnant me her little room while she took the kitchen couch. The boys slept on broad shelves in a shed, where Thora lingered to chat until sharply recalled. Effie was not all that fussy later when we all went to a fair and David stayed behind to keep Thora company while she minded the fry. Effie just laughed. But David only worshipped with his eyes, and his overhand crawl in the lake was no good. A bored Thora moved off. Nothing dampened, he wrote to her later while Helge wrote to him. Their first letters crossed. Helge was avid to know what David and Thora had been up to on the night of the fair.

Joan had little to do during the visit but wander the highway with the small ones, looking for mice trapped in holes ready for telephone poles. She thought the mice should be rescued but got bitten when she tried it. The boys filled Effie's pot with grouse. I had offered financial recompense for the larder, which was well stocked, but was refused.

My boys were amazed at the continuous supply of moose meat, jar after jar sometimes mixed with ground pork. Joan was astounded by big pots full of moose stew. Vegetables and fruit were also bottled. The whole thing so impressed David he moulded his holidays and bush trips accordingly, for several years afterwards. Henry was pretty good with a gun, but this aptitude made him more likely to win cups at rifle shoots.

The Song of Gunnar

Almost the first thing Effie had said to me on arrival was "You know Gunnar's in hospital?" It was two or three months after his visit to Smithers.

"I'm not surprised. He could hardly swallow."

"He came back raving about the dinner you give him. Poor old guy."

"All I did was mince up his meat and mash his vegetables."

"I got to tell you what he did for us only it will have to wait until there aren't any kids around."

Now there was a story about Gunnar, apart from what Effie would reveal. He had been well known in that country and they called him the "2300 Swede." On that first night with the men Bob heard all about it and often laughed over it. Harry had got Gunnar to tell the tale himself.

"D'you know this guy is a wanted man?" Harry had begun. "And he can teach you more about trapping than anyone around. Tell him, Gunnar."

"Well I had lines all ofer. De biggest went from Whitesail to Ootsa." He meant the big lakes that are at the top end of what is now Tweedsmuir Park. "Then I had to get out and leave it all. Holy Yeesus how I hate being old!" Bob had then asked him cheekily how old he was.

"What's dat to you? Fresh young bugger. I am seventy-five and nobody hauls my wood, see? Aye look after myself in everytink." Bob had calmed him down by saying he knew of a man of seventy-five who could jump off roofs. Harry told Gunnar to get on with why he was a wanted man.

"Yimminy! Dose were my CNR days. Came up from the States to work on the railway."

"One time I was workin' on de tracks by de Skeena wid a bunch of udder Swedes and we spent six munce dere drillin' and loadin' rocks." His English was always thick with Swedish difficulties when he got excited. He had no problem with the first person singular unless he took a breath to begin a sentence, when it came out "ay."

"Den de whole damting fell in the river. Yeesus! We was workin' along de Skeena Valley a lot and one time dey was gettin' mean about our wages. Nobody gyps me. So I vowed to get efen. Ay was so mad I clean forgot it was near payday and I sneaked into one of dere warehouses wid some dynamite from de last site and blew her up. God did I run! And never stopped runnin' until I was out of town. Only den did I remember dey still had my pay."

Bob had been impressed. "But what's this about you being the Twenty-Three Hundred Swede?"

Gunnar slapped his knee. "By Yee! You would remind me of dat! It was when I sold my line— real rich territory. When I'm troo I'm troo and I take what I can get. So I took de train to Rupert and dey say I spent de whole twenty-tree hunnert in one night."

It transpired that Gunnar went into partnership with a man from Kamloops in buying forty acres outside Burns Lake. "We wasn't squatters. We owned it all. He was cleverer than me about land. What do I know about such tings? He got me to sign sometink, I dunno what, and he took off wid de money from our parcel because he'd sold it. He left me dis one acre on de lake because I guess he figured a old guy like me wouldn't need more." Bob snorted. He did in people who did in old men, if he could find them.

So Gunnar had lived the usual northern bachelor's transient life, taking jobs and friends and women wherever he found them. Such men liked to make a good haul but never worried when there wasn't one as long as they could get by. His cabin remained spotless and you always took off your shoes.

Now Effie was telling me of Gunnar's last kind act before being struck down. Her eyes filled with tears.

"I was in the store one day and there was this old bag, Mrs. Boyd, with her usual couple of hangers-on. You know the type. Pretending to be somebody and showing off with good works. She belongs to the Ladies of the Royal Purple..." I hooted and she waited for me to get over it. I was new to women allied to fraternal lodges but she didn't bother to explain.

"And she brown noses the parson." Effie could be explicit but she demanded a clean floor and a clean mouth in her house. "These women looked at me, nothing new. But this time she did me in."

"I was puttin' in our order when I heard her say she was going to send the welfare woman up to see if my kids were treated right and that we were a disgrace to the community having all those kids and not married." Now she and Harry were living common-law of necessity due to Effie' s unfortunate marriage at sixteen to a young Native who took off, never to be traced. It had ceased to matter.

Gunnar had gone over to her house that day and found her crying after the ordeal at the store. She who never cried. His face became engorged.

"Ay'll fix 'em. You stay quiet. You won't be troubled again. More decent folk never breaved."

He returned to his cabin with no idea of what he would do but knew he would have to get something on somebody. He had just been into Burns Lake having beer with some jokers who, strangely enough, had mentioned Harry's brood and his unwed state. They thought it very funny and disclosed that this woman, Mrs. Boyd, had been raking the story up locally. One said she had a nose as long as part of his anatomy. Gunnar had stood up, put money on the table, dispensed a few threats, and then left. He'd had no intention of relaying the gossip to Larsens but now he might put it to good use.

After seeing Effie and going back to the same men, he asked in a roundabout fashion if Mrs. Boyd had any relatives. He hit the jackpot. Yes, she had a kid brother up in Williams Lake who had put two girls up the spout. From that far away Burns Lakers knew nothing of it. Gunnar now had a weapon.

One train ride later he had looked around Williams Lake and had seen for himself a little boy entitled to call Mrs. Boyd his auntie. Armed with names and addresses he returned to his beer buddies and told them how they could spike the Boyd's guns. Intimidated by Gunnar they swore they had meant the Larsens no harm as they were just gossiping about Mrs. Boyd's latest. They promised to get on it right away.

Gunnar was too late to prevent the visit of the welfare woman, who had been very understanding. She told Effie to ignore local talk and carry on. The woman had been amazed. She said she had been into many "regular" homes that were not worthy of the name.

"Gunnar'd told me to keep going to the store like nothing ever happened and I'd soon see why. I sure did. Mrs. Boyd's lodge mates were in there one day and they said hello to me. When she came in they turned their backs suddenly and began orderin.' They say she had nothing to say at lodge meetings and pretty soon she stopped goin' to them. I couldn't figure what caused the change at the store until Gunnar came in slappin' his sides. She was the only person giving us trouble. Nobody else cares that much.

"Now I don't know what will happen to the poor old man. It's got to be the end. The kids will miss him like crazy."

CHAPTER · V

‖‖

The Wrong Highway

Athabasca

The farmlands of Alberta in the height of the haying season stretched before us as our three-quarter-ton red Dodge truck bounced and swayed along the approach to the Alaska Highway. It was the only route to Mile Zero by car in those days and the Highway might have been said to start at Edmonton.

As far as we knew, we were making for Dawson Creek as our first big stop and breather, but first we had to fill the larder. That fact was the only one in which we were in accord. Bob and I wanted to search for a good romantic destination in which to work—in the Yukon or not—and to make the most of this expedition as a hunting and camping trip. His brother Tom, who did most of the driving since it was his truck, was after jobs and making money and getting to them as soon as possible. He was looking for bigger centres and kept his foot to the floor when we suggested dalliance.

As we had outfitted the truck with every sort of spare, our finances were fairly low but our spirits were away up. The men peeled out at the first likely lakeside and joked to each other about people who shot ducks when they were sitting. They were going to get food every way they could, whether

88

it was flying or hiding in bushes, but it would be a little cool swimming to retrieve birds.

The road went due north to St. Albert through four small settlements to Athabasca on the Athabasca River. Over the fields and marshes misty wraiths levelled through the trees and across the waters. The very air spoke of prime hunting time.

We made our first camp at Ghost Lake, just outside Athabasca. The lake was pretty and very still, except for moose-like splashings in the reeds beyond the mist.

Bob and I set up our pup tent and I made a fire while the men went off hunting. They were skunked for duck but came back with some grouse, which were soon roasting over the coals. The idea was to live off the country where possible and save our food supply. The rest from work was good for them and it gave me time to ponder.

My thoughts were clean and clear of doubt once more, apart from a general sadness I did not try to analyse. Adventures are very exhilarating and not to be taken too seriously. The three of us had been joking along the way, exchanging "ruderies" as the road hurled us about and at times Bob took turns at driving. This first day out of Edmonton was the real revelation of what I had done and I could not help brooding into the embers while the men drank coffee and made plans.

Retrospect

In the week that followed after the children left I'd had plenty of time to think about the life I had wrought.

Happy as kings, the children had gone off together with the bounding dog. A train journey and a sea voyage lay ahead of them. The oldest boys had surveyed me sadly but I doubt the other two even glanced back, so glad they were to be going to the land of money with their brothers. As I walked about the empty rooms a storm had raged about my head and my insides felt like a bottomless pit. It was as if the circumstances I had set in motion were squeezing me in a vise.

Things had moved swiftly once Bob had arrived. It was

September at the opening of the hunting season and he was anxious to get rolling before snow flew. With his brother Tom along things could not go too wrong, he reasoned; Tom was always the business brains of any enterprise.

In no time at all the most vital things I had bought were condensed into a couple of small crates which, together with my steamer trunk and personal luggage, would have to fit with Bob's kit bag, guns and packboard, and God knew what of Tom's belongings as well as food supplies, into the back of a small truck. Very soon we were stowed on the CNR train for Edmonton.

My leave of the agency was no special occasion except that they were wisecracking and non-committal. But the engineer, after shaking hands and bidding Godspeed, had turned away and added under his breath "and to hell with getting someone without shorthand after this." All the same, I had served them well.

On the train Bob started to be smart about my tummy and promised me his son was going to get a prenatal start at the rough life, sleeping under the stars on the hard, hard ground. Nothing could have been more true. We were going to camp when possible.

He could not fail to notice my sad silences on the train journey, for my face, people told me, was an open book. Eventually my outlook got through to him and things came to a head in our hotel room in Edmonton. We were both tired and strained, having sat up all the previous night in a day coach. He shut the door ominously and came at me livid.

"Are you coming with me willingly? Or do I have to drag you by the hair all the way? Because if you can't come gladly I'll give you your train fare back and you can go straight home."

His language when he was angry was flawless. He forgot to copy his friends and drop his g's. He was a terrific mimic when he copied anyone and mischievous with it. Now I was getting a sample of his heavy side.

The thought of going home pregnant and defeated was not to be borne, or the trouble and fuss of moving children around and the probable glee of their stepmother at my downfall.

Also I had just given some vows. Bob might forget that but I couldn't.

"I'm coming with you," I replied icily. "Naturally."

I was shaken that he could think otherwise. A deal was a deal. His was a guilt reaction, but I did not realize it then.

The deal was sealed permanently when we met Tom for dinner in a cafe, after visiting a jeweller. When we were married the Smithers jeweller had been away and prior to that Bob had not known my ring size; we had to make do with my old wedding band.

"Do you mind very much?" he had asked. "I don't."

Yes, I had minded very much; it had seemed like a travesty. Also I was afraid it would bring bad luck. Now a fine conspicuous gold band was chosen. As we slithered in opposite Tom in the cafe, I was told, "Stick out your hand."

He slipped on the ring, looked at his brother and said, "Now you're a witness that I've made an honest woman of her." I did not think it was funny and Tom didn't either. Tom didn't think anything Bob did to tease people was funny; Tom never risked hurting people. He and I were too serious by far.

These brothers were like Damon and Pythias, the legendary friends that stood as hostage for each other, or better yet, David and Jonathan, whose brotherly friendship was "surpassing the love of women." Some women found it tiresome.

It was the oddest love/hate relationship I had ever seen. They were complete opposites in every sense. Tom was my height, about five-eight, slight, dark and handsome in a fleshy sort of way compared with the pale, tight classic features of his brother. He was very serious, kind and thoughtful, and very generous; an instant ally I felt. He was also as lazy as sin, sloppy and unreliable like as not, although he could work very hard when he felt like it and never let down a friend.

Studying them kept me greatly diverted. Tom's shortcomings drove Bob up the wall. Bob's bush gear was always cinched, tamped and neatened off, with any jags or tears carefully mended. Tom's was a pile of belongings just chucked into the truck. One man lived by the labour of his hands and the other by the working of his mind.

They were juxtaposed from every angle: height, colouring, aptitudes and natures, rank and choice of armed service. Bob had thrown away university after one year to become a commando on a Normandy beach; there had been no university for Tom but a year of banking before becoming an officer in the RCAF. But when they got together they stuck like Siamese twins.

In any mutual venture, like the hotel they bought in Purcell Mountain country with their combined veterans' grants, Tom supplied the plans and financial arrangements, handled staff and did some dog work. Bob supplied the energetic labour, plus all the cooking and any artistic effects needed such as rustic work. He had a secret complex about Tom's brains versus his, and Tom's height versus his five foot two and a half. That was the height accorded him by navy doctors when he enlisted. On any applications he filled out himself, he always listed his height as five feet *four* inches.

When working together and in doubt about any problem they would repair to the nearest beer table, away from women and cares, to reassure each other and plot earnestly. This habit went a long way towards ruining Tom's marriage as no woman can compete with a David and Jonathan team. At least some women can't; I thought they were cute.

They would fight physically like Kilkenny cats, the claret flowing freely, to the point at one time when Tom's eye was little short of hanging out due to some smart remark he had made. They would sit together afterwards side-by-side and holding hands, saying "Sorry, brother."

"I've never seen anything in my life like you two," I would tell them.

"No Stella, I guess you haven't," they would reply.

Mist and Mud

During the night at Ghost Lake it rained and we were snug in the tent, but Tom, who had not provided himself with one, thinking to tough out our nights on the ground but mostly to sleep in motels, had simply put down a ground sheet, spread his sleeping bag and had disappeared under a tarpaulin that he had pulled over his head. He had not noticed that he was sleeping on the side of a small rise and woke in the morning to find he was lying in a large puddle that had crept over the ground sheet instead of under it.

Laughing ourselves silly at his appearance, we told him not to despair, as there was a handy little Public Works hut nearby where we lit the stove, made breakfast and dried him out. We left everything the way it was, doing a little cleaning for good measure, and with that experience we were broken in.

From Athabasca to Slave Lake was good duck country. Sloughs and ponds stayed with us for the day's traveling, much to our joy. At times I felt I was the only one watching the road. The two men kept hopping out and scored a grouse, a teal and two widgeon that day. But a siege of wet weather was setting in and before we got to Slave Lake the highway was pretty sticky.

The Alberta section of the road was in very fine shape for an unpaved artificial thoroughfare. As it got nearer and nearer to Peace country it appeared to be dead straight to the horizon, as far as the eye could see. It had a three-lane traffic width in the centre of a roadbed built wide enough for five. The wide canal drainage system on each side was impressive, where culverts had mosaics of stones packed around the mouth of each pipe.

We were winging along, making tremendous time, passing great fertile fallow fields where not an inch of ground was wasted. All was care and order until the road began to get greasy. We started to slide a little. As we passed the odd truck ditched, our apprehension mounted until we reached Great Slave Village with the first feelings of wear and tear. We listened to the locals in a pub until we felt better, then moved into a steamy little den where we huddled over hot meat pie and left it to pour outside. That was the first sensible meal since the memorable ring ceremony dinner in Edmonton.

Things dried up along the shore of Lesser Slave Lake and the disappointment to me was in not being able to linger. There were fields going down to the lake, sand dunes, poplar trees, animal tracks and a Roman Catholic mission that reeked of history. There were moose and grizzlies around somewhere. We were flying by sites where early explorers and traders had landed and where a couple of HBC trading posts had been in operation. The road today goes along the lake about a hundred miles through settlements to come out at High Prairie.

We had four days all told of rain and mud, putting our opinion of the highway on a different level to that held by later cheerful tourists when the road had dried up. This mud was the tacky, sticky kind that plastered the inside of the cab and was all over our pants and boots. We got used to steady skidding.

High Prairie then was not on any map that we had, but it was a rising centre with a big new hotel and several garages among other new buildings. It was the usual toss-up between beer and coffee before ploughing on to Grande Prairie before nightfall.

Half way between High Prairie and Grande Prairie was Sturgeon Lake; we were crossing the area dominated by the Peace River's southern branches, the Little Smokey and the main Smokey. At Sturgeon Lake was another Roman Catholic settlement. The lake was impressive enough, though not one of those inland seas like Lesser Slave. A great imposing brick edifice, fronted by a statue of Christ, was built on a rise facing the water and overlooking considerable properties. At the water's edge were rafts for swimming and boats drawn up on the beach, all part of some plan for housing and training Indian children only. It took forty years to find out what went on in these places.

Although adorned with wireless stations and field-like airstrips, Grande Prairie was obviously an old pioneer terminus. We found this out for a fact. Clerks eyed us so dubiously, as we came into the main hotel late and spattered with mud from head to foot, that the place was instantly "full up." We were directed to the hotel's annex, which was the real old time thing.

There was the usual square gap over the room door in lieu

of a transom. Ladies and gents shared the same bathroom, simultaneously by the plan of it. I got trapped in a cubicle when a man came in to clean his teeth at a basin. If the bathroom was busy you washed in the community hand basin in the upper hall while people went up and down stairs beside you.

My being trapped in the bathroom and having to wash on the landing caused the tittering "twins" a great deal of glee. It seemed I was to be comic relief on the journey. If I held up well it would be something to brag about, but God help me if I went wimpy. They were glad of my presence; I could see that, even if I slowed them down here and there.

There was one thing about Alberta that infuriated me and amused the men. Every time they went into a beer parlour I had to either sit alone in the ladies section or wait in the truck, as Alberta segregated the sexes completely. I longed for BC, which in those days only "partially" segregated beer parlours, having both "men's" and "ladies & escorts" sections.

Stemming from provincial repeals of Prohibition in the 1920s, a number of jurisdictions implemented laws that required licensed beer parlours to have a separate entrance for women, or to actually have separate rooms for the sexes. Alberta repealed Prohibition in 1924 but then banned mixed drinking in 1928. In "Question B" of the 1957 Alberta Liquor Plebiscite, voters in the Calgary and Edmonton areas were asked to vote on repealing segregation in beer parlours; rural areas did not receive "Question B" on their plebiscite ballots. The urban-only vote passed by a margin of four to one, finally allowing mixed drinking in those cities; however, province-wide segregation was not abolished until 1967. Hotel lounges in BC received approval to remove the separation between the "men's" and "ladies and escorts" sides of beer parlours in 1963 or 1964.

There was no job prospect to hold us in Grande Prairie. Mud again became part of our traveling day. Soon we hit the BC border and were back with BC's road problems. From here until Dawson Creek required great artistry in driving. We wanted to get there before the employment office closed at noon. Many cars were stuck on the side of the road awaiting a tow, though most people drove trucks and got by.

The Peace District was open and majestic, broad bosomed, with mile on mile of farmlands visible from the slow grade.

As it was fall when we went through we were treated to a study in pale green, yellow and gold, which crowded out the darker trees.

We headed straight for Dawson Creek, ignoring Pouce Coupe. Then as we were starting to make good time, close to Dawson at ten minutes to noon, a small car passed us coming from Pouce Coupe. One of our troubles was the lake system in the middle of the road, into which we usually plunged head on, stopping only once to dry off the distributor. This oncoming little menace had the same plunging technique and suddenly a solid curtain of mud hung before our eyes and we were blinded to a dead stop. It was like someone throwing a pail full of brown cream. Some of it was still up behind the driver's seat a month later.

At Dawson Creek we just about broke up our trio.

"There has to be work here," decided Tom. "This'll do for me. Far enough."

"Northward, ever northward," murmured Bob.

"Well, don't you think so? Place is big enough."

"Northward, ever northward," chanted Bob.

"Use your head, man," snapped Tom as he got out of the cab. The front tire had developed a slow leak. A more bleak and open vista full of nothing than Dawson Creek we had not seen.

We seemed to wait all day for that tire to be changed. Bob went reluctantly with Tom to find labour information but they drew a blank. I changed into high boots and waded around and around the Mile Zero marker, which stood in a sea of mud. Tired of that, I sat fascinated in the truck watching some hopeful idiot having his car washed off.

A few miles out of Dawson the same tire blew. When we pulled up Bob took out the little .22 and handed it to me. "Here. Make yourself useful," he ordered in facetious mood.

It was the little gun bought as a boy from the sale of squirrel skins, which he used to keep broken down and strapped to his leg inside his pants in game warden territory. Now it was mine by courtesy. He carried the .410 shotgun and a Winchester 30.30; also at hand were a ".22 long" cartridge rifle and a dreadful old 12-gauge pump gun he called Betsy that had been in and out of hock frequently.

Apart from the whiskey jacks, the bush was dead. We had yet to learn that animals seldom came near the highway by choice, unless they were migrating. We knew of no restrictions against hunting the verges and perhaps there were none.

At Fort St. John another tire had to be fixed and the argument arose again as to work versus the lure of the north. Bob knew someone trapping at Charlie Lake, just outside of Fort St. John, and we would have liked to explore around, but once we were in the truck our brain's trust simply put his foot to the floor.

"The longer we stay on the Alcan the more food we'll eat," lectured Tom, "and the more money we'll spend. Better to fly along on an empty belly and trust for grouse at nightfall."

Something we had not provided for properly was water. Keeping a wet canvas bag full and dripping on the side of the truck was efficient, for the canvas swelled and oozed without leaking and chilled itself off, but it didn't go far in making tea, and besides, we needed it in case the engine boiled over which it did more than once.

Table Mountains

There were still about 850 miles ahead of us to Whitehorse and at least 250 to Fort Nelson. In 1949 the road was as wide as it is now but the surface was all potholes and slime. After a rain storm trucks would pass without slacking speed, throwing more buckets of mud, which had to be wiped off by hand as the windshield wipers were useless. Unless it was raining there was no water for washing it off except when passing an accessible river. The dry stretches were a waste of dust in spite of gravelling, and dust too spurted off the tires like poured cream. This was a feature you came to know in the north when it was not freezing, runny brown cream you got in the rain and pouring brown particles you got in the heat.

The last tire went flat before reaching Fort Nelson. We were in real trouble, using only mended spares. Tires took our money, not the cost of food. All four original tires had gone and we were running on those mended ones with no usable spares.

When the last good tire blew we parked on a shady verge, with a faint slope to it that followed the grade of the road. I noticed this slope with some apprehension and was ignored when I mentioned it because, being a mere woman, I was not supposed to have opinions on mechanical matters when real men were about.

They got the jack under the front wheel with great assurance and speed but when I suggested chocking the rear wheels they ignored me again. "Stand back and look at the view" was their general attitude. I watched the great jack as it slowly, slowly sank forward and the nude wheelbase just as slowly slid into the ground with the full weight of the loaded truck behind it. My nerves gave out.

"I knew it! I knew it!" I cried, dancing up and down.

Those crazy guys frightened me. Both of them stared at me. They were red-faced with exertion, fatigue and fury. "Why the hell didn't you say so?"

Why indeed?

We were getting ourselves into a jam and no one wanted to think about it. No money, little food and a truck asking for repairs. Soon after the jack catastrophe we camped to cool down the engine and stop making time on the last tires. Tom thought we should work for a week or so at Fort Nelson to replenish our resources. Arriving destitute in Whitehorse would be no way to start.

We came down one hair-raiser called Suicide Hill at Mile 158, which originally had a one-in-ten gradient and got its name from a joke road sign saying "Prepare to meet thy God."

We were some way between Pink Mountain and Trutch. The scenery from Mile 158 to 200 (Suicide Hill to Trutch) has been described as passing "range after blue range." Seen from the air those ranges are so many that looking down on an ocean of peaks gives a plateau effect. Some peaks actually had plateaus upon them and could be called table mountains.

At Mile 159 we dropped down to the Sikhanni Chief,

which runs between Pink Mountain and Trutch; then at Mile 175, fourteen miles further, we reached the Buckinghorse River. A government bulletin (#98, Museum of Canada, Biological Series #27, 1944) describes the area: "The Sikhanni is rapid, shallow, 75–100 yards across and full of boulders. The valley sides are grey earth and rock, with spruces and poplars up to 60 feet high along the banks."

Between there and the Buckinghorse, goats lived along the cliffs with the cliff swallows and Harlequin ducks in the river below. The Buckinghorse itself was ten to fifteen yards across with a rocky bottom making cut banks of dark shale from ten to thirty feet high. Willows and spruce thirty to forty feet high lined the stream, which was full of grayling in the 1940s. All this country sheltered moose, caribou, wolves, fox, lynx and marten. Rabbits got squished on the highway.

We had not lingered and somewhere around the Minaker River we were on the climb to Trutch, a stopping place with a lodge that accommodated big game hunters.

As the miles went by the boys were having a bad time bemoaning all the hunting they were missing, for hereabouts were sheep, goats and grizzlies, but there was nowhere to stow, cook or keep big game. By the time we had chosen a campsite halfway up to Trutch and got a fire going, they had recovered their spirits. They went off in different directions to look for small game for the pot. Bob did not go far before shooting at something and came back with four grouse in his hands and looking stunned.

"Just shot one and look what I got! They were all behind it in the bush." He was using the .410 of course. Tom returned with one bird and his .22 and was snide about buckshot.

"Jealousy will get you nowhere. Takes me. At least we will eat tonight." We usually made bannock in the frying pan and that filled us too. You could call it a scone or hot biscuit. On the wedding trip Bob had simply poured lake water into an indentation in the salted flour right in the sack. After puddling up a nice little ball of dough he would stand his frying pan on end beside the coals. Sometimes he might twiddle a little baking powder into the sack and let the 'bread' rise up the slope.

But now we were on a hillock with no water for coffee and no running water for miles. It had rained heavily not long before and although the raised ground had dried off there were still big potholes down in the road, full of water. I dipped a billycan gently under the surface of the biggest of these to collect enough water for three. Boiled up with coffee, canned milk and sugar added it wasn't so bad. Our theory was that along that lonely stretch any germs in it would belong to nature and not to man.

It was a beautiful light fall evening. Stars were visible but it was not really dark. Our sleeping bags were thrown down on the hardpan with burnt grass on it that smelled of straw, so that I spent my first shelterless night, as prophecied on the train. Naturally I ached and couldn't find a decent position, but eventually weariness from all the jouncing and anxiety had us all asleep before we knew what had happened. Also, I was quietly getting tougher.

The next stop, Fort Nelson, had to produce jobs. We dare not think that work might not be found.

Next morning, after gathering up pots and bags from the inhospitable burnt hay, we continued the high climb to Trutch. There were road signs advertising packhorse trips with guides.

"This is for me," quoth Bob speculatively, as he surveyed the mountainous terrain. "Sheep, caribou, elk, moose. See that light ram against the rocks? By winter he'll be snow white. The Stone sheep are darker but they've got a white rump. And thin little spiral horns—nothing like those big curls on Rocky Mountain ones."

We were in a contemplative mood calmed by grandeur during the break at Trutch. Bob went on explaining the game to Tom, who had not been north before. It seemed that most far northern animals are darker than BC ones, the Alaska moose being bigger, darker and glossier than ours. He went on about the bears: black, cinnamon, and grizzly. Wolves were in variety: the enormous McKinley timber wolf, the gray wolf and the tundra timber wolf, all of them living on small game like mink or marten. "As for the foxes! They've got white Arctic, red, silver, cross-fox and black. How do I know? I've talked to the guys up here, don't forget."

Even the squirrels and mice were different—squirrels with red backs and mice with white feet. The country seemed partial to white feet, white tails, white noses or backsides, and pretty soon I was to have an "unfond" memory of a housefly with white feet.

The north from that point onwards had a primeval feeling until after Muncho Lake. There are higher mountains in BC, but those through this area have to be seen to get the impact. They have a look about them that suggests they arose majestically out of primordial ooze and that you, who are no more than a bit of protozoa, had better keep still. We became silent.

Before reaching Fort Nelson we encountered three more rivers: the Beaver River at Mile 206, the Prophet at Mile 222, and the Muskwa outside Fort Nelson at Mile 296. The Prophet River valley was five miles wide with the Rockies' snows in the distance and the river paralleled the highway all the way to Fort Nelson. The Muskwa ran east–west nearby; the Muskwa River was actually on the lowest level of the Alaska Highway, at 1,000 feet and was prone to making flash floods.

These mountainous scenes would continue until after Lower Post, BC, near the Yukon border, where the landscape changed and became almost tundra. Tundra has its own sweeping grandeur, but it lies in far away stretches and the trees are short, sparse and far between.

In 1949, as we went by, a typical roadside stand consisted of a steel Quonset hut left by the US Army, which was an elongated metal igloo with a central passage through its rooms that converged at the rear. Supposedly bear-proof garbage cans swung high on chains, and a gas pump sat out front. Coffee could be had inside. Some had a few crude guest cabins and there were signs about bears on the loose. Places like Ma's Kitchen and Somebody's Garage did not exist at every stopping place. Our truck carried jerry cans of gas, which we refilled at the main settlements. Water and gas, water and gas; and tires, tires, tires, for on the first run up the Highway in those days one did not know where the stops were, or if there were any.

From Trutch Lodge to Fort Nelson was roughly one hundred miles. The flat top hills in the east were a thousand feet higher than the road, which had been built on muskeg bogs' bald burns (probably reforested now) and stretched for miles. The Minaker River meandered into the Prophet. Hill country appeared with birch and aspen gleaming against dark spruce. Mossy verges hosted bunchberry and twin flower and there were small coppery streams. By Mile 250 we came into the Fort Nelson area with a view east of the Nelson River, which seems to become the Muskwa on the other side of town.

We made Fort Nelson in the dark and nosed meekly among the transports and tankers in front of the hotel. We were made to wait until the BYN bus came in, its passengers having priority over the rooms. The British Yukon Navigation Company operated the bus and ran passenger and freight lines between the Yukon and Dawson Creek, as well as paddle-wheelers on the northern river waterways.

Dinner was eaten in the dining room of one of the ex-army mess halls that was also a hotel. These buildings were nearly all the same. Rather like Quonset huts in plan, the entrance and office were in front—just as in a barracks—before a long corridor like a ship's with rooms off it, said corridor leading into the dining hall. Sometimes one was led through the dining room into the kitchen and then into a line of rooms behind.

When finally accommodated, we dropped everything and headed for hot baths, but as luck would have it all the water was off for that night.

We thought the prices scandalous for food and rooms in the upper reaches of the Alcan. Store keepers and lunch counter operators soaked us without turning a hair because they had terrific freight bills and felt justified. Furthermore, in that mushrooming world it was dog-eat-dog and to hell with your competitor. As in Gold Rush days, the necessity for survival ruled everything. One night many tourists in Fort Nelson were told at a certain garage that the whole town was out of gas. They were not told that the man across the street still had his tanks full.

Of course in most small places in BC and the Yukon the

feeling was just the opposite, it being mandatory to help one's neighbour. The Alcan did serve such places or would when future cut-offs were finished. The Alaska Highway had a life of its own with news and good friends passing from settlement to settlement along its length. It did not need British Columbia or the Yukon or Alaska. It was its own thing and probably is still.

The next day brought a "Balkan mix-up," as when Middle-Europeans had differences in understanding. Staying at the army camp hotel for more than one night was impossible. We did not know at this juncture if accommodation or finding jobs should have priority, until a chance inquiry ran us into a Ukrainian dishwasher for the army who told us in indistinct English that his house was available. His wife was leaving for work out at the airport and a girl who also lived there would be back to pack up that afternoon. We were welcome to make ourselves at home right away.

CHAPTER VI

Trading Posts

Short Order Cook

In those days Fort Nelson had one main street, close to the highway, very wide and all gumbo with small wooden houses on each side of it. Added to this were the inevitable maintenance camp, repeater station and garages. Six miles out of town the airport was just being extended and you took the road through it to get to Old Fort Nelson across the Muskwa where Indians traded.

First we drove out to the airport, where the boys were lucky enough to be signed on for construction work, and on return we found the Ukrainian's shack, after a lot of false starts, among the army quarters. Row on row of similar huts.

Our new home appeared as if someone had left in haste, but there was no evidence of moving. We made a meal with slight feelings of uneasiness. Then the men left for work, leaving me with the guns and baggage to face the surprised girl when she came home to pack. But what burst in was a lad of twelve who listened to my stumblings with nonchalance while he darted about playing with the puppy and three cats. He chattered away and then said in sudden illumination, "Oh, I get it. You're in the wrong house." I elicited information from him as to what might be the right house, wearily packed the cook kit we had just used, put the bags together in a corner and walked out. His father had another house and to it through the mud I went.

Earlier we had aroused a sleepy young woman onto the bottle-laden porch of this second house to ask her where the first place was. She didn't seem to realize she was in the one we were supposed to have. She opened the door again and said no, she was not moving and had no intention of moving. She was very annoyed and back I strode to get Sir Balkan out of his kitchen.

He was still unintelligible and somewhat amused at me, so I took what was close to our last dime and blew it on coffee and more information about housing. Drawing a blank I started walking the six miles to the airport. There was nowhere left to sit down in Fort Nelson and at least I could rest in the truck.

During the first five hundred yards out of town I did just spot an empty house and snooped. Half way out to the airport construction site I got a ride, and when the boys saw me walking up to them their faces were a study. They gave me the car key and, after three hours of wading and questioning in Fort Nelson, I fell asleep on the truck seat. So much for pioneering.

The following morning we awoke in our sleeping bags on the floor of the empty house, which had become ours for a week, with all our trunks and boxes piled around us. Light dawned on me.

"What on earth am I supposed to be doing while you are both away all day?" From 8:00 a.m. until 4:30 p.m. alone in the heat and dust, or rain and gumbo. No one to talk to.

"Get a job too." Smirking, Bob added, "Think you're getting a free ride?"

"Where?"

"Look around."

My one thought was "I'll fix you." I should have thought of it first.

It was not easy. The first day passed slowly while the men were away and I didn't know what to do with myself. There was a sort of diner at the end of the street near the highway, at an obvious place for travellers to turn in. There was no such thing as a restaurant on the Alcan. You just got fed.

The man at the diner was slightly hesitant. He couldn't tell from my bush clothes if I'd be adequate to work there and the general cut of my jib seemed to indicate not.

His wife came into it. "Sure," she said. "If you can fry chips and keep the orders coming I could use the help. Can you get into this?" She held up a white coverall.

That afternoon I was frying steaks and making short orders and deep frying chips in between.

"Takes me," I told the boys that night. They were relieved to think I would not be sitting around all day. They had been worrying about what to do with me.

The couple running the diner were American and had brought proper equipment with them. All I had to do was peel endless potatoes and push them through a coarse French-fry cutter that turned out square sides. While the chips were seething away I fried steaks with eggs and made sandwiches. The wife made pies galore and dinner features; my job was strictly short orders and counter service.

Various characters came in and out of the diner and sat at the counter. We catered to men from the maintenance camp and airport, American tourists, GIs, mechanics, truckers and transport drivers. I was cursed for a crook over steak prices and subjected to queer requests. One girl shyly asked me for a needle and thread. Her only slacks were ripped and she was en route for Fairbanks from Montana. When I peered outside I saw their trailer was as long as a city block and as high as a house. They were under contract to haul the freight inside it and she was a weary little thing along for the ride. When they reached Fairbanks, she said, they would head back to New York with the same rig.

A sight like that was as common an occurrence as it is now. The road signs were little different: Sharp Turn, Gear Down, Dangerous Curve. Most corners and unexpected places had diagrams on the signs to show what one would find, essential for the slow-moving vans. Some of the greater trailer trucks had several trucks each piled on their backs, a precarious mess to pass.

Temptation presented itself once. While I worked in the kitchen a soft-voiced Scot sometimes sat on a box and talked to me. He was awaiting transportation to "Outside" and was fresh from the bush of the Liard country where he operated a trading post. He would have leased it to my employers if they'd wanted it as he had not left it for twenty years and needed a break. It was two hundred miles by boat, he said, down the Nelson (Muskwa) River to Fort Liard, where were only an HBC post, the RCMP post, a game warden, his own store and home. The population was almost exclusively Indian, and mail came by plane and dog team. The Indians paid for most of their supplies in the late spring when they hauled in their beaver catch.

My heart was jumping for Bob's sake but I could not bring myself to tell him about this frontier site. He might have settled for it. The trader said he was not popular in a place like that, operating in competition—to the HBC presumably—but one could run into the same problems operating a store in Fort Nelson. It was Robert Service's law of the north, the survival of the roughest and toughest. Robert Service was quoted a lot in those days by northerners, and my two were no exception. But separating from Tom and staying behind to have a baby born at Fort Liard was not in the cards.

In the diner not all customers were pleasant. We sometimes got sheer riff-raff off the highway.

"Gimme some coffee, will ya? I want steak and eggs and I want the eggs sunnyside and not all leather."

My face went into its usual mask at this man's crassness but his seatmate had something to say.

"Don't talk to her like that. Can't you see she's a lady?"

How nice. All the same I didn't want my boss hearing them, as "ladyship" was the last thing they needed behind that counter. Or so I thought. In days to come I was to meet many a civilized woman living and working in crude circumstances. The boys had met some of these and knew well enough how such women managed, which was why they didn't mind throwing me to the wolves. It wasn't "mean" of them; they considered me an equal partner and had every confidence I would learn to cope. And had it looked like I might not win my own battle, they could and would have waded right in.

But it would be a long time yet before I would see a softly spoken Mrs. Rancher with a stable full of wranglers at her dinner table or an aquiline blonde Mrs. Pollard from the Three-Bar on horseback as she took a noisy bunch of dudes by trail to her lake. These ladies simply ignored anything vulgar or untoward and stayed true to themselves. The wranglers and ranch guests liked that and respected them for it.

The Road Again

After a full week at Fort Nelson we had all earned enough to allow us to roll on again, so we left that Sunday morning. It had been hot at the airport as the weather had not yet broken into coming winter and we were afraid that it would. Quitting for the men was no bother as labour was transient, but I felt very red-faced at the diner. Yet they were unperturbed, as help abounded and the season was closing down.

With the week's lapse of time a lot of scarlet had crept into the scenery. The truck was now in good shape, we were refreshed and not so tense with half the highway behind us and the grandest part of the Alcan still before us: Steamboat Mountain, Summit, Toad River and Muncho Lake—one hundred and fifty miles of sheerest wilderness.

It was all curves and muskeg for twenty-five miles and then we started up a long grade of twenty-one miles. Half way up we were on the slopes of Steamboat Mountain, which the Indians thought looked like a steamboat hull. Steamboat is compelling, as it does look like a mammoth boat hull. Higher and higher went the highway in the Northern Rocky Range. Forest growth was looking more arctic, of the kind seen when approaching tundra country. Such trees belong with muskeg also—white spruce or swamp spruce most likely. What the trees lost in appeal the mountains gained: mountains of smooth unblemished stone.

At the foot of all these monsters were very clear lakes of deep bright blue.

When we reached Summit Lake Bob said we were at an elevation of 4,256 feet.

"That's higher than the White Pass. The one the Klondikers went over."

"How d'you know how high it is here?" I asked.

"Because I keep my eyes open and read signs."

I was bemused by all this. The territory became prehistoric: granite peaks and squared off blocks, as if pushed up by a giant hand. They either went straight up or over at an angle, stark in their bareness. Some one hundred four miles of this went right into Lower Liard country past many mileposts. This silent wilderness was getting to me.

"You feel like an intruder," I muttered, "and that ancient gods are watching you."

The men said nothing. No jibes. Now I was one with them. In fact they had been peculiarly calm, united as always, tensions and worries put aside as they recalled boyhood dreams of exploration.

Between McDonald River and Stone Mountain at Mile 403, if you could see up through the cloud banks, you would likely see a cloud streaming like a pennant from one of the peaks. We saw that the watercourses were all dried up, but in spring they would be a sight. Except for summer dry-up there are hundreds of waterfalls.

Racing River introduced us to a hundred miles of Liard country.

We rested at Toad River, which ran beside the highway for fifteen miles and was full of Dolly Varden trout. Eight miles inland from the road are Toad River Hot Springs, all fifteen of them, from small to large. They are a long walk in, to the junction of the Toad and Racing Rivers. We gave it a miss and pushed on, past a glacier near the road, then Hoosier Falls, then got our first glimpse of Muncho Lake.

This lake I was never to forget. The road came down and hugged its shoreline around a cliff for nine miles. It was turquoise blue with a rocky mountain face behind it that came right down into the waterline. Its walls were stained red and yellow with mineral deposits and the contrast of these colours with the turquoise waters, through which one could see to immeasurable depths, made one ache with its grandeur. Furthermore, there were the remains of a burst of little yellow flowers along the banks of the cliff hugging the roadside.

Halfway along the lake was Muncho Lake Lodge, big even in those days. I longed to stay there, but we could not possibly afford it.

"Some day maybe," said Bob.

We went onto the promontory where the lodge was sited and wished we had a boat. By now we guessed what such lakes contained: Dolly Varden trout, arctic grayling, lake trout, whitefish and pike. We could at least have changed our diet with some fish frying over our campfire that night. Our trouble was time and Tom's anxious foot on the gas pedal. We sighed and went off to feed ourselves at a stand on the corner of the Muncho cutoff. The owner told us fish stories and his wife regaled us with her hired help problem.

"I got a lake trout this summer weighing thirty-two pounds, the biggest on record here except for a fifty-three-pounder some GI caught once."

"And I can't keep help," wailed his wife. "I got an Indian girl from the missionaries didn't know nothing but camping and tenting. I taught her to speak English and do housework but as soon as she was worth her hire the lodge offered her more money."

We did not stop again until we reached Lower Post, 160 miles further on. We kept seeing mountain goats, caribou herds on the move and the odd Stone or Dall ram. There were salt licks on the roadside and we saw animals busy as we whizzed by.

Even with two fresh drivers trying to keep the vehicle out of holes and from swerving in gravel as we made time, the whole stretch out of Nelson was extremely tiring. Dust was always on the windshield, on everything we owned, and every riverbank was a blessed relief for washing off, drinking and filling the radiator. Flying gravel and bits of rock were another trial and the glass on the truck had its share of pits and holes.

Trout River followed the road for thirty miles, then we crossed the Liard on a suspension bridge. The Liard River follows the Alcan for roughly 100 miles and for most of its course it is lined with giant cottonwoods (from which the river gets its name in French.) The water was greyish and full of silt, and one could look upstream from the bridge towards Whirlpool Canyon and downstream towards the Rapids of the Drowned. My skin crawled at the latter implication and towards similar road signs. In addition to suicide hills and constant fatal rapids we saw blown-out tires placed in gruesome piles—not to mention some macabre warnings like "Prepare to Meet Thy God," intended to scare motorists. These were home-made signs, erected by road buffs, not by maintenance crews.

About half a mile beyond the suspension bridge crossing were Theresa Hotsprings, which had two pools, one encased by army workers and reached by a trail and footbridge. Again we did not investigate but heard the place was full of dense vegetation, wild flowers and berries.

Somewhere farther along, the Liard is entered by the Coal River, which had left lumps of anthracite coal on its sandbars.

At Mile 496 was the lodge for Lower Liard; at Mile 513 was a bridge over the Smith River, at Mile 543 was Fireside, BC, and finally, at Mile 588, Contact Creek.

Here is the point where southbound road construction out of Whitehorse met the northbound road building up from Dawson Creek. Today a signpost commemorates the event. Where in 1949 the earth still lay in bulldozed heaps, now there are soft mounds covered in blue lupins and wild roses.

Mile 606 brings the Hyland River, named after Bob Hyland of Telegraph Creek and Spatzizi development. At Mile 620 we reached Lower Post.

HBC Country

From the beginning Bob and I had kept Lower Post in our heads as a possible trapping site, a thriving hub in the heart of big game country. Going on to the Yukon simply meant going farther north and more travel. The Lower Post area was rich and it made a settlement we could stay in. It looked like something out of a Nelson Eddy movie and was clearly a Hudson's Bay post with its red-trimmed white stores and white hotel. In the hotel lobby lay a huge snow-white husky who barely opened his eyes when we stepped over him. Raw fur hung on the walls on coat hangers, all for sale. The young woman in attendance at the Post was smart and cheerful. A big school was being built in the compound behind.

We stayed overnight, and Bob and I talked things over out of Tom's earshot.

"I'm sick of feeling at his mercy all the time," Bob said. "When we have to decide something he always wins out. He's so damn sensible all the time, won't take a chance." Why was Tom with us if he wouldn't take a risk? "Let's get up early and look around in the morning and case the area and tell him we're going to stay." I was all for that.

At daybreak we walked along the Liard waterfront and past the row of snug little log houses facing it. Some river boats were pulled up on the bank, one being a Game Department launch. From here we could see the mouth of the Dease River where boats go upstream but south to Dease Lake, another new and enterprising scenic place where there was a mining community. The Liard was also an unofficial takeoff site for floatplanes.

We found no work at Lower Post, so hopes were useless and we had to carry on with Tom. We said nothing about our romantic lurch, afraid of his ridicule. As it turned out, the immediate area was sparse locally for game and logging so we did not feel too regretful about leaving; Watson Lake was an alternative only a few miles away.

At Lower Post the livings were made outside the community and likely grubstaked to get started. We needed capital. The Indians were Cascas who brought their furs to the post, as did other trappers. Miners hung around. Lower Post was on the Telegraph–Stikine route and was the jumping off spot by plane for Cassiar country and the Nahanni Valley. It was used by the BYN—the British Yukon Navigation Company—as an overnight stop for their buses; nowadays they stop only for food and keep going night and day with relief drivers. We had slept in one of the lodge's white-painted barrack huts and the noise and commerce went on all night. There were three hundred miles to go to Whitehorse if Watson Lake wasn't any good.

Seven miles out of Lower Post the Alcan started to zig-zag, ploughing due north. I had read somewhere that all this zig-zagging had been deliberate to prevent strafing by war planes. Present day documentaries now reveal they were just dodging around muskeg.

Twelve miles from the Post we came upon the Watson Lake community where the highway forms a "Y" junction. The Alcan carried on more or less straight ahead from the fork. At the centre of the "Y" was a wireless station, maintenance camp and hotel. The other fork to the right went eight miles down to the lake and village and airport. At this junction was the Message Post. People had tacked up licence plates and signs to show where they came from, all over the world but usually the States. It gave us an inadequate feeling.

"Look at that, will you?" I exclaimed. "We should say we're from Okefenokee. Is that in Florida?"

We had just pulled in near the hotel, undecided, and were watching a group of packhorses and a man with them, when Bob gasped and leaned out the window.

"Slim!" he yelled. A tall thin cowboy sauntered towards us, an old friend of theirs from Interior days, and there followed the usual "What the hell you doin' here?" exchange.

Slim was six foot six, without exaggeration, wearing a ten-gallon hat, knotted kerchief; a cowhide jacket and high boots. He had fourteen packhorses with him that he was taking to a winter range after coming off a summer surveying job about forty

For over one hundred years, packtrains were used to freight supplies between waterways and railway headings throughout BC, especially for prospecting and highway surveying. Slim was both a wrangler and a big game guide; he later worked in the Chilcotin country with Bob's brother Tom, big game outfitting and guiding in the mid 1960s.

miles from the road. He had had great good fortune in hunting grizzly, sheep, moose and caribou, presumably as a guide.

It was from him we learned all that we needed to know about Watson Lake and its possibilities. You'd need a good stake until you made money off the land. By this time we knew we were headed for Whitehorse if we wanted to make money of any sort. We skipped Watson Lake.

So the country abounded with big game but not within a day's journey of the road, which was never still for long, day or night. Once or twice we met little groups of packhorses wandering unattended along the road's side. They stood politely in little knots awaiting our passing, quite traffic conscious and just the opposite of cows.

Home Stretch

We were within a day and a half of Whitehorse, another three hundred miles, and could not seem to rush getting there. We would have to make camp again, though sick of that. On we went, working through jack pine country, which rolled forever towards the rounded mountains further north. Ahead lay the route through the Cassiars. Beside the highway ran the Rancheria River for many miles, with brown water swirling between rock canyons. Here and there were small marshy lakes.

Once we were into the Yukon, tourist camps appeared, situated about every twenty-five miles at pretty, strategic waterholes, whether lake or stream. Some were simply picnic grounds with barbecue pits, but others had shelter houses painted government green with white trim and containing cook stoves with firewood neatly stacked, tables and benches, and outdoor privies. After other experiences we wished we could have stayed a week at Morley River camp.

By Mile 752, out of sight the eighty-odd miles of Teslin Lake, the waterway had begun to be parallel to the highway. By Mile 800 the road now ran beside it.

Bob was back in Shorty Johnson territory, the guide who had ferried him to the head of the Telegraph Trail. A previous Shorty Johnson had died of flu in 1920—not our man.

Teslin Village is down on the waterfront at the end of the 1900-foot Nisutlin Bay bridge and was there before the Alcan went through. Teslin dates back to gold rush days with log cabins and missions both Roman Catholic and Anglican. We took this in for a while. Then the men asked questions and had a brief walk around in the hope of finding Shorty. Bob wanted to prove he'd made it to Telegraph Creek, and wasn't "nuts" for attempting the hike, but there was no Shorty and Tom couldn't wait.

Thirty miles further on, Teslin Lake ended at Johnsons Crossing where the Canol Road reached east to Norman Wells. It was closed due to bridges washed out, but was going to make a quiet hunting-into-game-territory road not far from Whitehorse.

A stone's throw away, towards Whitehorse, the lake became the Teslin River. BYN paddle-wheelers had had to steam north all the way down the Yukon from Whitehorse into the Teslin River, then back south (and upstream) into the big lake with supplies for Teslin Village. They stopped the service in 1942. Where the Teslin River met the Yukon River was Hootalinqua, a natural berthing place.

Flying along we came to Squanga Lake, then Jake's Corner, a junction. The pre-Alcan road used to go left and west (as you traveled north) from Jake's Corner, then down around the bottom end of the 26-mile long Marsh Lake which, when added to Tagish Lake and Lake Bennett, made a continuous waterway. From that

The completion of the Alaska Highway in November 1942 made the Yukon accessible by road for the first time. Previously, most goods had come by sea to Skagway, narrow-gauge railway to Whitehorse and then to the river communities by steamer. Dawson City and Mayo remained supplied by river and winter road until 1955 and the completion of the Dawson-Mayo Road, now part of the North Klondike Highway.

old road, down which you had come and which then curved north, upwards and east, along the other side of Marsh Lake and back to the Alcan, you could branch off to Carcross and Lake Bennett, which would feature in our future.

Marsh Lake Lodge, near the Alcan Highway, was a place Bob wanted to show us quite badly as an example of what he wanted to own. Before deciding to walk the Telegraph Trail, he had been in Whitehorse sounding out any possibilities that would be like the hotel they had given up. He heard of the lodge and went to see it. (Theirs had been a three-storey old-timer on the Columbia near the Monashees and they had made everything look rustic with a rustic bar and stools, with bear skins on the floors and stuffed animal heads (left by previous owners) on the walls. They'd been fools to let it go when Tom's marriage broke up.) The Marsh Lake owner went in for guiding in a big way. The place had everything one would require in a dream hunting lodge. The licensed premises alone were like the lounge of some big log hotel and luxurious with furs and souvenirs of the northern life. It reminded the men painfully of their own lost lodge and how they might have improved it.

Marsh Lake Lodge was beyond their wildest dreams, with its setting by the shore. The main lounge was decorated with the heads of mountain sheep and goats, with great white pelts for hangings. It faced the lake with a view of cabins, boats and floats. The lodge walls were built of mill-cut logs, square on two sides, to lie flat without chinking. There were plenty of log houses and cabins in the north that had logs taken from the bush, peeled and chinked with everything from cement and mud to moss. Except for trading posts and offices, none of the buildings ever used paint. No one seemed to have heard of it.

As for young dreams, we wanderers were to find back then what the Yukon had to say about plain survival and what it took to be a sourdough, but we needed the hope of owning such a place as that lodge to egg us on. Today Marsh Lake Lodge is gone, burned down, and the site is surrounded by a bedroom community to the urban sprawl of Whitehorse. The highway we knew has vanished in many places and has either been covered over, rerouted, or become a heritage trail.

CHAPTER · VII

IIIIIIIIIIIIIIIIIIIIIIIIIIIIIIIIIIIIIIIIIIIIIIIIIIIIIIIIIIIIIIIIIIIIIIIIIIIIIIIIIIIIIIIIIIIIIIIIIIIIIIIIIIIIIIIIIIIIIIIIIIIIIIIIIIIIIIIIIIIIII

The Kee Bird

Moccasin Flats

Bypassing Miles Canyon, we soon skidded down the long Two-Mile Hill into Whitehorse. We had not stopped to admire the panorama from the top. Whitehorse was much smaller than the size it is now with a bare bones population of about eight hundred, which was rapidly escalating towards the thirty-five hundred it would be in two year's time when it became the capital of the Yukon Territory.

We selected at once our usual information bureau, which had to be the oldest bar on Main Street. We were in Robert Service country, the end of the road for many people. Six paddle-wheelers towered over the town, shored up by railway ties on the banks of the Yukon River after being hauled out of the water up a ramp of greased timbers prior to freeze-up. Huskies howled at night and the whole town hummed along to the furtherance of military purposes and moneymaking schemes. The stores were full of good things and shoppers sometimes dressed in expensive northern fashions; the pubs were still bustling with uniforms and pretty women, and the sky was full of planes.

Before I knew it I was being shepherded down to Moccasin

Flats to an Indian compound where there was an empty shack. After unloading our gear Tom left the two of us and went off to make a life of his own. He'd had enough of "playing gooseberry," as we called it, meaning the odd man out. Thus began our married life proper.

The shack had a dry acrid sort of smell, but we got used to it. During the night the owner's friends would bang on the door, not knowing we were in there. The outhouse needs no description except to say it leaned a little and when snow came it was ringed outside with "oysters," the ghastly expectorations of phlegm-filled chests and committed tobacco chewers. In fact my whole impression of Whitehorse that winter was coloured by oysters in the snow and yellow holes created by uplifted husky legs. And not always by huskies, either.

Moccasin Flats was down beside the Yukon River. We were not on an Indian reserve but in an Indian settlement. The road to it followed the riverbank out of town from the big White Pass and Yukon Railway station at the end of Main Street, to wind up in a US Army camp a short distance down the river where GIs remained in a sort of mopping up action. (They were not the only military people. The RCASC [Royal Canadian Army Service Corps] were in Whitehorse, as was an RCAF [Royal Canadian Air Force] base with radio operators and other personnel). The flats were busy with camps or yards or other compounds but it was not all industrial there; along the river there were also several small shacks and cabins.

The men found work right away in a Public Works yard and rather than stick around, soon I was working too, in a laundry somewhere in a dusty stretch between our shack and the BYN depot. There I sorted men's' dirty socks and underwear and ironed shirts. The equipment was just as good as at home in Victoria and all drying was hung on the line outside. I was good at ironing shirts. As a kid I'd been made to iron my own school shirts, the kind worn under a tunic, and there had been nothing but men and boys' shirts ever since. The theme would continue.

It was very hot and steamy inside the laundry, with the last of the fall sun outside, and I wore shorts to work—at first.

While pegging up a row of washing I felt a nasty bite on my thigh and espied the aforementioned housefly with white feet making a meal. The sore suppurated in no time. Next day, not having learned, I let it get me again. The odd thing was that the fly, or its mate, went right to the wound and ate it anew. After that I didn't wear shorts for four years.

By now the air was chill with the feel of snow. It was still hunting season, but we had no transportation to a hunting site. Tom was off somewhere and Bob did not want to bother him. In Whitehorse in 1949, a sack of potatoes cost ten dollars and a can of milk one dollar, before inflation became general in Canada.

"Don't worry. We'll soon get a house but we've got to beat these food prices." Nothing daunted my hero, because he always found a way, and before long we were in a boat crossing the Yukon—my first experience of going upstream full out, to land exactly opposite our starting point. The Yukon was faster than the Skeena but it must have been crossed almost daily, as a little road went straight up a cliff from the place where we would land.

By now I was heavy with child and challenged, but if the Indian women could climb this sort of thing while carrying then I could. A great deal of scrambling took place. Following my leader up the cliff I was told that a couple of miles through the bush there was a small lake, supposedly studded with ducks and geese. We found it, but not before I had crawled up leaf-covered slopes on hands and knees to reach it. I'd given up caring what I looked like and did actually make Bob humorously remorseful and a little anxious.

The lake was small and close to freezing, while a chill wind swept through the trees. Bob did get a duck all right but it plummeted into the water. He swore but said he'd have to go after it; we could not afford to lose it. Stripping off he made a long dive and came up beside the duck with a yell of agony and was back with it in a wild thrash of spray. He was already turning blue. We returned to the river as fast as I could keep up. Our boatman was waiting across the water for our signal.

The next day, sitting alone in the shack, I didn't know what to do with the duck. Nor did I know how to cook one properly. I was waiting for Bob to come home and pluck it, as he did the grouse always, and to show me the ropes as he'd cooked enough ducks for himself. Come home he did.

"Where's the duck?" He stared at the supper I had scraped together. "Do you mean to say you haven't even plucked it?" He was furious. "I've been thinking of duck for dinner all day."

His anger was some time in subsiding and I knew I was letting him down in his idea of Indian-like virtues, but the crummy shack and the crummier outhouse that we shared with our neighbours was taking its toll of my resolve. Pride dammed my tears as he seized the bird and systematically started plucking.

'Kee-rist It's Cold'

It is always darkest before the dawn. Within forty-eight hours of that new low we had our house. Its absentee landlord was working "Outside." For years afterwards we referred to it as the "house with the moosehorns" because of the set of antlers over the front door.

Two small one-room houses had been set together like a duplex with a door cut through the mutual wall. A kitchen was built along the back of both rooms with a door cut into the main room and another to the outside. The main room and bedroom were sparsely furnished. The whole place was whistle clean; white outside and white enamel paint inside, with waxed lino floors and a fat little airtight heater in the living room. The wallboards were white, with skimpy cretonne at the windows; the bedroom was panelled in white tongue-and-groove and big roses decorated its white curtains. Water was delivered by the pail and the honey bucket system prevailed outside. With a baby due soon, our relief at finding this shelter was enormous.

Our house was on the road to the army camp, on the river side of the road but not close to the river. Snow covered all sights. After shopping in town I would walk back towards the station, turn left and cross the tracks to pass the big paddle-wheeler steamboats lined up side by side on the banks. They were, for the sake of history, *Keno, Klondike, Yukoner, Aksala, Whitehorse* and *Casca*. The *Casca* was closest to the river. *Yukoner* and *Aksala* were taken apart after I left. To my great grief the *Whitehorse* and *Casca* went up in flames years later, in 1974, the others having been moved. It had been such a thrill to walk past them every day or so, feeling a part of the country. They towered over my head, peopled with the ghosts of Klondike passengers, and yet that life was still going on.

|||||||||||||||||||||||||||||||||||||||||||||||||||
While navigation on the Teslin and upper Yukon Rivers ended with completion of the highway, steamers still plied the Yukon and Stewart Rivers between Whitehorse, Mayo and Dawson until they were retired in 1955. The last voyage of a Yukon River steamboat occurred in August 1960 with the voyage of the *Keno,* when it was moved from Whitehorse to Dawson City to become a National Historic Site.

We were now settled down. I was too fatigued to handle laundry anymore and the boys were both working in a maintenance camp nearby. Bob's money was good even if the prices took it all away. Tom was holed up somewhere and spent his evenings with what company he could, but at times he'd come desperately to us.

"I come here to get intellectual conversation. There isn't any in Whitehorse." He was at loose ends but Bob was very busy cozying himself down with projects. Winter would be long and hotel bars were only for fun and gathering information.

First, a load of logs arrived and he spent hours in the snow bucking them on a sawhorse he'd knocked together, with a big swede saw going and his beard full of icicles. Growing a beard had been another thing. *De rigueur* today, it was anathema then, as only rubby–dubs (a drunkard who drinks rubbing alcohol) grew them. He was fifty years too late for being the sort of pioneer he wanted to be and forty years too soon to be what men are now, willingly running around in the bush as environmentalists.

The next projects would be a cradle and buggy. Our son, whose gender was never questioned, had to have accommodation. What developed was a heavy five-ply box, cradle-shaped, with deep sides that cold could not penetrate and with nicely cut out hand-holds head and foot. A simpler version copied it and was attached to a sled that had iron runners.

That done, Bob turned his attention towards building a boat, right inside our living room, a duck skiff for fishing and hunting. The room seemed big enough to have a boat yard at one end and a dining area in the other. Most of the time nobody sat anywhere but beside the heater. The white room looked out into the white snow, the winter sun was blinding, and our smoke went straight up for miles.

The radio was a blessing. We could hug hot cocoa mugs appreciatively while listening to *Baby, It's Cold Outside*. Bob liked to get the Ink Spots and Spike Jones. We would go into fits at the sound of "night shades falling." Anything for laughs. Another was "Heap big smoke and no fyah! Him second-class Indian." And then there was Edith Josie broadcasting by phone from Old Crow, the Yukon's northernmost settlement, who announced seriously every day "Here are the news."

Old Crow is the northernmost Yukon community, home to the Vuntut G'Wich'in First Nation. Edith and her radio program *Here Are the News* became a newspaper column for many years, and for which she was invested with the Order of Canada. It was published from the 1960s to the 1990s.

Sometimes we would go out with Tom in the truck on weekends to forage for wood. On one of these days we had come back into town and I was left in the truck, idly watching the passing scene, when I saw a jeep come whizzing on to the main street from off the hill and circle deliriously to a fast stop near the shops. Out got a very tall aristocratic old woman with thick white hair, who was sheathed in a beautiful long black fur coat, her feet encased in snow boots. Obviously a pioneer-somebody by her manner. Some Indian women greeted her; clustered would be a better word to apply to the three or four of them around her. She called them all by their Christian names and they stood there confabulating, then she went off arm in arm with one of them.

I sat in the truck very small. My own view of Indians at

that time was that they were okay as long as they behaved in a civilized manner, but of course most of them didn't, couldn't or wouldn't. It never occurred to me to meet them like this woman, on their own terms.

On the other hand there were many whites in town—drunks or drifters that the Indians despised—and they practiced their eccentricities in the bars and streets. Bob and I thought some of these characters were an absolute gas; they all had nicknames like "Wigwam Harry," whom we met. In fact one couldn't remain in that country for twenty years without becoming a legend oneself.

Meanwhile, I never moved from the heater except to go shopping in town or to cook meals. I learned to make bread so that lunches should not consist of white sawdust at Whitehorse prices. Bob had a typewriter, with vague ideas of writing some day. On this I typed a bread recipe for my mother, hoping to fire her up into an understanding of pioneer life.

Alone during the day, all my thoughts were of home and Christmas. Somehow longings for my children and parents welled into a rosy fantasy of them as I sat in the warmth of the heater. The real panic was what to do about them for Christmas with no money to spare. Consequently I bought bags of wool and instead of knitting baby things, which could be done later, from November 1 to mailing time I knitted endless mitts, mufflers and slippers. Finally, after the parcels were mailed, by knitting until 2:00 a.m. on Christmas morning, I finished a ski pullover for Bob with a skier poling down his back, which I'd kept hidden. In retrospect I don't know how I did any of it.

We were very isolated—Bob with his projects and I with my heavy condition—and there were things going on that we had to miss. There were Saturday movie matinees and Sunday midnight shows, and at New Year's they featured *The Great Gatsby* and *The Arch of Triumph*. I couldn't go alone and Bob hated movies.

When we went anywhere it was usually to the Whitehorse Inn or the Legion Hall. There was fun everywhere. During the war I'd heard of a certain bird that chased himself in ever-decreasing circles over the North Pole crying, "Kee, Kee, Keerist

||||||||||||||||||||||||||||||||||||||||||

It is a common misconception
that Robert Service wrote
*The Face on the Barroom
Floor,* but it was actually
written by Hugh Antoine
D'Arcy in 1887 and titled
The Face Upon the Floor. It
was put to music by country
music stars Tex Ritter and
Hank Snow.

it's cold!" There he was, the Kee Bird, hanging over the jewellery and novelty shop. Little placards in windows held poems and ballads about cheechakos who had not the guts to be sourdoughs, about what it took to be a sourdough (unabridged) and about the perils of the Alcan. My two men would sip beer and recite *The Face on the Barroom Floor* and *The Shooting of Dan McGrew.* Their father treasured a little green suede volume of Robert Service poems. A little known one that intrigued them was *The Men Who Don't Fit In.*

"That's us," they said.

We shared Christmas with Tom, a bird and a bottle of rum and were jolly enough.

More winter wore on. It was a long wait for the baby, and God knew what the hospital would be like. We heard it was okay.

Once I walked home from town carrying groceries and facing the wind. My parka hood was up but I didn't realize it was fifty below. When I reached our house Bob was bucking three-foot lengths of stove wood amid clouds of steam. His beard was a mass of icicles. He regarded me awhile then told me my nose was frozen. It looked rather white in the mirror, then thawed.

Two other freezing events added to our enlightenment. I was sitting knitting when I heard a buzzing sound. Two "dead" flies, frozen to some thawing planks by the heater, suddenly stretched their feet and wings and were soon flying around the room. So flies can survive fifty below and that's where they go in the wintertime!

The other lesson was the frozen fecal spike rising out in the privy with the honey-bucket man long overdue. He simply didn't come and we didn't know how on earth to manage.

"There's no help for it," Bob decided wide-eyed. "We're just going to have to thaw it out and empty it."

Being the sort of man who turned green at anything like

that—especially, I foresaw, diapers—it was obvious what the decision cost him. Donning heavy work gloves he went outside and manfully grasped the bucket handle, jostled the noisome thing past me as I held open the door, and got it onto the heater, which was holding a good fire. His face was damp and pale with nausea while I, with a much stronger stomach, was in stitches again. One would think that very shortly the whole house would become uninhabitable. Nothing of the sort happened.

In a short time the fire had done its work well enough and putting on gloves again Bob went through the process in reverse. I did not ask him what he meant to do with his burden. Pick axe a hole near the riverbank? Eventually he came into the house again, threw the gloves into the flames, and sat down shivering and crying "Ugh!" every few minutes until he got over it. In the heat of the summer the water pail service might fail, and in the dead of winter—that.

By now some old men had crept back into Bob's life but I didn't often get to meet them. I think it was because by visiting with them they kept his dreams alive. There was one old prospector with a jar full of nuggets who promised the baby a nice one. There were old men at the Legion Hall where women were not allowed.

Tom decided we were not having this; he knew I needed to get out and have some fun.

After taking thought Tom and Bob smuggled me—parka hood up, "bay window" and all (that is, with a tummy jutting out like a bow window on a house front)—into a hidden seat behind an open door off the lounge. At a piano in the lounge a man was playing ragtime and looking, swaying and jerking just like someone I knew back home.

One of my erstwhile brothers-in-law, Jack, was not only adept at ragtime (and Chopin) but could do an excellent Cab Calloway undulation with his long body. My nostalgic tears oozed pleasurably. There were so many people I missed, like this man and his brother, and their brother my ex, all three, whom I had known since childhood. If I could have seen into the future I would have found that my Calloway type was to become a pillar of Whitehorse for twenty years after we left it, that he would play ragtime on that same piano, and that two of my sons would make waves in that city thirty years later.

Harry Lauder Keeping On

The pains began one night close to twelve and Bob went out to fetch a ride. We still had no transportation but it was next on the list after settling with doctor and hospital.

The latter was large and clean for the type of town and everything went normally until they put me in the case room. There was little delicacy in the north and the case room was directly across the hall from the old men's "bullpen," as the nurses called it. One hoped the old boys were deaf and didn't walk in their sleep.

Their nearness didn't bother me at first. All I thought about during that confinement was the loss of two sons and about how I was going to get the other children back. My tears flowed and flowed.

"It will soon be over," soothed the nurses.

"Who gives a damn!" I yelped. One could not very well say, "It's not that, you fool, it's my kids!" As I laboured and laboured the old men took over to drown me out. A gramophone began to play very loudly in the bullpen with a rendition by the Scottish comedian, Harry Lauder.

And so, with contractions timed to "Keep right on to the end of the road, keep right on to the end," our little sourdough was born.

The song played on. "Though your heart be weary, still journey on, 'til you come to your happy abode." Not only did I have a new little blessing to look over, but the old dears had raised my spirits too. Later I wished I could have gone to see who they were and ask them what was the big idea of turning on a gramophone in the early hours of the morning, and to thank them for it.

Bob came bustling in before work to sit on the edge of my bed.

"I know what we're going to call him. Mark. Just one short

B.C. Wildlife Park
9077 Dallas Drive
Kamloops BC
V2C 6V1
(250) 573 3242

Date/Time   : Jun 25 2013 15:55:34
Txn #   : 350571

Card Number : ***************4534
Auth. #   : 066618
Order ID   : 05-0625131555511
Ref #   : 20872104001574009Q C
APP LABEL   : VISA
EMV AID   : A0000000031010
ARQC TVR   : 0000008000
ARQC   : F96211B1BDFAB5D6

Visa

Purchase
Amount $49.54

VERIFIED BY PIN

01 APPROVED - THANK YOU 027

IMPORTANT
retain this copy for your records

Customer Copy

B.C. Wildlife Park
9077 Dallas Drive
Kamloops BC
V2C 6V1
(250) 573-3242

Bus. # 119 298 149
GST 5% # 119298149
PST 7% # 30571B

Inv #	: 350571	Jun 25 2013
		3:55:45 PM
Cashier #	: GIFTSHOP BREAK	05
Cust #	: 1	Cash Sales

TSHIRT ADULT MIN S,M,L,XL OR 21.95 GP
BOOK HP WRONG HIGHWAY 24.95

	Subtotal	46.90
	GST 5%	1.10
	PST 7%	1.54

	Total	49.54
	Visa	49.54
	*************4534	

Thank you for supporting the BC Wildlife
Park. All profits from your purchases
will be used to support the Vision and
Mission of the BC Wildlife Park.

syllable that no one can mess around with." Bob's father was to remark, "Why didn't you call him Luke while you were at it." The winter stretched endlessly and Mark throve. When he was a few weeks old I began to worry about him not getting fresh air and put him outside in his sleigh bed. The sides were deep and windproof but it was still around zero down on the flats. A sort of arctic sun shone all around. A string of diapers flapped into boards on the line before being damp proofed by the heater. Our neighbour's two huskies, looking like wolves, moved up to see what the box contained, then settled down in the snow, one on each side of Mark's bed, on guard. Later I heard of an Alsatian down on the coast that had eaten a barracks baby but I feared nothing, for in those days there was an instinctive rapport between the dogs, the baby, the north and me.

Pretty soon Mark and I were going to town using the sled. I had no idea how we looked until one day two American tourists wanted to take our picture. Highly amused, and standing there in my brick coloured parka, holding the long wooden handle of the sled, I waited graciously. It never occurred to me that we looked and behaved like natives.

Depression about my children still lay on me like a pall, in spite of Mark. I used him as a comforter with his sturdy little body against me, and that role, somehow of his own accord, he has never dropped. He was the calmest, most cheerful baby though he evinced a stronger will than my others. But his little presence was not enough just then.

One Sunday morning, as the sun was out and enticing, Bob decided to take a walk down to the river. We went right out onto the river ice, which was thick enough to support a car but you could see the green water flowing beneath its whitish green cover. I was not frightened. Instead I was feeling so low that, except for the baby, I wished the ice would open up and swallow us. It was the lowest low of my life so far and I muttered to myself that if I were to die and they opened me up they would find written on my heart, as Queen Mary of England said they would find written on hers the name of her lost City of Calais, the names "David and Henry." I would never get them back. The two youngest would return, not their brothers.

Bob knew nothing of postpartum blues but sensed I was being a wet blanket. He left the ice for town, leaving us to come along behind him, and headed for a friend's house and some cheer.

This couple proved to be not exactly my cup of tea, but were okay; they meant well. Also they were living common-law. I was quite put off and thought do we really have to be with people like this all the time? By now it was obvious that the north was a sinkhole for drifters, runaways and illicit relationships.

We were made welcome with coffee and the conversation got a little personal. I was sitting with Mark on my knee and the man, who was tall and corpulent, stood over me surveying us and blowing smoke.

"They are all right," he said, indicating with his head his wife and Bob who were laughing about something. "It's you and I who are the fallen ones."

"Speak for yourself!" I retorted, puffing with indignation, big gold wedding band and all.

"Is he bothering you?" asked his wife. She came over and sat down beside me. "Don't pay any attention to him."

The man's probing perception, like a poking finger, had jabbed my innermost sore spot, the stigma of being divorced. You had to get used to that up north where nobody bothered about the amenities and said straight out what they thought. You ran into it everywhere and finally developed a tough hide.

While the men talked, the woman questioned me in a kindly way about my life and finally drew me out. I got around to the "wishing-I-were-dead" bit on the river ice. She looked at me thoughtfully.

"You'll get them back," she said at last. "SHE won't want them."

From then on I was cured of melancholia. Where the hell had been my faith? It was just a question of time. It could be said that from that moment on I began to settle down. On the way home Bob remarked that my new friend seemed to be good for me.

But we were not quite through with northern uppercuts. Before reaching our house we dropped in on the old prospector with the nuggets because Bob wanted to show him our son.

"Well," said the old boy, as he looked the three of us over, "can't be much wrong with a relationship that produces something like that." And he took the baby into his arms.

Where do they get the bloody nerve, I wondered, to say the things they do and do it with such charm? Bob must have been talking too much or giving false impressions. We were taken into the prospector's cabin and offered more coffee, which we declined. Then the old man went to a cupboard and produced a jam jar full of nuggets, which he set down on the oilcloth in front of Mark. Reaching in, the prospector fumbled for a while, retrieving between thumb and forefinger a small round piece of gold about the size of his little finger nail. The baby took it solemnly and the nugget was to become the centre of Mark's signet ring.

Sons of a Miner

Spring was still a long time coming.

A little green boat made of plywood mostly, but with expert grace, had grown in our living room. It was a flat-bottomed skiff with squared ends, lightly curved so that the bow and stern would just clear the water. The bow was closed over with a pleasant plywood arc, for stowing gear out of the wet, and a slatted deck covered the bilge of the little craft. Any steaming of wood in order to bend it had been done ingeniously outside in the snow with old iron pipes and bits of culvert for cauldron and conduits. It was a first class job, but now we needed something on which to haul it.

The men's spring fever knew no bounds and they were getting spongy-footed with it. The American army was still in town residually and planes, theirs and ours, were still going overhead constantly. As related, near the house with the moosehorns was the US Army camp complete with GIs and Quonset huts where they were barracked.

One icy Sunday, when the Yukon was still frozen solid, the two men, with nothing to do, were getting more pop-eyed and restless than ever. They had not had a good physical scrap in months. They could not take off to hunt or fish and still hold on to jobs and were generally stranded.

"Let's go have some fun," put forth Tom, his dark eyes dancing as he rubbed his hands together. "Let's visit some GIs and stir up something."

They did in spite of my protests. They were gone about an hour or so and came back half plastered, laughing themselves senseless and more or less on the run. They were also carrying something. They laid it at my feet and I saw it was a small windup gramophone in a neat little carrying case.

"For you," they said.

"Where the hell did you get that?"

They collapsed around the room, laughing and weeping.

"Jeez. Haven't had so much fun in years."

They had gone over to the camp and had scraped acquaintance with a couple of American soldiers who had invited them into their quarters for some poker and American beer. This would have been in a Quonset hut full of off-duty soldiers while some were asleep in the rear. All went well for a while. Eventually the Americans got a little expansive about the USA's part in the war, wielding the construction of the Alcan as an extra weapon. They had of course been led neatly into it and fell into the trap. Our veterans gave them to know unto whom they were speaking. Beery in the head because they had started drinking a little earlier than my commando and flyboy, the two GI poker partners made mock. All was as planned. The poker kitty lay on the table forgotten as the two solemn wags looked at each other.

"Shall we teach them a lesson?"

Without further ado young Whitehot Whiteknuckles flew in at both GIs at once, with more deliberate punches coming from Tom at strategic spots. They always fought this way, with Bob doing the cheeking and assaulting and Tom doing the final punching. They did it rather well. Their opponents had been relaxed and off guard while their buddies, who were resting at the back of the long hut but paying no attention to the poker game, were not immediately available.

At first the men in the back refused to let their Sunday be disturbed by the fistfight that had broken out. But when the Americans heard how Canada was in the war first and heard their two mates being described between yells and thumps they rose to their elbows. Suddenly the honour of the United States of America came into question and the two warriors had to clear out as the whole hive came alive.

"This'll do for our winnings!" Tom had cried, grabbing the little gramophone case as they ran hell for leather.

I could see there was not much point in ordering them to take it back. They were not amenable to female coercion and I was young and chicken.

"You ought to go back and face the music instead of swiping it," was my feeble response. This brought fresh paroxysms as they slapped each other's shoulders and fell down in chairs, ground to a halt.

Contained inside the lid were a couple of .78 records. There was one in particular that had *Son of a Miner* on one side and *Headin' Down the Wrong Highway* on the flip side. One would guess what the highway song did for me.

> Too many heartaches and too many tears,
> Crowded too much into just a few years.
> I want to go right but I've lost my way,
> Headin' down the wrong highway.

The boys were overcome with love for the miner's song. Deep drunken baritones would assail me at festive times. "Oh I am the son of a miner. My father's father was a miner too." There was something about "a whole lot finer" and the rest escapes me. The other record played the *Flying Eagle Polka*, an appropriate trophy.

In such ways did you make your own fun in Whitehorse. Naturally there were many kindred souls doing the same disreputable things. In fact, apart from being sore about their gramophone, the GIs had probably enjoyed their Sunday too. They had said plenty that they wanted to say and should not have, which makes any man feel good.

Bob was always looking for sport and someone to tease although sometimes he went too far and had to be sat on. At one time we were in a bar that was very popular, likely the Whitehorse Inn. It was before Mark was born as babysitters were out of the question afterwards. The three of us were having a merry time, even though half a glass of beer was all that I dared. And as the bulgy part of me was under the table I didn't mind being seen in a pub.

Sitting alone near us was a venerable figure, yet another of those in the north determined to die with their boots on—her boots in this case. She was an old nurse, at least seventy-five years old. She wore a wool cape lined with scarlet and her nurse's formidable navy felt hat, the crest on which dated her right back to the Boer War. Beside her was a gnarled walking stick. We heard later that she came to this spot every night.

She started to question us from a distance, rather brashly I thought, and addressed herself solely to Bob. She told him he looked like a fine specimen and where did he get that red hair? She was an old nympho, though I did not believe it of her at first. I just thought the woman had had too much.

"Auburn 'aired Charlie," they calls me." He smirked. "Won't you join us?" he added courteously, through thin smiling lips with eyes wide. He'd spotted another one.

"Don't!" ordered Tom under his breath, thumping Bob hard on the thigh. But up she got and I was made to move over as a chair was placed cozily next to my husband. Another round was ordered and during the time spent drinking it Bob listened to all sorts of sprightly adulations that bespoke the wiles she used to mete out for the comfort of British Tommies in the early 1900s. It was fascinating to me when viewed clinically and without bashing the creature with my beer glass. Every age has its courting techniques and language and this was how they had done it in South Africa. "Fine figure of a man" was one expression, but even my mother had used that to describe a Mountie.

Bob looked across at me poker-faced, his eyes as always getting bigger and bigger with mischief. I glared right back.

"You don't mind if I talk to him?" The nurse noticed me finally. Neither beggar explained that I was not just a date, but a wife. At last Bob had bitten off more than he could digest and began to lean away from the old girl, eyes rolling in real revulsion. Game over. I was delighted. The woman began to be explicit about Bob's imagined prowess.

"Time to go!" shouted Tom, as he and I rose together. Out on the street Bob inquired of him what was it that was eating his backside?

"I just can't stand making fun of people, that's all!" yelled Tom as he strode off down the street towards his truck.

I felt sad that the brave soul should have made such a right royal ass of herself when led astray, and had no doubt that when her time came she would go with her cape wrapped around her and the felt hat pulled down over her eyes. It would have been nice to hear the story of her life.

The Balaclava Experience

Close to the moosehorn house was a yard full of army surplus cars and equipment. We could see from our window a row of big Dodge carryalls, military station wagons much larger than usual, with hefty wheels and a winch on each front fender. These vehicles would go over almost any terrain using low range, also sometimes called "bull low," and could winch themselves out of any bog or hole. A new dream had begun to form.

There lay the rub. In the north every cent you earned went against living expenses. It was impossible on a labourer's wage to buy transportation or leave the country, short of hitching a ride. We could not pay our way out.

We had all begun to realize that we were too far north for the sort of lush green country the men were used to for living and working purposes. In short we were all bona fide British Columbians. In spite of the attraction of Yukon living, we were not the right material. Tom in any case had visions of ranching and had only come this far north to see what was going on. We found the life entertaining but barren for our own purposes. My men folk did not wallow in gold rush history; they liked to make history. They were *Grass Beyond the Mountains* boys.

This was not the sort of place to leave a wife and baby; that never came up. Bob and I were in things together and were really stuck. To get a carryall we would have to make double the money. The wagons were 1942 models and it took three hundred dollars down to hold one.

Jeeps were popular in the Yukon, but anything that small would not carry our boat, crates and trunks. While we debated this Tom decided to go home, driving his truck down the highway.

"You can't," I protested. "If anything goes wrong with that old thing you'll freeze to death!"

"No I won't. If I have to stop and rest I'll climb into the mummy bag and close the zipper. They're made for sub-zero temperatures."

He went in spite of all our fervid remonstrations.

"It's all very well for you guys. You've got each other and the baby. Something to live for and you should be damn thankful. You'll get on here eventually, but there's nothing here for me."

Bob was fearfully worried about him but knew how stubborn his brother could be. I gave Tom two of my most cherished possessions, a navy muffler and a navy balaclava that had saved my face from freezing more than once. Also for some reason he took the little gramophone. Perhaps it was really his.

Just over a week later he walked back in through our door. He said the muffler and balaclava had saved his life. "If I had not had them my head would have frozen."

He had made fairly good time on the ploughed road and had stayed overnight at Teslin. The next night he toughed out by dint of keeping the motor running and the heater going for short periods. It was after that, on one of those long deserted stretches where there is no stop for what seems hundreds of miles, the truck broke down. The engine would not start and without it there was no heater.

Sunk into the mummy bag, with only his eyes showing through the balaclava helmet, and his head swathed around and around with navy wool, he had waited and waited for rescue. By dawn he was in a stupor when somebody came alongside, the first vehicle through after he had broken down. Nobody passed any car in trouble on the Alcan in winter and perhaps they still don't. The upshot was that he was taken by this man to stay with his family at some outpost until his truck could be towed and fixed, which took all his money. So he gave his hosts the gramophone.

"Stella, your *Wrong Highway* is down the highway. There were kids there and they loved the machine so much what could I do? It was the least return for their kindness to a stranger." We were so glad to see him safe, but oh how we mourned *Son of a Miner* on the record's reverse.

While Tom was away someone told us that the White Pass and Yukon was looking for a section cook at a railway camp somewhere in the mountains. I could cook somewhat. The finger pointed at me inexorably.

"What if," said Bob, "they'd let me work on the line and you do the cooking? Even with a bunch of men and no other women you couldn't come to any harm if I was there. Think you could do it? Of course you could."

Right here was an example of Bob's belief that you had to try things, experience them. His quixotic orneriness, braced against refusal, was a challenge to me. I rose to the bait every time.

We simply had to have two wage packets to get back to BC. There was no recourse other than staying and Bob's working forever to save slowly. He couldn't do it without me and besides, there were my children as a burning incentive.

As the railway was affiliated with the BYN we found ourselves in the office of the BYN's chief steward, who worked out of the building down by the Yukon River, near the beached paddle-wheelers hibernating on the banks. He hired us at once— man, wife and child—subject to interrogation by and subsequent instructions of the railway superintendent. We were to see him closer to the time our services would be required.

"Can you make bread?" the chief steward had asked. I replied yes, turning pale. Onto the company books we would go as cook, gandy man and mascot. Also, by company rules Cook was to reign supreme.

"You take nothing from anyone, remember! You report only to me," admonished the steward. Cook wouldn't have reigned supreme over anyone without the help of our next dear old friend.

CHAPTER VIII

The Train Is By

Cooking for the Cannonball

The train stood steaming quietly as our possessions were piled in a heap. This was a place where man had no real business to be. Innumerable animal tracks crossed the silent white fields and ice caps towered foursquare around the big red section house. As far as the eye could see was magnificent arctic loneliness. Back in Whitehorse the Yukon had gone out, all its ice had disappeared and summer had begun. Here, although May, it was winter again, with snow from hill to doorsill.

Proud and forlorn, we watched our fate sealed as bags were put down. The train moved ahead slowly. Sharp jets of steam and a shrill cacophony resolved into "shave-and-a-haircut-six-bits," rolling in falling echoes around the impervious peaks. A blonde in the section house doorway waved at the train with vigorous abandon until the last coach vanished around the rock face.

"Hi," she said to us then. "I'm Marge."

We said hello to Marge and followed her in, the new cook and section hand for Log Cabin.

"I've been holding up dinner for the train. You'd better come straight into the kitchen as soon as you have your things off and watch me serve."

Four men were sitting at a table in the middle of the huge room, which was the kitchen. It had a row of windows along the outer wall, two cold storage lockers were built in across one end of the room and a big iron stove filled up the other end, save for a door into the dining room. Sinks and dish racks were under and beside the windows that faced down the tracks, and a great square work table, at which the men were now eating supper, sat in the middle of the room. The remaining side of the kitchen held three doors: one into the hall, one into the cook's quarters, and one near the lockers that covered the rear wall, which went into a large pantry store room.

The glances of the men were frankly hostile, as well as curious. One by one they looked up at us newcomers then looked down again to continue with their soup. I felt the usual angry rise of gorge induced by challenge from those that might not take to me, the new chef.

Marge fixed that by introducing us to each man in turn: the foreman, two section men and a spare hand. Then Bob was told to sit in with them. I was to eat later after a lecture tour, as Marge had eaten ahead of me prior to her takeoff.

One crammed and voluble hour after that found Marge changed out of her floury whites and putting on her coat. Outside on the track was the "casey" to bear her away, with her boxes strapped to it and a man waiting. The casey, which was used a lot, was a "speeder" that carried three men at most; a "crummy" was a small "troop transport" that carried up to eight crewmen sitting back to back. There was not much hopping off.

Rapid-fire reports on ordering, rules and instructions had followed the opening of each door and drawer. My head was whirling and I was stiff with fright. In our bedroom was a big office desk and on it were order books, requisition pads and enough papers and carbons to keep a trained clerk busy. On the wall of the narrow entry hall was a big country telephone with bells on top and a handle to crank. We had been told by the superintendent, who had interviewed us more fully, that all I had to do was cook "just like at home" (we had envisioned some sort of log structure beside the railway). But, I was to be the train dispatcher also.

As the freights passed by I was to lift the telephone receiver, crank the handle around a couple of times, sing into the phone, "The train is by the Cabin," and then hang up. The phone in each section house rang accordingly when I did that. If the train was running north it was a signal for putting potatoes on to boil down the line at Lake Bennett, which was a feeding stop for passengers. If the train was running southwest to Skagway, the phone bell was a warning to the next section to have someone ready on the platform at Fraser for whatever prevailed. Rarely did the section houses speak to each other unless the foreman had something to transact.

Another thing I had to do for the company was dispatch the rolling stock from other places that went through. When the foreman was around he would do it, but when they were all working on the line I had to keep my ears open and it was probably no coincidence that the kitchen windows gave a clear view of the tracks. Anyone going through on a casey or crummy had to blow a whistle to get my attention or hop off and come to clear himself over the phone. I had to keep strict records of every piece of wheeled equipment to ensure they were always off on a siding and not impeding traffic on the single rail line.

The little casey soon clicked and rattled towards the western pass then on south to Skagway, carrying the excited bundle that was Marge away to liberty. I stared from the windows of the deserted kitchen until she was out of sight. Bob had gone to his fate with the foreman; the fire was going down and there was cleaning up to do. I seized a long iron hook, inserted it into a slot in the centre of the gigantic range, and dragged off the fifteen-pound manhole cover they called a stove lid, and started up.

A week's nightmare followed. We had to be up at six to get the huge coal stove going. Bob did it while I fed Mark and put him back in his box. Next I had to make a vast amount of hot cake batter. The top of the stove had a great polished steel surface and straight onto this went bacon, eggs and flapjacks all at once, to be lifted to huge platters and carried into the dining room, which seated eight to ten men. At the moment we were short of bodies and the four men left on the crew were using the kitchen. I hated that because they were under my feet and I had to wait to eat.

These four men, or five with Bob, ate as much as ten men; I had never seen anything like it. The storage lockers were full of half sides of beef, lamb and pork, as well as chickens and ham. The pantry shelves and cupboards held hotel-sized cans of tomatoes, vegetables and all kinds of fruit. They were spoiled with peaches, cherries, fruit salad; everything that we ourselves could never have afforded, like pie filling, came in these great big tins.

I soon got used to requisitioning as the men whittled down my supplies with ease. Everything had to go on one form, which went into the mailbag for the northbound train to Whitehorse. With it I gathered up any mail from the men and put it into a bag that was tied with a trick knot then held it out on a forked stick from our platform. As the next train or freight came by the baggage boy leaned out to hook his arm through the Y of the stick, which somehow transferred the loop of the mailbag to his forearm, while the train thundered by at great speed nearly sucking me in. There was no signal that the mail would be ready. Somebody just watched for my forked stick as the train came around the bend.

Usually the supplies came on the first train to Skagway the day after my order. Sometimes I had to wait another day, so there was no question of allowing myself to run out; we always ordered well ahead and lived in a constant state of glut at BYN expense, since that company catered the White Pass Railway food. The glut was not just my doing; the pressure on me to keep it coming was immense. It was also my job to take inventory of everything once a month and to keep supplies on hand to cover snow slides and isolation.

The supplies would be unloaded onto the platform, case by case, sack by sack, and carcass by carcass. If the men were not there when things came I had to haul everything out of the sun that would spoil and hump sides of beef into the kitchen myself. On top of that I was supposed to butcher the meat and clean any chickens or turkeys, as well as pull out all tendons with pliers.

How Marge had managed I do not know. It is likely she was on intimate terms with somebody and sweet-talked him into helping. Perhaps nobody offered to help me because I had a husband. At any rate, Bob's hotel experience was handy. Since we were a couple he was allowed into the kitchen while off duty to help me with anything heavy, and he knew perfectly well how to cut up moose or beef and make steaks, chops and roasts. Once a week at least, usually on Sunday, he would set to work to butcher the next week's supply using meat saw, cleaver and murderous knives. He kept all knives sharp and lugged in coal, but as he was not around most of the time when I needed him, I grew muscles from dragging off the manhole cover and heaving up the heavy scuttle. My grim-lipped motto was "if that Marge kid can do it, I can."

Meanwhile out on the line the men had their hardships. The foreman could expect a complement of six hands to deal with his section, which covered, I think, about fifteen miles of rail. The system was that early patrols discovered any trouble, which was reported at breakfast and worked on at once. The main job was to replace the ties as needed. Under the most primitive circumstances they dealt with falling rock, slides and ground heaves; every day brought something new. The track was like a live thing, always thinking up mischief.

After each trip and road mending session the foreman would phone in his report. He had also to maintain subsidiary buildings that housed various iron-wheeled types of rolling stock, keep the water supply full in the tower, and keep the section house heating plant running.

A new face was like gold. According to White Pass rules we were to be stuck there until the next snow fly without seeing anybody or taking a holiday of any sort.

Sam the Turk

We had arrived at the Cabin on a Friday afternoon and on that first hopeless Saturday by myself, with lunch over, I had known I would have to make bread before morning. In Whitehorse I had made a loaf or two out of our little mixing bowl, but here I was supposed to start up a small bakery making bread and rolls.

When I had put out a triple amount of flour and had pulled out a huge bowl I heard a noise from the stairs that came down into the kitchen, near the dining room door. Stealing softly in slippers, and where he was not supposed to be, came Sam the Turk to rescue me.

He was not old by ordinary standards, but he was very senior by active working requirements. He was a bull of a man in his mid-fifties or even older, a Russian calling himself Turkish or a Turk, which meant coming from around the Black Sea. To us he was old, but frightening. We couldn't predict a Mediterranean type.

Well over two hundred pounds, with a "bay window," he was grizzled, had thin mobile lips with a wide greasy smile, a big flattened nose with a hook in it, and rather nice eyes suggesting finer feelings. He walked like a cat and later we saw that he danced like a feather, he was crazy about children and deeply emotional. He was full of information and thoughtful manners. When he came in after work he always changed into a fresh white shirt, black pants and slippers. He was always so immaculately clean he would endear himself to any cook. We learned that he liked to spend money in ridiculous sums and liked to have little luxuries around. He was very, very dangerous if you got his temper up, and my first impression was that a woman would not be safe with him on a dark night. He turned out to be a pussycat. This then was my saviour. He watched me start to cut up bits of shortening.

"Ach! You can't do it like that!"

He had known I'd be an amateur mess and had come down to help. He knew what the men would do to me if the product did not look professional. He got me to melt the shortening and soak the yeast while he washed his hands at the sink. Then when I had dealt with appropriate amounts of flour, water and salt we were off. His huge fists got busy when I had done the initial blending.

"You see how easy it is? You gotta attack it in a cheerful manner and don't be afraid of results. You have to dump it all together and punch it around. Get rough with it. Here, you try it."

I flung into it and the great bowlful of dough started to feel soft and airy. In no time at all, in half the time I would have taken, the bread was rising in pans under cloths on the shelf above the range.

Sam became quite batty about the baby. When we'd arrived, in the middle of May, Mark was four months old. He had a folding table over by the storage lockers. By July he was sitting up in his portable bed in rompers. When I let him, Sam would cradle Mark in his arms and beam fatuous rubbish at him. He disapproved of bottle-feeding. The boy was getting Pablum and baby foods topped off with his bottle. While Sam watched this I was given a dissertation on breast-feeding.

"In Turkey where I come from the children are still at their mother's breast when they are walking around. You see everywhere the mothers sitting on their doorstep nursing their babies, and then a little one will come running up and say, 'I want some,' and she will say, 'Sure, help yourself.'" I was treated to the sight of a hand inside his shirtfront, which he withdrew imaginatively while I averted my eyes, half expecting to see the real thing.

The men followed Sam's example and called the infant Baby Boy. On that first full working day, while serving lunch, I saw Sam through the window, along with the foreman and another man, bending over Mark's box and lifting the net for a closer look. It was nerve-wracking trying to dish up and watch that they did not put their grubby fingers instead of his teething ring into his mouth. But really I was delighted. If they had a soft spot for babies, maybe they would be lenient about his cries.

Upstairs were the men's quarters where they slept, washed their clothes, talked and fought. This area was strictly out of bounds for the cook, who kept the downstairs presentable, while the men upstairs were responsible for cleaning their own quarters. The crew never knew when the chief steward was going to pay a surprise visit while they were on the tracks—he being the god of bunkhouses—but in any case the section foreman had his eye on everything.

I never knew how well or ill they were fixed up there and Bob did not go up unless specifically invited. His position was precarious as the husband of the cook and he kept strictly neutral in all that happened. Getting out of the Yukon depended on this job, and Bob became a very good boy indeed. What it cost him to hold down inner explosions I couldn't imagine.

Fights did break out. Sam had a rival for overtime in the person of Mallory, another section man. Their welfare hung upon who was foreman. Mallory was favoured by the present incumbent, Joe, but Sam was waiting for his old friend Karl to replace Joe and look after Sam's interests. Nepotism in corporations was nothing compared with this. Sam had a radio and deliberately kept it louder than Mallory could stand.

"You don't need a radio with that baby downstairs!"

There were three other men who did not come up to these two in causing trouble. There was a man called Paddy, out from Ireland, who was very anxious to make a good impression and a mite obsequious with me.

"Yes lady. Can I carry anything for you, lady?" He seemed to be the usual drifter; it did not occur to me to wonder what *we* were.

The spare hand was nondescript in looks and deeds but the last man on the team they called The Boo. The poor boy was a little simple and tried hard and the men were quite good to him. Every time the crummy came to take them all away to the trouble site he would hold up the gang by saying, "Excuse me, I gotta go and boo." This meant a trip right through the section house and out the back door to blow his nose. As many noses in the north were blown between thumb and forefinger it had to be done outside and in private. The foreman would sigh and they would all wait patiently. They had not the heart to fire him. Drifters came and drifters went, but the Boo faithfully stayed and stayed.

They used the casey, or speeder, for patrols from about two miles north beyond the next section house to about three miles south past the other house; in all some fifteen miles. Their section contained many bends and one long steep grade on the Skagway side that occasioned two engines if the train was long enough. When they got to the Cabin they'd drop off the surplus engine and there was often a locomotive on the siding to spoil my view.

In mid-winter it sometimes took twelve hours for the snowplough to blow a hundred feet of snow off the track, and slides came without warning. Drifts could be thirty or forty feet deep.

Once, before our time, an engine had not made it and slid backwards. There was a story of oranges and lettuces all over the place but I never heard how they got out of that. We could hear the little loco chuffing and straining up the grade a long way off, as sound carried far. I was put in mind of the ditty that so closely resembled it: "I-think-I-can. I-think-I-can. I think, I can. I thought I could. I-thought-I-could (faster) I-thought-I-could-I thought-I-could-I-thought-I-could."

The red section house had a large platform before it, but no passenger was allowed to alight. Nearby were various red buildings for tools and rolling stock, and a little telegraph shed near the line. Under the lengthy stretch of the kitchen window spread the field with the siding that could hold an entire train.

When the snow went we were surrounded by meadows full of scrub bush and far off from them, on the south side and out of sight, lay a chain of shallow lakes. To the north was Lake Bennett, to the southwest was the route to Skagway. North towards Bennett was a morass of tundra and muskeg, and to the south was a wall of mountains hiding God knew what. These compass-point summations are my own and not necessarily accurate. It seemed so isolated back then, miles and miles from anywhere, yet today what was known as Log Cabin is just a few hundred yards off the South Klondike Highway where the rails cross the roadbed, a few miles north of Canada Customs at Fraser, BC; if you know what to look for you can see it from the road. Nothing remains of the section house, only memories; there is just one small siding and a tool shed across from where it stood. The area is popular as a marshalling point where hikers from the Chilkoot Pass are picked up.

Down from the north every day came the line superintendent, a Mr. Andy Knutson, who had given us our job instructions. He came on any available transportation, stopping off here and there to check with each foreman. The big graniteware coffee pot was always on at the Cabin when he came in and there were always cinnamon rolls and pie at the ready.

Such visitors seldom ate, but walked around, mug in hand, asking questions and hearing complaints. Knutson was a windblown character in parka and storm clothing, serious, well educated, and believing in working himself to death night and day as if some personal devil were on his back. He spoke little but to the point. I liked him, but he was only concerned with the line and not with problems in the section house. In any case I had been warned by Bob not to start up anything but to bear as much as I could because, if he had to take my part, there would be trouble and we'd be done for. Still, I was getting by with the men and Bob was holding his own easily, being used to frontier life if not to railway conditions.

At night, with the coal oil lamp set on the kitchen table and the empty counters clean and shining in its glow, Sam would leave the muttering men upstairs and come down and sit with us—with conscious graciousness on his part and as a special concession on mine. Close fraternizing was not encouraged, but it happened. He would sit there in his clean white shirt, beaming at us with his loose smile, and commence to go over the day's affairs and gossip, a benign sultan with belly and slippers. Bob never committed himself with opinions during these sessions but listened wide-eyed as usual, his trick for drawing out people. Sam could never go back upstairs claiming he had been agreed with on any particular point. Sam was a "sea lawyer" of the rails, but could not write a word of English.

One night he complained of all the overtime going to this Mallory who was the foreman's pet. Overtime was obtained by going on early morning patrols and by pumping water via the pump house after meals and on holidays. Someone also had to stay in the house to check when the tank was full or be outside when the overflow pipe started to run, to give the signal to shut off pumping.

Fights broke out on the track and Joe wasn't much good at stopping them. But Joe was leaving and Sam was ecstatic.

"Everything will be all right when that guy goes and my friend Karl comes. Work's much better when Karl's around. He gets things done and he's fun."

We did not regard this as much of a recommendation until the super, Knutson, told me likewise. It was expedient to keep the cook posted equally with the foreman. She was queen of the section house and he was king of the line. Power battles were not wanted.

After Mr. James, the steward, had interviewed us in Whitehorse, Mr. Knutson had gone over us for suitability. We had known we were not expected to swallow his easy preamble about our duties, but the fact that he'd worked that section himself carried a lot of weight in our acceptance. We also met his wife and decided that if the Knutsons could stand that sort of life then we could.

I was inclined to accept as gospel everything Knutson said when he came stamping in for coffee with his parka full of ice, after battling mountain gales while ducked down behind the shield of his gas car. Therefore, if the super said things would be better upstairs and in the dining room when the new foreman came, they would be. Everything depended on the foreman; the men reflected his attitude almost directly. He controlled everything outside the cook's domain and it was imperative that the two of them get along for the good of the camp.

Finally, Joe went and Karl was on his way.

Karl the Boss

Dinner was over one night and I had just started a great soapy clatter. I was also putting a cake into the oven to utilize the heat. A train with the new arrival on it had been and gone and Knutson the super, who had come with it, dispatched it himself so that there had been no need for me to dart about and view this new paragon. Nor had I been interested.

A strange dark man walked into the kitchen. I was just

straightening up from the oven flushed with heat. He was short and sallow, dressed in a dark suit and dark top coat with a black snap-brimmed felt pushed back on his head. His too-familiar swagger into my world halted uncertainly, as he stopped with his hands in his pockets, coat tails flaring. Anything less likely to be in charge of a section you would never see. He looked like a mobster. The suave cocksure smile set on his face when he saw the choice of cook for the Cannonball camp. His astonishment matched mine at what passed for a railway foreman. Neither of us found words.

Then a friendly bulk filled the doorway.

"Dis is Karl," proffered Sam proudly. "Maybe you got some coffee for him. I gotta go."

Karl recovered first and sat himself down in an expansive manner. He pushed the hat a little further back on his head and thanked me with kingly condescension for the cup I slid in front of him. He sat there stirring for awhile and a ring flashed on his hand.

"So you are Mrs. Smith." His voice was husky but even. He sucked in his breath and looked around. "I trust you are making out here."

"Quite well thanks."

I had gone back to the suds but I could not very well turn away to finish the dishes so I faced him, pressed hard against the sink and fighting for something to say. His face was pocked and emaciated and there were dark circles under his eyes. Nothing but a gangster, I thought, and a cheap one at that. Trembling I invented an errand and excused myself; when I came back he was gone. What an awful, awful beginning to mandatory cooperation.

Six o'clock the next morning found Bob rattling down the coals. I heard scraping chairs with the clink of cups and men's voices. Nobody was supposed to be in the kitchen and I peered out in alarm. There was Karl in his underwear washing at the sink. Breakfast was due at seven and I had not even made the hotcake batter. The other foreman had always slipped in quietly to take a big jug of hot water up to his room. Waiting tactfully until Karl had gone made me late.

"What on earth did you want to give him coffee for?"

"Just wanted to get off to a good start and size up the guy," snapped Bob, always trying to make me look toffee-nosed. "He could be okay. But what a voice! Sounds like an anchor chain running over velvet."

I was not about to have the place turned into a farmhouse or be held up in my work. Since the addition of Bob and a new spare hand all the meals had been served in the dining room; it was an unwritten rule that the men were to stay out of the cook's way except at her discretion, as once in the kitchen she would never get rid of them.

It was very worrying because I knew this man would pick holes in everything and make trouble for me. It was written all over him. He had a lot of straightening out to do if the section was going to be run his way, and there was no doubt from his manner that the entire Log Cabin section, house and all, was to come under his jurisdiction. He was not accustomed to any other experience. He got things done, certainly, and with dispatch.

When Knutson and other company chiefs came through they were greeted with a long list of his accomplishments and put-downs of other men's efforts. His enemies to a man were the men he supervised and perhaps his main enemy was Knutson, to whom he ran mostly with his tale bearing. The super of course would never have hinted of his dislike to the cook. Certainly Karl was not too well supported, except by Sam.

The days passed and Karl shifted his morning ablutions to fifteen minutes earlier and acknowledged me grudgingly whenever we met, but he still drew in his breath impatiently, holding his mouth in a thin, mean line. It was not long before I found out what was brewing.

The attack began one raw wet afternoon with a request for coffee. He was waiting for the roadmaster, another visiting god, who would come in cold and wet with half an hour to kill. Dragging a chair before the stove, Karl turned it around companionably and sat astride. His heavy wool work pants were tucked into his hunting boots and did give him an air, even if the habit encouraged snow to get inside. He wore the railroader's short striped denim jacket with a striped engineer's cap pulled down over his eyes.

"You must be lonely here," he purred.

"Oh yes," I sighed, off guard, "but really I'm too busy to notice it."

"You should get Sam or someone to take you down to see the cook at Fraser. There's a nice woman. Always, any time you go in, she puts so much stuff in front of you. She and the woman we had before Marge were real good friends.

"Look," he gestured authoritatively, "do you mind if I give you some good advice? The woman that we had here that I'm talking about, she had the place real nice." I began to bristle. "At meals she had a cloth and flowers. You know what you should do? Come in and sit with us, just like in your own home. Sit at the head of the table and see who needs another helping and all that. Mother us, like."

I felt cheap. It must be lonely for them too, especially without a woman's touch. It was little enough to do if that's what they wanted. So, at noon the next day, blushing furiously, I eased in opposite Bob amid stunned silence. Sam still went on expanding his latest views and did not move from his end of the table and the other end was the foreman's by custom, so there was no presiding by me; besides I longed to be near the kitchen door and inconspicuous.

Karl began talking shop, but to deaf ears. Then Sam reared out of his spaghetti and saved the day with lively diversions and I turned to him. Forgetting my lunch, I was intensely absorbed in how he had batched down at Fraser section house one winter, when I felt Bob studying me. When I looked at him across the table my blood boiled because he was grinning like a Cheshire cat. He gave me a slow wink.

The experiment was not a success. I was as out of place as any woman in a mess hall full of men, and they could not talk naturally. I stuck it for several days, feeling my growing unpopularity. The conversation began to include cracks about the food and if it was not to their liking, pampered and overglutted as they were, they would say so to my face and slap it onto their plates in disgust. I pretended to lack of appetite due to all the cooking and from then on ate alone. What a dupe! "Mother us, like."

Karl took to shaping me in other ways. It was customary for the men to take their plates out after eating or to come to the kitchen door to ask for anything extra they needed. Karl had other plans.

"Mrs. Smith," he would call, not moving a muscle from his chair.

I would peer in coolly, eyebrows raised, and he would point to the salt.

"May we have the shaker filled please, Mrs. Smith?" It was never less than half full.

"Of course." I was always agreeable.

No sooner was the salt back on the table and myself in the kitchen than it was, "AN' the pickles, if you please, Mrs. Smith!"

This type of episode was repeated several times. I had no idea how to handle him. Soft soap never occurred to me.

"If you start a war," said Bob in anguish, "then he'll say something rotten about you and I'll have to hit him. He's just waiting for me to say something now. It's up to you if you're game or not." Bob was absolutely right, although he burned with embarrassment at staying neutral. We had signed on purely to finance leaving the country and my one thought was to get back to my kids. Without funds we were stuck. We were two hundred and fifty short of the money for that power wagon with which to leave the country. It was sitting back in Whitehorse with a deposit on it. In any case I would not have run at any price.

Karl soon had other things to think about besides me. There was trouble on the tracks one day, manifesting the long-standing feud between Sam and Mallory. They bickered almost every night upstairs, which was why Sam came down to visit. Added to his radio selections he was now the foreman's pet and collecting the coveted overtime. Mallory's dander was aroused in earnest. On this day Sam was vainly trying to pry up a stubborn section of rail while Mallory taunted him. Sam heaved the crowbar and it landed at Mallory's feet.

"Try it yourself!"

"You bohunk bastard!" yelled Mallory. He picked up the crowbar and charged at Sam, point first.

"Stop!" Karl came running down the tracks. "Stop that!"

The fracas did nothing to sweeten his temper. His prestige was wearing thin also. It had become only too obvious he was toadying to his superiors, more immediately the road master. He also kept the men working in the rain when it was customary to seek shelter. Then there were other labour worries.

The spare hand had drifted off to be replaced by an ex GI who was very good looking and hooked on vanilla extract. Some cook had ordered him a whole case of it when he'd worked on another section. He would come into the kitchen pleading, "Aw come on, don't be hard to get along with," as he followed me around and into the pantry until I threatened to tell the line superintendent. In the end he went AWOL to town overnight, ending his spree at Lake Bennett where he frightened some women, then quit before he could be fired. Heaven knew who would replace him.

Visiting Olympians

One day my confidence was really shaken.

The only sound to be heard in the mountains was that of rumbling trains and echoing-steam whistles, the doleful wails that bring tears to the eyes of railway buffs. Even then they filled the heart with longing for nameless adventure.

This day there was a sound in the mountains that was impossible: an automobile horn. There was no road within hundreds of miles. I listened as it came again, nearer this time. Rushing outside to the platform I saw a station wagon approaching along the track, fitted with narrow-gauge iron wheels instead of tires, which turned out to be a specialty ordered for directors and advertising men of the White Pass Railway. I could not believe what I saw as it stopped in front of me.

Out stepped an executive type wearing a new brown station wagon coat with a fur collar, underneath which was his business suit. He was sporting a smooth new Stetson and fur-lined gloves for driving and he handed out a woman companion who was dressed to kill and wearing spiked heels. They said this man was given to piloting ladies to Skagway, combining his examination trips with sightseeing tours. The cook was usually tipped off to these visits so that she could have a good tea on hand, but nobody had said a word to me about it.

These visitors meant fresh tea or coffee, as the stuff on the stove wouldn't do. I had been about to cook pies and rolls for the next day and there was nothing to offer that wouldn't cheat the men. Also, I was furious and crestfallen that some chick in furs should see how I looked in baggy slacks under a white coverall and no hairdo for the past few years. I led the way down the hall and then nearly went into convulsions. The kitchen radio that I had left blaring gave out with, "If I knew you were coming, I'd have baked a cake. Howdy do, howdy do, howdy do."

The visit was not entirely a social one, although they could have fooled anyone on that score. He was pretending to show the lady around. There must have been rumours about Log Cabin for this particular guy to be here. He was the one I had to worry about the most.

He presented me as something out of the Ozarks to his girlfriend and suggested I tell her a few tall bush tales while I cut sandwiches. There must have been a lot of background about Bob and me on the company files for the man to know that I could. Nothing loathe, I regaled the blonde with a few revelations of life in the bush while trying not to be conscious of the administrator burbling with Karl out in the hall. Karl was doing fine, sixty to the dozen.

"Alright then," urged the brass, "how's the food? Everyone happy?"

That much I heard and then Karl's husky murmuring going on, giving his anchor chain a smooth lying run. One up for him, doubtless.

But, the next score was for the cook. The report the executive turned in brought "The James," the chief steward A.E. James, down for a visit.

A.E. James was in charge of supplies and food for hostels,

boarding houses, resorts and paddle-wheelers owned by the BYN, because the British Yukon Navigation Company was the CPR of the north. He supplied passengers on the steamers with menus and fare, he supplied meals for rail passengers at Lake Bennett—a resort as well as a food stop—and he fed all crews everywhere. He was extremely courtly, with white hair and a monocle on a black ribbon, a ladies' man with an arm ever ready to encircle and protect. The vast domain covered by Mr. James' eyeglass and his sudden entrances left no doubt about his ability to handle anything. He was a thorn in the flesh of railway men who said, "But he's a steamboat man." He was responsible for every item personally, down to the deep fry skillet I had been nattering about to Supplies over the phone.

Another company prince. He arrived and it was me he had come to rescue.

Every time the men didn't like what they were getting they would mutter, "I'm going to tell The James," making sure they were heard in the kitchen. Here it must be said that my hot cakes were fat and feather light, my coffee rolls were excellent, my cakes wholesome and not too bad, and at last I was achieving a rich short pastry crust. One cannot help being good when one is turning out the same baking over and over. The men did not want fancy variations in anything in their meat and potatoes world. No made-up dishes or casseroles. Variation was supplied by the BYN with its great tins of fruits and vegetables. My bread was good too, and my roasts. Cooks like Marge served standard luncheon dishes and these I supplied, when I found her notes, for fear of censure at any change.

At one time the crew was going to tell The James because a freight had not delivered on a Friday the sides of meat ordered, and I was forced to feed them baked ham and huge chickens over the weekend. They whined like stuck pigs. The lack of beef was all my fault, they figured, although they had been fed like kings; the hams were beautiful and the chickens were fat capons, perfectly cooked. The even heat of the great stove helped, and the fact that I had no distractions. Mark gave no trouble, sitting on a huge cushion and tied to his chair, watching his mother.

"Tell me," began The James directly, "how do you find friend Karl to work with?"

Taken by surprise, my face was a study.

"Ah, I thought so. We have heard a lot about Mr. Karl before."

"The superintendent thinks a lot of him," I ventured, not to appear snivelling.

The chief slid an arm around my waist and said, "You leave the rascal to me." I was filled with an unholy glow. Then he cross-examined me for some time on food and ordering, how we butchered and so forth, how much baking I did. I was careful to blow my own horn a little and to point out that Bob kept his mouth shut at table, no matter what. I was trying generally to offset anything Karl might have said and Mr. James seemed satisfied.

Shortly after that I received a rather phony telephone call from him in Whitehorse about one of my requisitions. A clerk could have called me just as well.

"I see you ordered a new rack for your oven. Will you kindly give me the serial number of your stove."

It seemed odd he should call me or expect me to know the answer. Leaving the receiver hanging, I darted around front and back of the thing but no number was evident. I reported the fact.

"Is Karl around? Get him to look for you."

"He's outside, Mr. James, but I don't really like to…"

"Get the man to the phone! I'll talk to him."

Sticking my head out the front door I yelled, "Karl!" with the greatest glee. He looked busy and bothered. "Mr. James wants to talk to you on the phone."

"What the hell…" He threw his big gloves down and came striding over, giving me a black look. I retreated into the kitchen with my ears cocked.

"Yes, Mr. James." Bright as a honeybee.

Soon he was running as many rings as I had around the stove, but to no avail. He reported back and there was shouting and arguments. He returned to the kitchen almost running, to kneel on the floor and get his head inside the oven, scuttling around like a land crab for a better view. Temper and frustration made him look small and ridiculous squatting there. In the end he took measurements and left. For some reason I got no pleasure at all from his humiliation. The score was even. So what if it was? He was a small man only, and defenceless.

The following Sunday afternoon we were resting and reading in our room while Mark slept. Someone called my name. Karl was out there in the kitchen. What the devil now, we thought.

"Pretend you're asleep," offered Bob.

"I can't. I'd better see. Blast the man!" Apprehension mounted swiftly.

He was sitting at the kitchen table with an open mail order catalogue in front of him.

"Mrs. Smith, would you do me a favour I wonder?" He sounded tired and melted down. "I got something here needs a woman's advice." The open page featured clothing for little girls. He coughed and rasped his explanation with some embarrassment.

"There's some people in town I visit every time I go in. They've got two of the cutest kids you ever hope to see. They call me Uncle Karl and I always take them something, you understand. These people are so good to me, alone as I am, that I like to pay them back in some way."

I must have registered amazement for he looked more helpless still.

"Well look now, if you will. Here's two little outfits but I just can't seem…d'you think you could help me with the sizes and colours? I thought, both the same, see? But a red top and a blue skirt for one and a blue top and red skirt for the other? Then they won't fight over them."

I looked over his shoulder at the typical catalogue colour selections, which were pretty rank. What else but clashing blues and reds?

"What about a red top and a grey skirt for one and a grey top and red skirt for the other?" He was ecstatic. There followed a lot of imaginary measuring of heights, "so big" and "so high" and checking of ages against the catalogue sizes but we got something settled on the big side as the mother was "a dab hand at altering." With that we buried the hatchet.

It turned out that the need to be top dog had only been to appease his ego. He was in fact suffering from a real inferiority complex. The cause of his behaviour had not been at first apparent. He had been bitter and unhappy inside. If he got drunk, he was careful of example and did it in town; he was never hung over on the job.

Violet Time

The mountain passes could keep summer away no longer. Everyone burned to get out and see something. Wild flowers took over before the snow had taken leave and pushed right through it. Then one day a lone locomotive shunted into the siding instead of going straight through, which it was supposed to do. I watched as the engineer got out and started to walk across the fields.

"What on earth is he doing?" I asked Sam.

"Picking violets. They often do it. Don't hurt none because it only takes a few minutes and they make up their time."

The summer that struck was summer indeed and early one morning I heard cat squalls and looked out. Sitting on a big rock in the scrub meadow outside our quarters in the new sunlight was a red fox. He was looking down his nose with tranquility at the station cat who was making a frightful din and trying to claw him, though too timid to make a flying attack. The cat went around and around the rock and the fox just sat there, merely following the cat with his nose.

That cat was a mouser outside and not friendly inside. But I had a pet of my own. The kitchen windows stood open and were fitted with screens, to which one day a fat squirrel came to make inquiries. He was very big and his little nose wanted food. He flew when I opened the screen to put out some cookie dough but he came back. Thereafter my mornings were cheered by his cheep, cheep as he ran up and down the shingles on the sides of the house and up the sides of the window casings. Every day he found something on the sill.

We had been at Log Cabin for two months without a day off, a seeming two years, with nowhere to go if we could. Sunday afternoons were free, for a few hours. Finally we found a way to break out of our prison on a Sunday. The only route we could take, in the few hours off we could snatch between cleaning up after the noon meal and starting supper, was up and down the track. But Sam said fishing for arctic grayling was great at some natural portage between two lakes nearby and there was another little lake if we wanted a swim. And in the bush right down the line near the next stop was a ghost town of which nothing remained but a garbage dump. Of course we were right in gold rush country. Bob was dying to look at the town site and thought we might fit in a swim.

With great ingenuity he devised a square box lashed to his packboard for stowing Baby Bunting. Once it was hoisted onto his back I settled Mark into it and we were off.

We were too bushed to let stories of grizzlies deter us and anyway the practice was to go out in twos and never alone. We never moved anywhere without a gun. A man had been completely scalped by a grizzly while hunting alone down the line. We had brought just the bird gun and the big game gun in the end, so we took the latter with us, the Winchester, the .30-30.

After about a mile of stumbling down the track we headed inland over tundra moss and lichens where bits of snow still lay unmelted. We found our lake, a little round mirror reflecting a very blue sky and puffy clouds and surrounded by wild flowers of every sort. Dragonflies flitted over the water. Bob did not wait but peeled down and dove in, emerging with a roar. Snow water, what else? I wanted to swim badly but the mosquito whine around me grew excessive and there was no place to park a baby even with a net drawn over him.

Then we sought the goldrush town site. Everywhere was tundra with sparse stunted pine forest, but we found it. Things do not disappear in the north as fast as they do in a warmer climate and each tent site had square footings now covered with moss. There was nothing to see in all the woods but little square green lumps laid out in streets. At the edge of the town on a slope lay the refuse pile and all that remained were long green bottles, dog sleds with wood bleached silver and runners corroded, and bits of harness. Tins and other artifacts had long since rotted. All through the woods were great white horse skulls but no skeletons. Very likely wolves and other animals had dragged the skulls around in play.

Climbing up on the heap I sat on a sled, fascinated. The bottles were mostly green but some were clear or brown. They were longer than our usual present ones and narrower, each with an indentation at the bottom. I knew they were collectors' items even then and fingered them lovingly.

"Oh no you don't!" admonished my spouse. "You tourist! We're only going to have room in that wagon for well packed crates and I'm not taking any junk." I had to content myself with a piece of leather dog harness with the buckle still attached. For years I regretted not taking a stand in the matter.

The Portage

Sam had said he would go fishing with us the next Sunday and show us the Portage. We did not have a rod, but he did, and the two men arranged to take turns. Mark had to go too of course in his back pack box. At such times in the heat we'd make a shelter of twigs, put a coat down inside it, place him on the tail of it and use the collar for a sunscreen.

We went a different way across the tundra this time, more to the southwest. Between us and the lake system lay a moraine, a long ridge of land pushed up evenly like a dike, about three miles long, on top of which was a natural flat road. We went along this in comfort, glad to be off the tracks. The lakes that lay ahead of us were in flat country with rough grey rock crumbling all around them; more moss and lichens were present but no grass. The lakes were stuffed with grayling. The easiest way to catch them was to stand at the portage and hook them as they funnelled through. Pretty soon we had a whole mess to take back for me to clean.

I hated them. They were slimy, they had sharp fins that cut you when you were trying to get a purchase on them for scaling or filleting, and when they were cooked they were delicate all right, enough to be tasteless, and a mess of bones. I longed for salmon.

The friendship with Sam grew that summer over fishing and storytelling, but one summer evening it nearly came to an abrupt end. Bob got over-confidential. They had just had a discussion about women in the north, which was concluding as Sam went up the stairs remarking upon my youth and verve. He thought I was a great deal younger than I was, by about ten years. This was too much for Bob.

"Hey! I'll tell you something."

Nipping smartly up the stairs to Sam's ear level he murmured things I couldn't hear, then leaned back in consternation when he saw Sam's face.

"No!" roared that worthy, "you lie! You kidding me. You better be kidding because if not I drop a whole load of ties on your head!" He descended a step or two as Bob retreated. Somehow Bob managed to look as if he had been kidding, in a sickly sort of way, as Sam turned and stomped upstairs.

"What on earth did you tell him?"

"Never you mind. Phew!"

Without any more said I guessed he had told Sam I was the mother of four more children. A man like that would immediately assume the worst. We got around it and things went back to normal. I didn't know whether Bob had resorted to bluff or whether he had taken Sam aside and explained all, and I didn't want to know.

It was not the only disturbing note from another life. A letter from my ex found me in the mountains. It shook me. I took it off to a far-off outhouse facing the tracks in order to get a first-hand grip unwatched on any trouble that might arise. It was only an account of the children's summer and growth. But in the margin he had written, "The radio is playing *Your Cheating Heart*. Reminds me of a saloon in Skagway." Skagway indeed. Just as if I didn't know all the words. "I walk the floor and call your name." Whose cheating heart? Did he mean his or mine? Was this his usual bleak form of apology for the runaround? Sure it was. The letter went into the huge stove, searing flames to searing flame, and had the manhole cover pulled over it. We both had to face the music and get on with it.

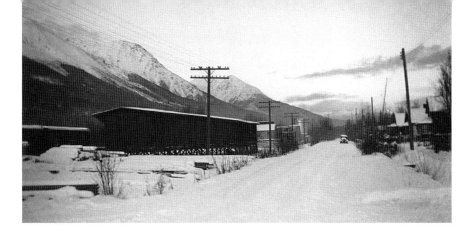

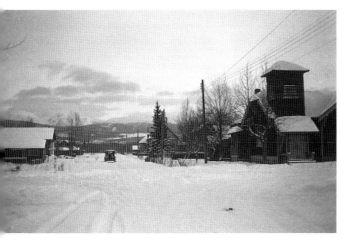

Smithers, BC, early winter 1948. Trading a warm climate and bustling city for the harsh winter environment in a small community like Smithers was bleak indeed. It was almost 50-below-zero. Ice crystals hung in the air, and winter felt like it stretched as far into the distance as this road.

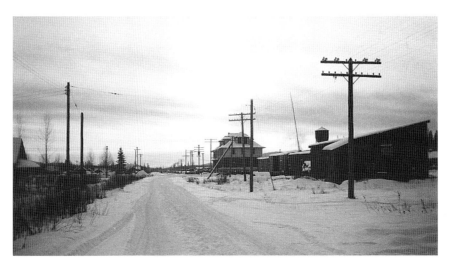

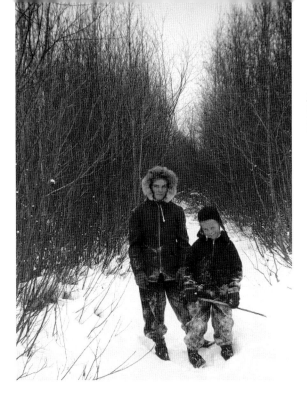

Joan and Robert looking for a Christmas tree, December 1948.

Exploring the Smithers' stockyard on a winter afternoon walk.

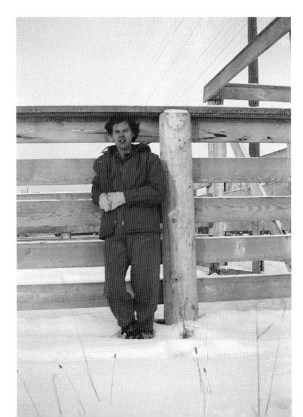

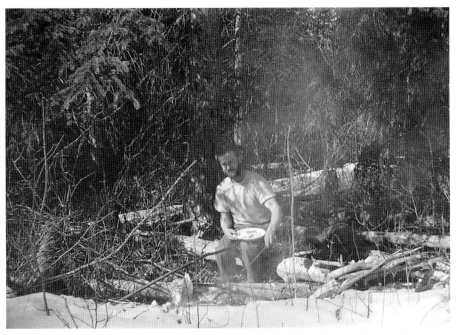

Our first spring bush hike, 1949. There was still a lot of snow on the ground but Bob was gleeful in short sleeves.

Bushwoman in training, 1949
—a long way from deportment
classes at St. Margaret's.

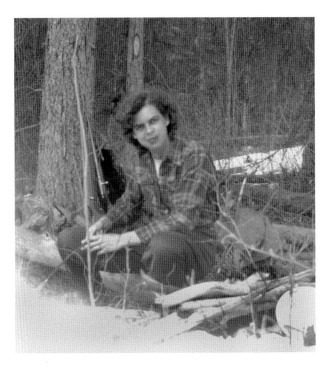

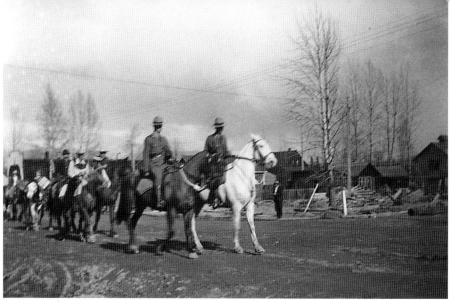

Smithers May Day parade, 1949.

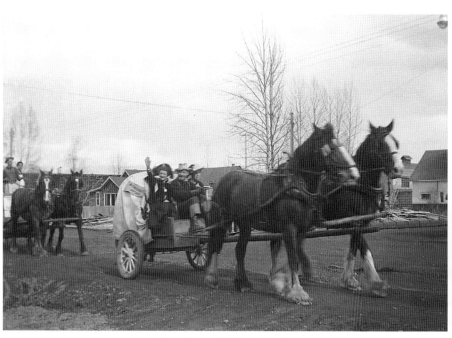

Pioneer float in the May Day parade.

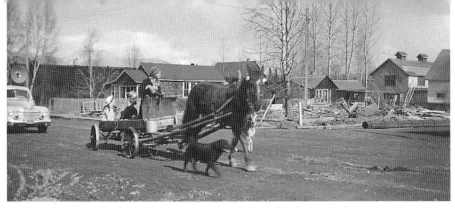

Kathleen Daisy Casler and her children in the May Day parade.

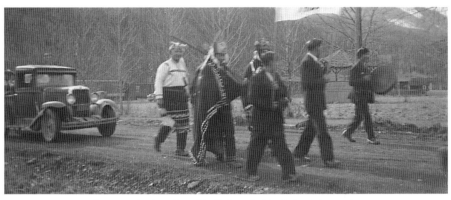

Moricetown Band members of the Wet'suwet'en First Nation in the parade.

The Elks Hall was transformed into the Dirty Shame Saloon for Klondike Day.

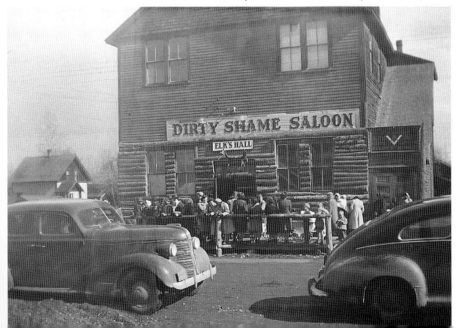

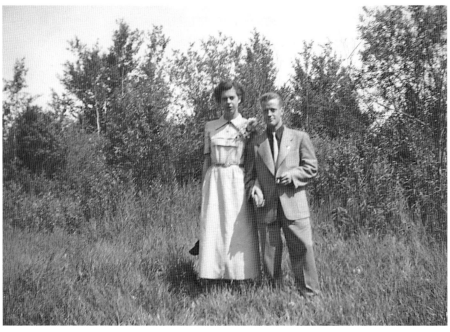

Wedding day, 1949. This was one of the very few pictures with both of us standing; Bob was very sensitive about his height.

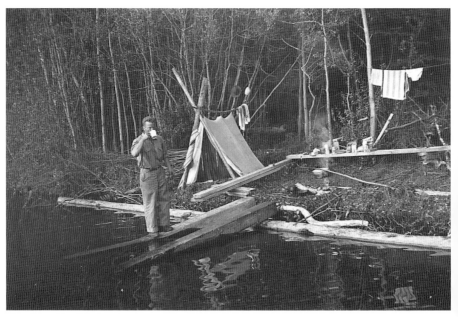

Honeymooning at Day Lake.

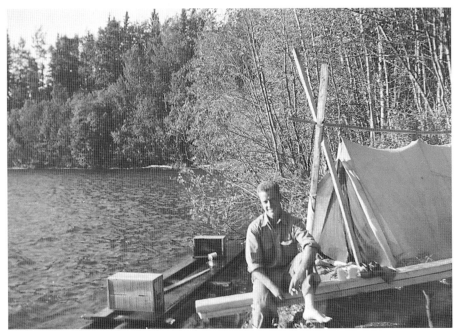

Bob made us an idyllic honeymoon campsite.

Stella with eldest son, David,
August 1949.

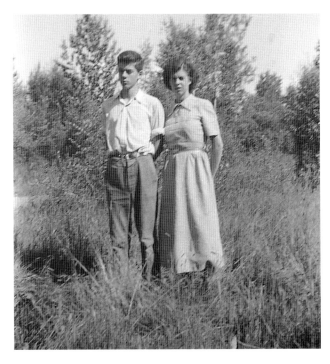

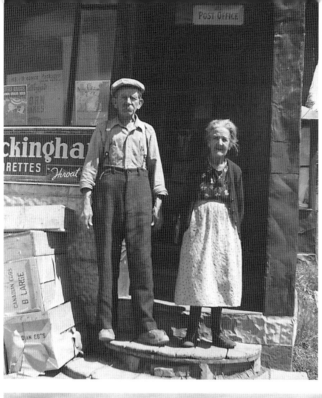

Albert and Cela Sturgeon, the storekeepers at Forestdale, July 1949.

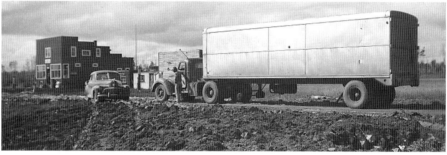

The highway into Fort Nelson, 1949.

Liard River Lodge at Mile 496 of the Alaska Highway,1949.

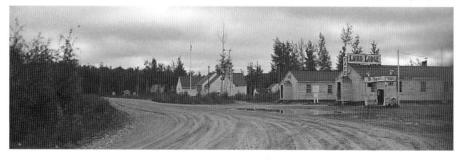

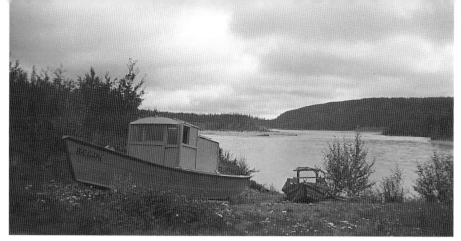

Liard River at Lower Post (Mile 620), 1949.

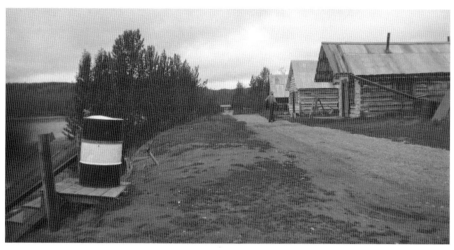

Lower Post—white buildings trimmed in red belonged to the Hudson's Bay Co. We liked the look of Lower Post and would have stayed if there had been work.

Moose horn cabin, Moccasin Flats, Whitehorse, 1949–50. It was spartan, but cozy and clean.

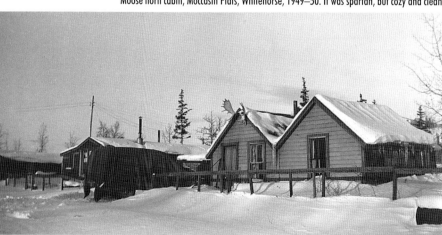

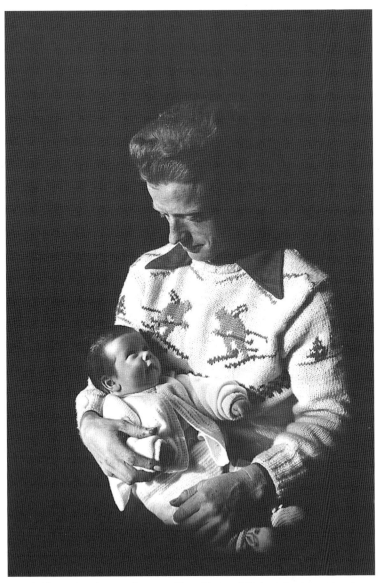

Bob holding Mark, and wearing the sweater I knitted for him, 1950. I took the picture with my box camera, a Brownie Hawkeye.

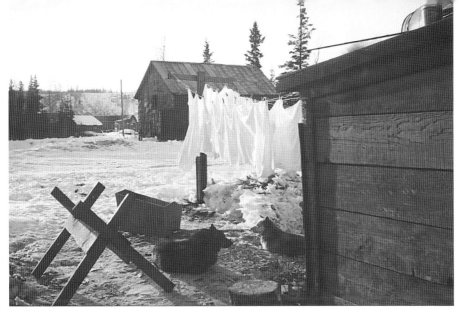

Prelude to Pampers. Huskies guard Mark's sleigh and his freeze-dried diapers.

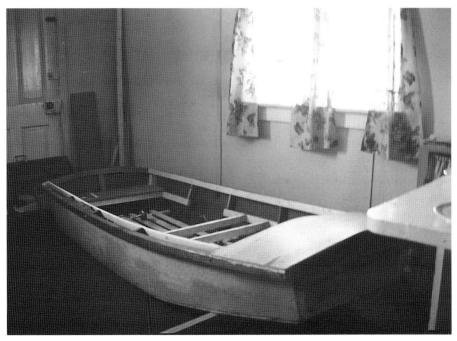

Bob's winter hobby: building a boat in the living room, Whitehorse 1950.

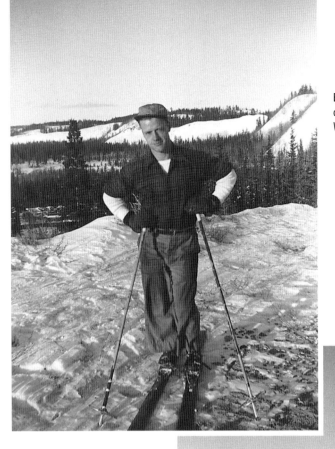

Bob cross-country skiing on Long Lake Trail, Whitehorse 1950.

A much longer stride than Bob's made cross-country easy!

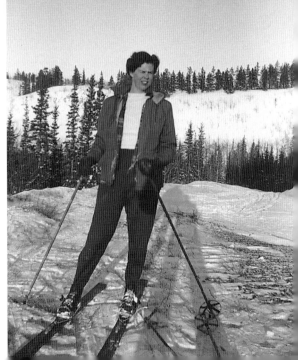

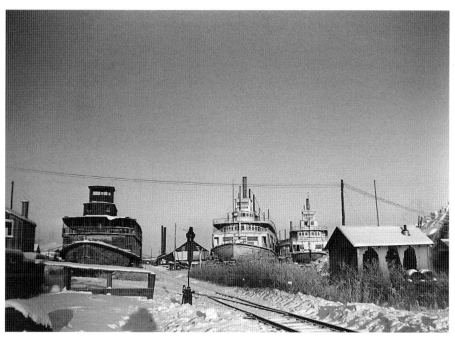

The beached steamboats, Whitehorse 1950.

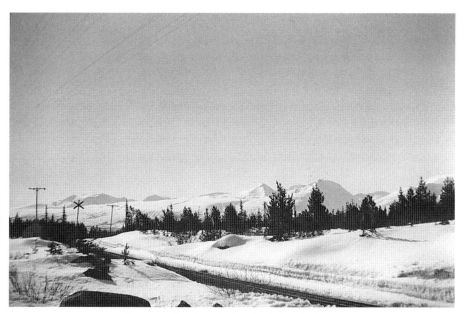

View south to Coast Mountains from Log Cabin section house.

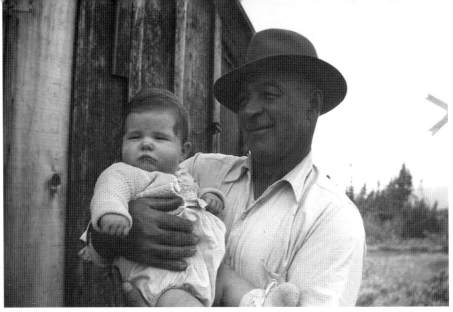

Sam the Turk with Mark at Log Cabin, BC, spring 1950.

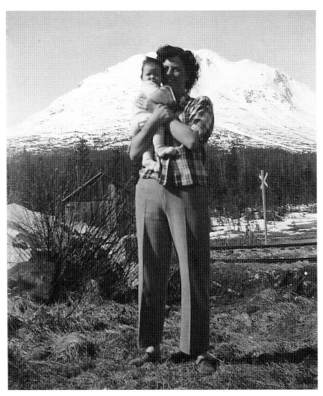

Stella with Mark, Log Cabin, BC, spring 1950.

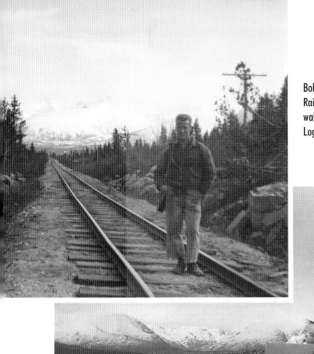

Bob, the White Pass Railway section man, walking along tracks near Log Cabin, spring 1950.

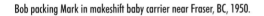

Bob packing Mark in makeshift baby carrier near Fraser, BC, 1950.

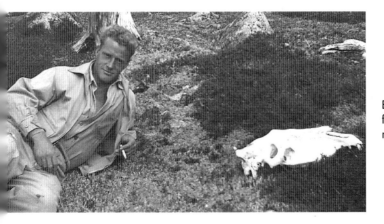

Bob with horse skull from Klondike gold rush era.

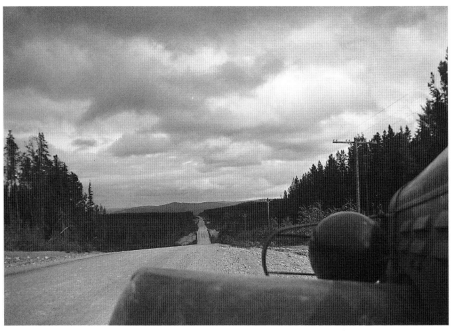

Heading "Outside" from Whitehorse on the Alaska Highway, fall 1950.

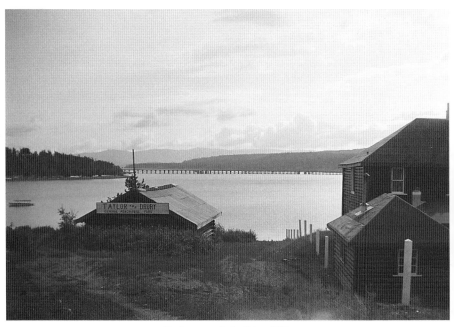

Trading post at Teslin, Yukon, 1950.

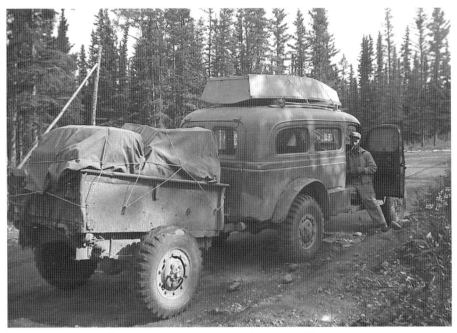

The $600 US Army carryall with trailer that held all our worldly possessions.

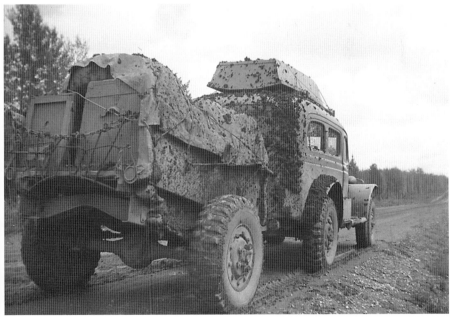

Gumbo cakes the carryall.

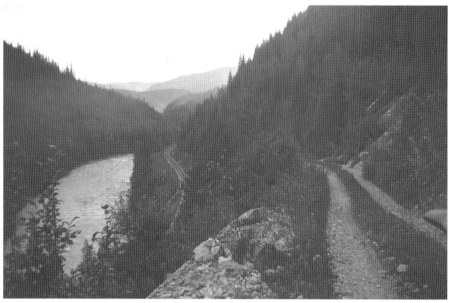

The future Yellowhead Highway (now highway 16).

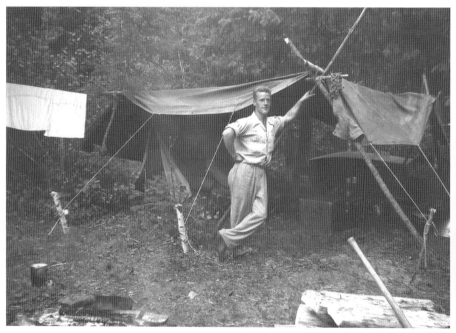

Raft River campsite, fall 1950.

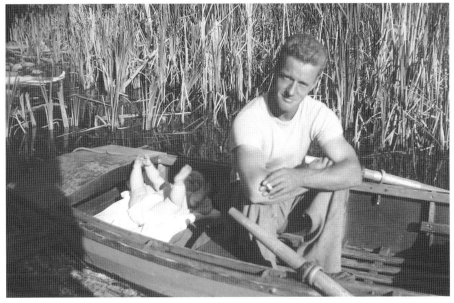

Bob and baby Mark both "pose" for the camera, near Barriere, fall 1950.

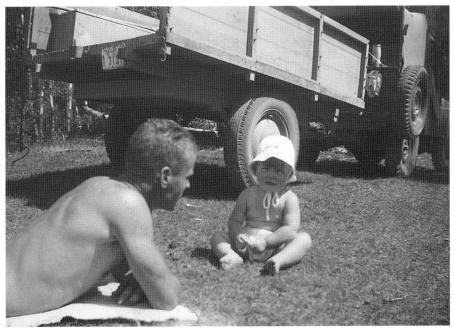

"A study in perfection" during the last days of summer 1950. When asked if he wanted another sibling for Mark, Bob said, "No, we broke the mold with this one."

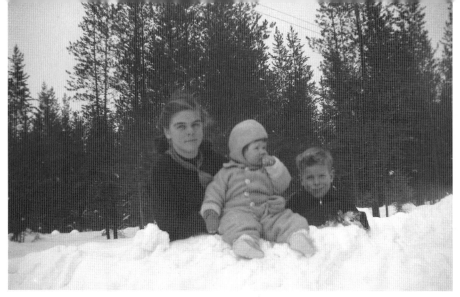

Joan, Mark and Robert, Barriere, early 1951.

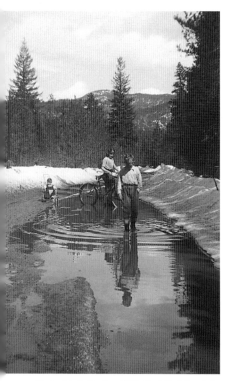

Springtime in Barriere, 1951. The kids dodge their way through the puddles.

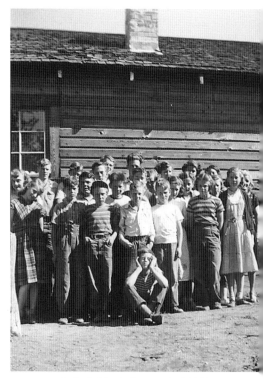

Grades 7–12 at the Barriere school, 1951.

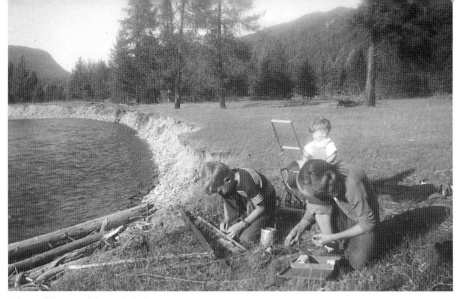

Robert and Joan river fishing with Mark,
summer Barriere 1951.

Skinny dipping in the swimming
lagoon, Barriere 1951.

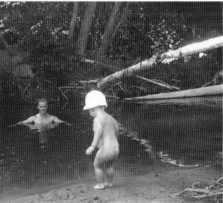

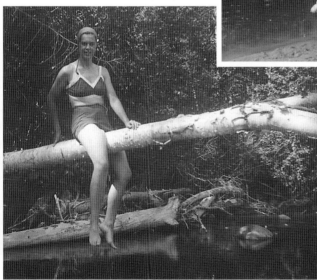

On the "bridge,"
Barriere 1951.

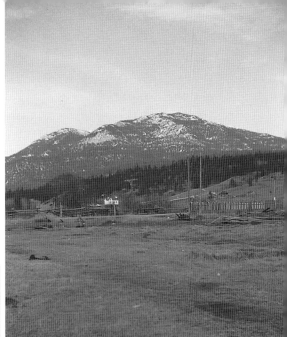

View from the house site in Clinton.

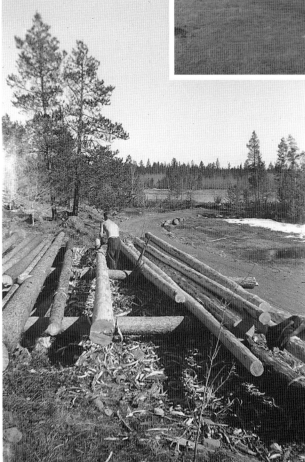

Bob peeling logs for the Clinton house on the log deck near 70 Mile, fall 1951.

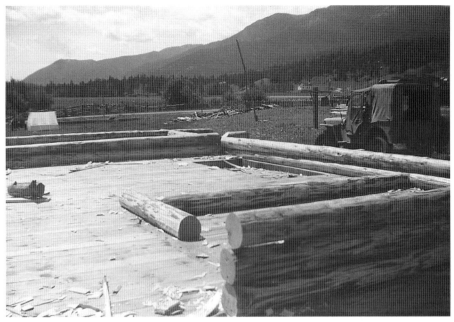

The house building begins, 1952.

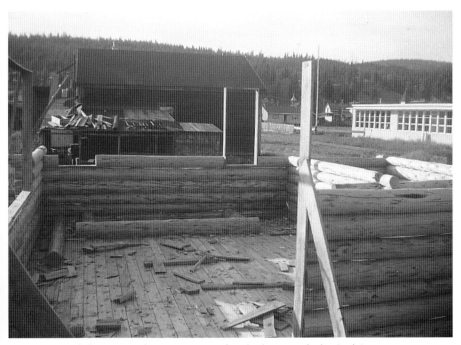

The living room under construction, across from the elementary school on Smith Avenue.

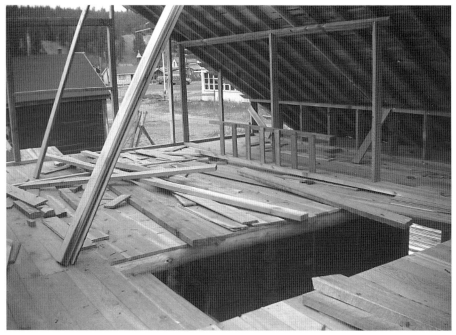

The second floor taking shape.

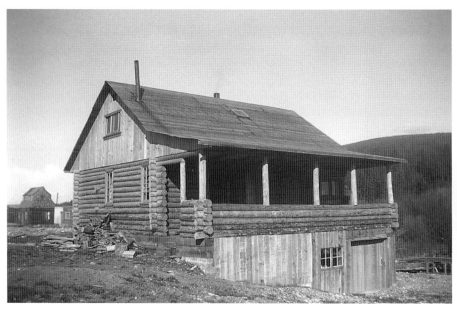

Finished!

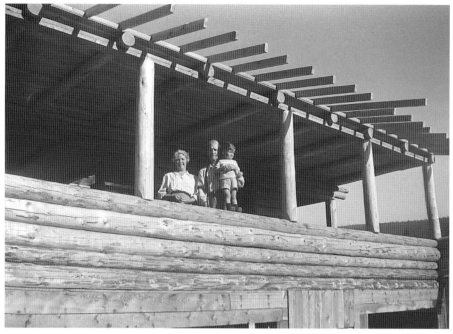

Bob's parents, Dorothy and Frank, with Mark on the completed porch.

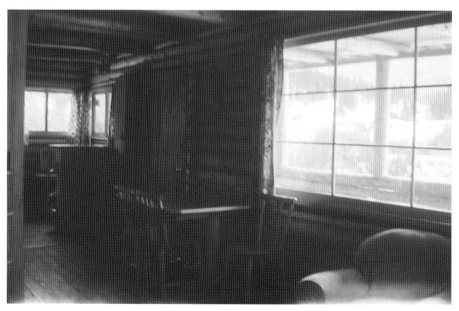

Bob's handmade table and chairs.

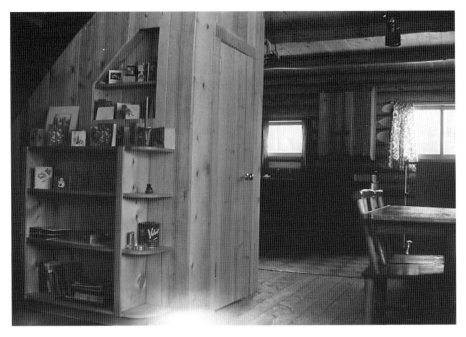

The view into the kitchen.

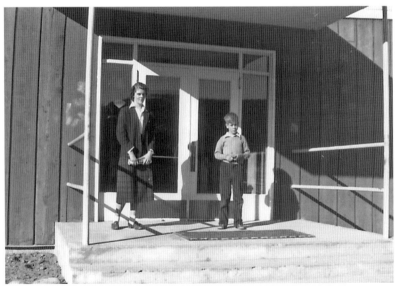

Joan starts grade 10, Robert grade 5, in 1952.

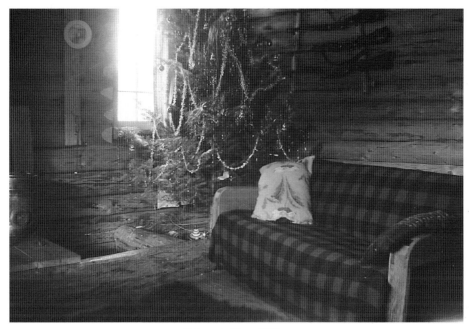

Christmas in Clinton, 1952.

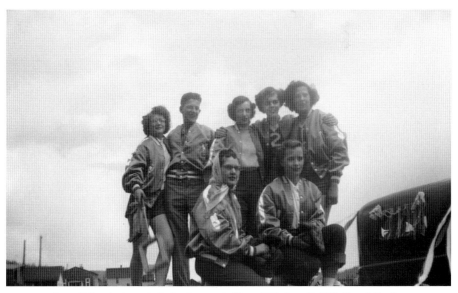

Joan with her school team in the May Day parade, Clinton 1953. Started in 1868, Clinton's May Day events are billed as the "oldest annual celebration in Canada."

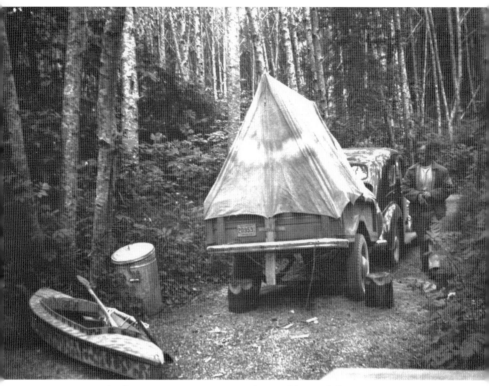

Bob at his getaway campsite at Quinsam Lake, west of the Campbell River airport, 1955.

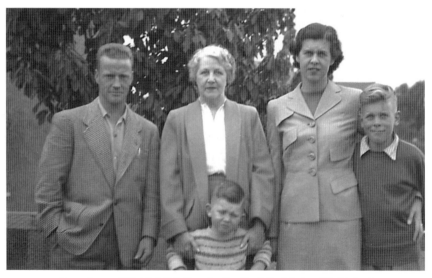

Oregon Avenue, 1956. L to R, Bob, his mother Dorothy, Stella, Robert, and Mark in front.

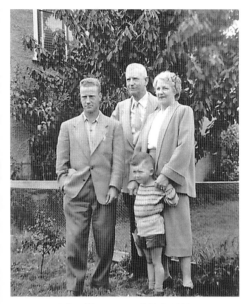

Bob and his parents with Mark, 1956.

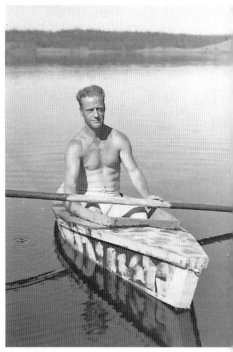

My last photograph of Bob, taken at 108 Mile in August 1956.

Family gathering at Oregon Avenue after Bob's death.

Standing: Henry, Robert, David. Seated, L to R: Joan (on stool), Stella's mother Nellie Cuming, Stella, Mark.

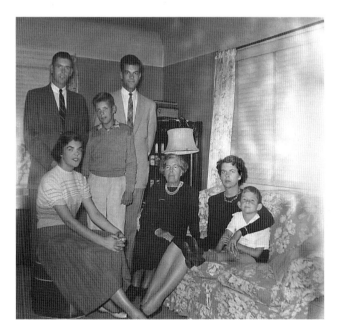

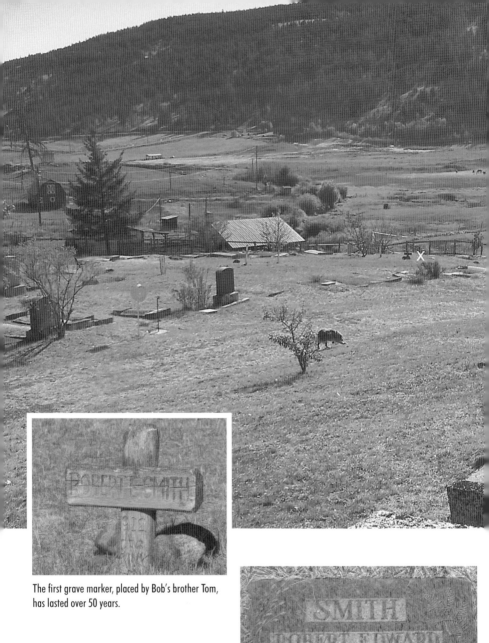

The first grave marker, placed by Bob's brother Tom, has lasted over 50 years.

The footstone on Bob's grave—"Gone Hunting."

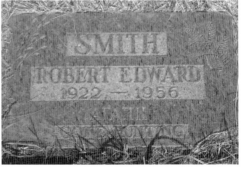

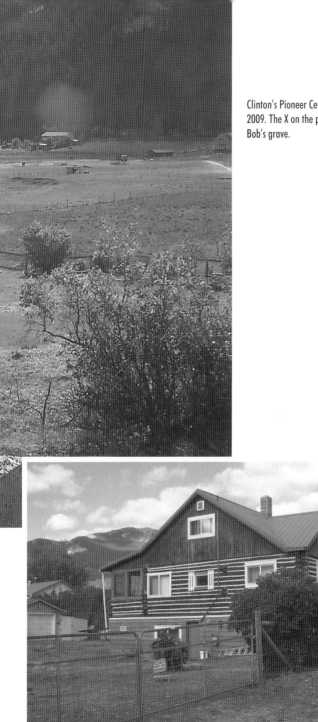

Clinton's Pioneer Cemetery ("Boot Hill") in 2009. The X on the photo shows the location of Bob's grave.

The beautifully maintained Clinton House in 2009.

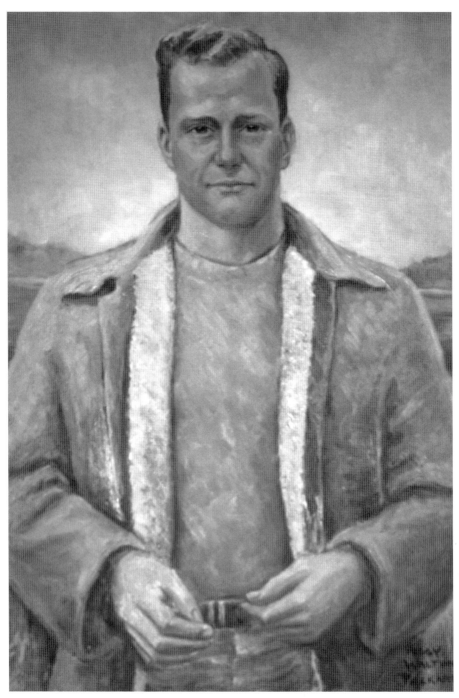

Bob in his prime. Oil painting by Peggy Walton Packard, 1957.

The Gandy Dancers

The men were feeling that summer had run out and they had had no fun. They were as confined and bushed as we were. Bob and I began to realize from some dark allusions that something was brewing among the men and it turned out that what they were all plotting was a Gandy Dancers' Ball. It was semi-legal because it was going to break many rules.

Karl and I had found out at about the same time. He had the sense to realize he was sitting on a keg of dynamite if he didn't go along with it; I envisioned a similar fate if I didn't provide some good things to eat. We pooled our resources of food and furnishings, digging in to make the thing a success.

The next night Marge reappeared from nowhere with a young male in tow. A case or two of liquor was brought downstairs and Sam brought his radio down into the dining room. The kitchen and dining room were now to be as one and the presence of Marge and I turned the event into a dance. Karl was getting a little lofty again and did not dance with me, but Sam's huge girth swung me light as thistledown. He took to bone-crushing bear hugs in his enthusiasm so that after a few turns with others I withdrew quite tired to get the coffee.

Karl came into the kitchen while I was busy and the others were whooping it up in the dining room. Bob was in there with them, perfectly happy with some beer. He always refused to dance unless he could waltz. Karl was no fool and like me had only taken one drink. The onus if things got out of hand was on him. He sat astride a chair again and began to talk of past days, as they all did. The loneliness outside the windows and the isolation seemed to bear down on their frolic.

Finally Karl's story unrolled. He had been a nightclub operator and was divorced, with one son. He had come from a big family and had worked his way up from the street corner to the management of a nightclub where he had met his wife. She had ambitions and more education than he possessed and had finally left him to better herself with another man, taking their son with her.

"Oh, what I found!" he moaned. Then, seeing himself outclassed, he had let them go, wanting his son to have those better things too. That was *his* story, but his pain was evident. I cursed myself for lack of insight as I watched him paw blindly through the teaspoons instead of picking one up for his coffee. To my horror two large tears slid down the sides of his nose to drop among the spoons.

"Maybe someday," I suggested lamely. A great smile and a new light illumined his face.

"That's what I keep hoping."

There was something about his expression that made me wonder if we were hoping for two different things. Alone again in the kitchen, I was left to ponder whether there would be reconciliation for Karl or a new ladylove. I shook my head at the frailty of men.

CHAPTER IX

Switchback Down the Thompson

Trailering

As Bob and I neared the end of our contract there was an option for renewal through the winter, but between us we already had made our grubstake—more than enough to buy the carryall and to pay our travel expenses to the Outside—and we were ready for more familiar climes.

Late August saw us back in the moosehorn house in Whitehorse where our gear had been stored while a friend of Bob's had moved in. We were packing for our exodus into friendly pastures and home hearths. We would cover the same Alcan terrain as before, only with a baby aboard; we'd do it in easy stages. We were also toying with the idea of following a perilous short cut beside the Thompson River to reach Kamloops.

In no time at all we found that an army carryall would not carry all. The Americans also called it a "power wagon," a cross between a jeep that could go anywhere and an army van with huge tires. It was necessary to get a trailer. Again the army obliged from out of their surplus and came up with one to match our vehicle.

The trailer took all the crates, trunks and boxes of things we would need until we settled down again. Our tent, sleeping bags and guns went into the wagon with suitcases and food boxes, along with jerry cans of gas and water bottles. There were a number of spare tires but we were not expecting these monsters to blow out in any terrain, especially as they would be no fun to take off and put on again. There was no helpful brother this time as Tom had gone ranching in Alberta.

The rig was quite a sight. At the last minute Bob swore as I ran out with a cardboard box of photos and memorabilia. He was too quick for me and had just finished nailing up the final crate.

"I'll just have to stuff it in here," he said determinedly, poking the box down in a corner by the tailgate, "and you'll just have to take a chance on how it survives."

The huge box trailer was securely covered with a tarpaulin. Any ropes or riggings were always secured navy style; at times I wondered if anyone brushed with salt for a few years ever got over it. The little green skiff was roped upside down on the roof of the power wagon. Inside, everything was packed in order of easy access from the front seats. Right behind my seat was Mark's bed box, which was to become his home for a month or so. He was a big baby, probably overfed, but had not reached the point where he scrambled around a lot or stood up, for which I thanked God. He took everything well.

People said we were "bound to come to trouble" in taking a trailer over the Alcan, but trouble was something we faced when we hit it. Bob believed that you didn't experience or learn anything if you didn't try it; it was better to try it yourself than ask people how, and better than sitting at home while others told their tales. I soon caught his spirit.

He did not recount his exploits much; he simply enjoyed them and went on to the next thing. Walking around BC was his forte. Before his Teslin–Telegraph hike he had tramped from Anahim Lake to Bella Coola—from the middle of BC to the West Coast. He was basically shy and modest underneath all the bluff, and although anecdotal to amuse others, he never bragged.

Dust plumes were soon flying again. The first stop was Teslin Village and again we could not find Shorty Johnson. Bob had wanted so very much to enlighten him about negotiating the Trail successfully after being called "nuts."

On the way out from Whitehorse we had bypassed Marsh Lake Lodge as a sad dream. Bob would drive by such places with a glazed look that to my suspicious mind read, "I'll be back"—if not to these places then to others like them. For now we had to settle down and he thought he wanted to do it in central BC.

It took roughly four days to get down to Mile Zero. We set up camp each day, with stops for food and leisurely inspections, depending on road conditions as to whether we could make time with such clumsy equipment or whether we should stop short of some goal. Seen in reverse, the highway looked different. Downhill grades were now uphill. The baby made a difference. For shelter we were not loath to enjoy a decent campsite instead of a makeshift one. Just under a hundred miles from Teslin, we made our first camp near the Rancheria River where we could get gas and water.

Nightfall towards the end of summer was around 7:00 p.m. Our usual travel procedure with the baby was to make camp at about 4:00 p.m. and break camp at 8:00 a.m., spending roughly eight hours on the road, with food stops.

The manner of our tenting was always the same. The site would have a grove of trees between which Bob would string another tarpaulin high enough to walk under and beneath which we pitched the small tent; a crate containing pots, fry pan and groceries was emptied and up-ended as a table; and a good cooking fire was started just outside the dwelling. It could rain hard during the night and we'd be dry, but it was bears we were afraid of. We sealed the food in our cook kit, either hung in a tree or taken into the tent with us. The last idea was not good. One night we heard a distinct scratching sound going on outside and very close to us. Bob woke me up.

"Listen!" The scratching sound seemed very close, in fact just on the other side of the canvas.

"Bears!" he hissed. I sat up in my sleeping bag terrified, only to see him convulsed into a ball and shaking with mirth. The devil had put his hand out under the tent wall and had been scrabbling his fingers in the gravel.

The day after, the Rancheria saw us through the Cassiars and Big Creek to Upper Liard Village then Watson Lake, where we took a breather and went into the hotel. After lunch there we decided to skip camping and put in the night at Lower Liard Lodge. And after that it was over the border and into BC at last, stopping at Lower Post for a beer. The trading activity around there held us and we did not leave easily. After Lower Post came the Hyland River, then Contact Creek, Smith River and the Liard, where we got a cabin.

We had crowed too soon about having no trouble with the trailer and carryall. We were heading for Fort Nelson again and would have to make time through at least one hundred sixty miles of Rockies from Muncho Lake, via those Stone Mountains up to the summit of 4,000-odd feet then drop down again. In there were some rough tests for the trailer even if the carryall was equal to everything. At the time there was no other route to the coast, except by rail or sea.

By now every single thing was plastered with lumps and gouts of mud, all over the trailer, the tarp, the hitch and the little boat's bottom inverted on top of the wagon: It seemed worse and messier than our experience on the way up. In fact mud flew so high that the tallest freight vans were studded with gobs from wheels to roof.

At Muncho it was early, too early to stay over, and once more we took coffee and wandered with no excuse to camp. I longed to stay there and drink it all in. All that beauty and blueness filtered into our souls but did not belong in our lives; we had to make real time through the mountains. Somewhere between Muncho and Summit Lakes on a flat stretch of road a car passed us with people flapping shirts and handkerchiefs to make us stop.

"Didn't you hear us? We've been honking at you for miles. You've left a trail of paper all down the highway."

They were my photographs and personal papers from the box inside the tailgate and had worked loose. It was useless to go back over a long, long road. As it happened I was able to replace much of it from copies held by relatives, but I was sick at my own carelessness.

It was downhill to Fort Nelson through forty-odd miles of spewing gravel and possible mountain squalls. We did not want to stay in that town again or renew acquaintanceships but we'd need to make use of its garages on the highway's edge, which would be closed when we got there. Haste being pointless we came down the long grade from Steamboat Mountain to make camp some twenty-five miles short of Fort Nelson. We had forgotten to carry water again, not being too worried about finding it. This time we were skunked. I had Mark's bottle to make up, not to mention tea for ourselves.

We had chosen a rather pretty place off a curve in the highway, which was now wending through muskeg. There was no stream in sight or any water save in small pools of runoff or groundwater among the lush grasses and flowers.

"You'll just have to boil the swamp water," advised Bob as he got busy with our fire. "To hell with this. Tomorrow we sleep in Dawson Creek."

It was a hasty camp using the small tent and the inside of the wagon for shelter. Gingerly I lowered the billycan into a little pool, being careful not to let bugs drop into the water. When it boiled and the time came to pour I was horrified to find the water full of tiny cooked shrimp. Bob laughed his head off.

"They're only crayfish. Freshwater shrimp. You could eat them." But I noticed he didn't. Taking a large clean white hanky I strained out the beastly things then reboiled the water. Like the good little sourdough he was, Mark drank swamp water with his canned milk.

Luck gradually deserted us after that. Arriving at the outskirts of Fort Nelson we found the highway lined with giant gumbo-covered vans, some pulling trailers the same size. Beside these our messy caravan did not look that insignificant compared with the cars and small trucks that were floundering around in the stew of sheer slime. We had never had to winch ourselves out of any holes, but might. Engine, radiator, trailer hitch and tires were checked. We loaded up with extra oil and gas.

Somewhere near Beaver River a car passed us with the occupants yelling, "Your trailer's gone! It's a way, way down the road. Couldn't you hear us?" No. The sound of the engine and the noise of the big tires on flying gravel made car horns remote unless they were right behind.

We turned the wagon around, saying our prayers. Everything we needed for living was in that trailer and even now somebody might be pilfering it. Or it might be upside down. Or down a cliff. Or was the hitch broken beyond repair?

Mercifully it was only a mile or two back and obligingly nestled upright but slightly canted on the shoulder of the road. The hitch was unharmed and the tarp intact. Somehow the hitch cap had jounced off its ball base and the strain had been too much on the emergency chain. We backed up to lift the shaft onto the hitch, wired the chain together, and bound the whole with stout rope. There was nothing we did not carry in the way of block and tackle, ropes, wire, repair kit, lantern and shovel.

"Just keep your fingers crossed until we get to Dawson. There's still mountain country ahead." And two hundred miles to Mile Zero.

Nothing worse happened. We got up to the 4,000-foot level at Trutch and down by the Bucking Horse and Sikhanni Chief Rivers. After Pink Mountain we were facing the worst ordeal of towing a trailer—that Suicide Hill again. With beads of sweat running down his face Bob eased the rig slowly over the downhill approach to prevent slewing and swaying, without mishap. Then we went into bull low and I sat with fists clenched as the wagon dragged the weight up the supposed one-foot-in-ten gradient.

Dawson Creek saw the hitch welded, some cable added, and supplies and fuel replenished. Now we had a decision to make. Should we play it safe and go home from Edmonton to the coast via Banff and the Columbia Highway, or take that shortcut we had heard about that went from Edmonton to Jasper and down to Blue River and Kamloops, known as the Yellowhead Road? In those days you had to go to Edmonton first, since the northern section of what is now Highway 97 from Vancouver to Prince George did not yet exist. Very few people knew of the Yellowhead's existence and we'd have to find out in Edmonton if it was passable. Ultimately we were going to the coast to pay respects and present our son before settling down.

Coming down south along the shores of Lesser Slave Lake again I took in what I could of missions, old posts and constant reminders of the Jesuits. No stopping for photos. What really frustrated me were the road banks on the Alaska Highway— and now here on the road to Edmonton—which were dripping with fat blueberries and other berries. The banks were alive with Michaelmas daisies and what I called brown-eyed Susans. No time to play with jam pots or flowers. It was just as bad for Bob in having to forego stepping out with his gun. The plentiful wildlife was everything he'd known. It would have made angels swear. We hoped passionately that soon we would live right among such gamey opportunities.

Information concerning the Yellowhead Road was sparse. We tried an information booth at Jasper Park's eastern gate, but were sent to the local ranger. He didn't know much. Our best bet, he said, was to get the lowdown this side of the Yellowhead Pass, and if the route looked too bad to give up and return via Jasper to Edmonton then head south. It was now the rainy season and the weather might not hold. We might find deep bogs in low-lying places, and washouts.

"It's just a trail, you know," said the ranger, "but with that winch and in low gear you are better off than most, and with trees along the road you should be able to wind yourselves out of any hole. You should be able to make it."

I was really afraid, especially with a baby in the car. Then I realized Bob was in no hurry to imperil us, or the expensive equipage for which he had so many plans, and so I left things to him. I would have done anything rather than have that little beast call me chicken, especially as he was doing his best to keep us upright.

The Yellowhead Route

"Proceed with caution," said the sign. "All who travel beyond this point do so at their own risk."

We were on a narrow road through Jasper Park and west of Jasper that was meant only for maintenance crews, pack-horses and the very adventurous. This was a much-contested short alternative to the Jasper–Banff and Big Bend route to the coast and purported to be the future connecting link between Jasper and the Trans-Canada Highway. It was a shortcut to Vancouver via Kamloops, where the Yellowhead Road ended, saving a distance of three hundred miles. Many years later, in 1970, the Yellowhead Highway would become Highway 16 and run all the way from Portage La Prairie in Manitoba to Masset in Haida Gwaii (the Queen Charlotte Islands), with a spur between Tête Jaune Cache and Kamloops now known as the South Yellowhead or Highway 5.

But the Yellowhead then was just a goat trail, mostly following the Canadian National Railway (CNR) south down the Thompson River at a great height above it, and was built by Japanese labour during the war when the Japanese had been interned. According to authorities at either end, the road was impassable and "you could take your life into your own hands." Two years after we went through better bridges were installed, so somebody must have been using it.

We found ourselves wandering through the pretty little world of the Miette River, which was small, flat and lazy among fields of grasses, creative oxbows for itself. Set back from the road was a sort of dubious hotel with a lot of long grass in front of it. The owners told us that the occasional car had come through, but we picked up no more details there than we had from the ranger. We were told to make it snappy before the weather changed, although they did remember one man who seemed to make it in all weathers when coming up from Kamloops to see his mother. That was good enough for Bob.

The little road was gravel and rutted, following every contour up, down and around, with no room to pass. Grass grew between the ruts for some miles. Save a few fields, the whole area was deeply forested. Some Americans were fishing hopefully along the river, with their cars backed into crevices or parked daringly along the bank. Absently swatting bugs with one hand while they fished with the other, they were the last signs of civilization we saw before reaching the western limits of Jasper Park.

Innumerable little trestles in the gravel trail were built over small streams. Our whole rig weighed three-plus tons and we passed the test of the first little bridge which had a posted weight limit of three tons, otherwise the whole expedition would have ended right there. The little road and river crossed each other endlessly via bridges, which were so low in some instances that the wood smacked the water under our weight. (Later torrential rains washed these bridges right out, but some were replaced.)

Jasper Park boundary came at Yellowhead Pass and the road then went into Mount Robson Park at the foot of the mountain. Soon we were following a trickling stream, which to our amazement was labelled "Fraser River." We couldn't believe the sign. It went under a little trestle and as we crossed it our weight again made the wood slap the water.

The pass we had come through did not affect us scenically after experiencing the Alcan, but might seem spectacular to others. Later we learned that the Overlanders, a group of explorers from eastern Canada, had used it in 1862. They had split into two parties after coming out of the Yellow-head pass, one to follow the Fraser River and the other the Thompson, down which went our goat trail.

Working south along the shore of Yellowhead Lake, we suddenly came upon a log-built lodge with cabins and campgrounds. Passing by the lodge we bumped along beside a bigger creek that contained the Fraser stream, to find it ended in Moose Lake. That new creek en-

||||||||||||||||||||||||||||||||||||||||||||||||||||||||||||||||||||

The Overlanders were a group of over 100 men and one woman, Catherine O'Hare Schubert, from eastern Canada heading for the Cariboo gold rush of the 1860s. Mrs. Schubert was the first European woman to enter British Columbia by land, following the southern route along the Thompson River on horseback and while pregnant, with her three other children slung in panniers on packhorses. Her baby, Rose, was said to be the first white child born at Fort Kamloops.

tering the lake actually was the Fraser River, for from the end of Moose Lake it flowed northward in a crescent to turn and drop down the centre of BC to Vancouver. All the other water in this country was running south to the Columbia River. In effect, both these great rivers could be said to arise from around Yellowhead Pass. We were slated to follow a river system southwards, involving the McLellan River, the Canoe River and finally the North Thompson, which does not become the Thompson proper until it hits the main river at Kamloops.

The mountain lakes in the Robson area were the scenic pride of the CNR, from its raised rail bed, but our little wagon road went right along their shores, as trains do not, and followed the whole wild waterway as the subsequent Highway 16 could never do. An arterial highway must use the easiest route and often had to give up the scenic one.

From Moose Lake the Fraser entered Fraser Lake to emerge as a boisterous little river not a dozen feet across. Still within Mount Robson Park we ran through forest and into Red Pass Junction, a jungle of tracks and red sheds. Until now we had been keeping abreast of the westbound CNR line from Jasper but it turned north at Red Pass, heading for Prince George and Prince Rupert, the train used so frequently by our Burns Lake people. We were pretty optimistic.

The way was now canopied overhead by the trees, which shut out light, and the rails beside it were not visible. The northbound CNR from Kamloops, unseen by us, had come up to join the southbound Rupert line at Red Pass, where both tracks merged to head back east towards Jasper. Red Pass Junction with all its rails was a remote, brave, empty little place in the middle of a lot of dark forest. The whole impact of the cart track from Yellowhead to this settlement had been one of overhanging gloom as we tunnelled under the evergreen canopy. The sun just did not get in except by the two lakeshore areas. Shortly, by contrast, we were to see one of the sights of our lives, which made up for fun lost on the Alcan.

The old carryall and its load were beating up a real animal track. Although we were still in Robson Park we could not see the mountain and thought we were on the side of it. We were gearing down a sudden torturous drop when suddenly we came out into the most breathtaking scene yet, a V-shaped river valley, flat and green and sandy, with gravel bars and the Fraser again, now turned seafoam by one of the many tributaries that fed it. Blocking the end of this valley and shutting out the sun was the menacing height of Mount Robson, exposed from base to peak. The sharp-cut tip towered over us and its angular, colourful rock faces came right down into the bright green meadow. At the foot of the mountain ran its own wide milky green river, the Robson, carrying glacial silt toward its confluence with the Fraser at Tête Jaune Cache.

"Here we stay," decided Bob.

It was paradise. We were at the rear of Robson and it was all ours. Nobody else was seeing what we were seeing or could, unless they had the courage to take the same road. The scene in its entirety was not visible from a train window, and in any case the line was further south. We made camp on a natural grassy site where hunters and back packers had left some small fire pits. Bob and I were now sixty miles from Jasper but it seemed like six hundred. And we were afraid of what lay ahead.

"Let's enjoy this while we can. I wish to God I had a river caster."

He meant the sort of line and lure that bounces enticingly off river boulders, the lure weighty enough not to pop up but not heavy enough to sink, which could be held behind a rock by fast water over any good fish sheltering there.

It was like finding Everest in your back yard, to crawl out in the morning and look up at the towering ridge. It was so close. Among the mountains in early fall with the dawning sunlight on it, Robson seemed a very local mountain, with colours and sharp ridges and flat rock walls rising to that sharp peak against the sky. Its rosy majesty at sunset gave an aura of far greater height than the 9,000 feet it towered above us. Its setting in a field of emerald grass, cut through by milk green rivers, enhanced its singleness. Mount Whitehorn and others are behind it but all we had eyes for was Mount Robson.

With great reluctance we left the heavenly place in the early morning and took to the little road. Ahead lay the unknown worst. Bob did not want to frighten me with his apprehensions and I did not want him to know how scared I was, so each said nothing. So far the hitch was holding.

Before the hitch did go we passed little places with names like Swift Current, Emperor and Swift Water. Before reaching Blue River there would be fifteen or twenty stops, but most of them were just nameplates and a siding down on the line. Our trail went through some groups of settlements but the others clustered down by the railway. Only a few of these survived Highway 16. We were seeing history and making it.

The hitch broke just before we reached the McBride cutoff at Tête Jaune Cache (pronounced "tee jon cash" by the locals). We lashed the trailer again with more chain but were afraid that constant friction would wear it through. The rest of the journey would have to be made at snail's pace. Without trailer trouble we might have gone through in one day; it took three because of the overload.

There were no welders afoot early Sunday morning when we crawled into Tête Jaune. We turned south with apprehension. The road, after a brave little start, became the usual two-wheeled track with grass down its centre, our lot for the next seventy miles. We saw abandoned trappers' cabins and beaver traps and some pole cutters' camps still in use by solitary souls, and construction camps left behind by the Japanese.

As we passed, Bob discussed his Japanese friends in Steveston who had been interned, and one of my friends had dated a Japanese man. It all came home to us now. Being logical, Bob said it was the fortunes of war and what could you do about it? Looking back at those days, some of us *were* afraid that some of our Japanese friends might just get mad enough to collaborate with Japan, the prevailing belief being that blood was thicker than water. In the camps the internees were paid twenty-five cents an hour for shovelling dirt and many, if not most, much preferred that to sitting around in a concentration camp. They were proud and industrious. What most of us thought was that it was only for a while and they'd get everything back. We trusted our government to be honourable. The

During World War II the War Measures Act was used to intern Canadians, and 26 internment camps were set up across Canada.

After the bombing of Pearl Harbor in 1942, the government passed an Order in Council authorizing the removal of "enemy aliens" within a 100-mile radius of the BC coast. On March 4, 1942, 22,000 Japanese Canadians were given 24 hours to pack before being interned. They were first incarcerated in a temporary facility at Hastings Park Race Track in Vancouver. Women, children and older people were sent to internment camps in the Interior. Others were forced into road construction camps.

The property of the Japanese Canadians—land, businesses, and other assets—were confiscated by the government and sold, and the proceeds used to pay for their internment. In 1945, the government extended the Order in Council to force the Japanese Canadians to go to Japan and lose their Canadian citizenship, or move to eastern Canada. Even though the war was over, it was illegal for Japanese Canadians to return to Vancouver until 1949. In 1988 Canada apologized for this miscarriage of justice, admitting that the actions of the government were influenced by racial discrimination. The government signed a redress agreement providing a small amount of money compensation.

Author: Diana Breti
Copyright © 1998 The Law Connection
Centre for Education, Law and Society (CELS)
Simon Fraser University, Vancouver, British Columbia

shock and shame came later over the sale of Japanese fishing boats and property. We interned other Axis-related Canadians as well, and people forget that.

Nevertheless, the Yellowhead Route was built almost entirely by Japanese Canadians, naturalized or native, and it is a memorial to them and should remain so conspicuously, even though buried under Highways 5 and 16.

Tête Jaune Cache was also the beginning of a branch road north through McBride to Prince George. It was said to be in the same shape as the Blue River route (where our Yellowhead Trail would end), lacking, some thought, about seventy miles to make the link between McBride and Prince George, said seventy miles being a goat trail like ours. In those days you could not get from Jasper to Prince George unless you went completely south to Banff and the Big Bend and back north again through the Cariboo. Rogers Pass Highway was non-existent. In 1950, in order to go north from McBride or south like us, you needed a jeep or 4-wheel drive and high ground clearance. Not to mention rope, shovel and axe.

The Corduroy Road

The wagon made it through cedar bogs and over corduroy railway ties quite well in bull low, through thick green gloom and damp foliage. Huge mosquitoes got into the car. Our goat trail was to lead to Blue River on the North Thompson.

What struck me vividly were the pioneer homesteads started by the Overlanders who had gone back after their trek to build log houses and little corrals, which were kept up right until we saw them, or at least until the big highway went through.

We passed many cabins and corrals deep in the woods but we didn't see a soul, except once when the trail at one place went right through a group of cabins that were on its verge. We were driving through a lane between wattle fences when we passed a house so close to the road we could look into the rooms and touch the porch from our car. A woman inside merely looked up and we stopped to ask her for directions. It was very awkward but the intrusion came about because we were sitting so high up in the power wagon, whereas an ordinary car seat would have placed us just below her vision. She didn't seem to mind. She thought we could get through and said there was a garage at Valemont, and a store.

We continued through the soggy shade—which hid great wallows of mud filled with branches and other signs of struggle—and over more corduroy without mishap until the car trail did come out at Valemont.

Bob's temper had been reigned in admirably during boggy stretches, but he was showing the strain. I tried not to show mine. For instance, in many places the corduroy had been covered with saplings over the worst wallows where crews from time to time had taken pity on us travellers. The saplings held and we often drove half in and half out of the bogs to keep traction. Once we winched ourselves out by fastening a cable around a trunk among a belt of firs whose shade kept the mire boggy. The winch system wound us out as neatly as one slides off a glove.

After much of this we would light a fire and eat. There was no fire hazard due to frequent rains and we were lucky enough to miss them when we stopped.

Valemont was a little settlement served by the CNR, with a general store, pub and garage. We left the bone breaker carryall, which seemed to have no shock absorbers, to be welded to its load, then gathered supplies and were finally on our way through bush.

Camp Creek ran past us to join the Canoe River heading south further over, but east of our route and unseen. Some thought the Yellowhead way should have come up the Canoe's valley but it would have wasted existing road.

At Albreda the road, enclosed by trees each side, dropped almost vertically down to the station, situated at the bottom of a horseshoe dip. There was no escaping it. We went down, and up, without pausing for a second, and saw nothing of either side. But that did it. The welding technique back at Valemont had been the rustic type. The swinging jounce at Albreda broke the hitch again just as we were about to sight the North Thompson. We ran off into a field. Fuming and even frightened, we wound the connection again with lengths of chain. All our worldly goods were in that trailer and there would be steep drops ahead. The whole seventy miles of goat trail averaged out at a speed of ten miles per hour. In the morning, from nine to noon, we could cover thirty miles. Afternoons, from about two to four, we'd cover about twenty miles.

After fixing the hitch we crawled along well into the dark until we found a spot to pull into near a stream at the bottom of a hill. We barely squeezed in. It was a black night and raining and we climbed into our sleeping bags and passed into oblivion. My last image was of the gas lamp set down in the middle of the road—while we'd tried to eat—which illumined the dripping branches overhead. We rescued and doused the lamp. Tomorrow looked unbearable. During the night bright lights and grinding gears woke us as a public works jeep went by. It was the only vehicle we met and must have been sent in from Jasper.

Stiff with cramp next morning we made coffee on the Coleman and pushed off. Mark always got his bottle and made no trouble. Wet plants hung over the road, loaded with some of the biggest berries we had ever seen. From there to Blue River the banks were full of them: blackberries, salmonberries, cranberries and blueberries. And sudden death over the brink.

We spent a terrifying morning driving around the edges and saying nothing while the usual BC grandeur rolled by. We were usually about five hundred feet above the railway track. After Albreda came whistle stops like Clemina and Gosnell down on the line. We used our lowest gear a great deal as we followed every curve and hump, up and down. The road disappeared entirely several times in great washouts but we skirted these edges safely through fields.

Down before us an incline was so sharp and steep we didn't know if the entire rig could go down without jack-knifing. If it did we'd go over the edge. To crawl ahead was easy but to crawl down vertically without a single stone dislodging the trailer's progress was pretty chancy. It was what we had to do.

I got Bob off to a good start by yelling, "Stop! Stop! Let me out to guide you." He knew my fears the second I grabbed the baby and took him with me down the slope. I did guide Bob with signs where the wheels must keep straight and he did ease the whole load down the grade to stop at a safe place. His face was lobster coloured and sweat was dripping off his nose.

"Some wife you are," he said quietly. "You were going to let me go over the cliff alone."

Right. Maternal instinct was uttermost and Mark was to survive. If there had been no baby I am not sure what I would have done. Stayed with him scared sick but afraid to lose face, most likely. In the end he would have had to let me guide him; thus one rationalizes. It was snatching the baby that had unnerved him.

The road flattened out through a cedar grove by early forenoon that day. The cedars were so old they resembled the California redwoods in size and antiquity. All the damp and bogginess disappeared as we drove out of the heat and glare of the upper reaches into the coolest fairytale lane floored with hard packed sand. We were safe. Whether or not the ordeal had been worth a saving of three hundred miles never entered my head. I did not hold post mortems over Bob's decisions.

The mountainous stretch we had left behind had gone through Pyramid, Lempriere and Thunder River. No cabins were visible at those sites, but cutters from abandoned camps must have placed their poles at the railway stops so designated. The next station, very appropriately labelled Red Sand, came where the groves petered out into a sandy waste bristling with jack pines and tire tracks going fruitlessly about. The road vanished completely here. Trusting to luck and hunches, we trailed ruts that seemed to lead straight ahead.

Suddenly we came upon the town of Blue River. The relief was enormous.

Flipping Salmon

Blue River was like some of the villages in the Fraser Canyon at that time. The houses were shingled with cedar shakes and there were dirt roads and pole fences. Women went about in cotton dresses and there was much activity. While I tried the stores Bob applied himself to the pursuit of information. We found we could get the hitch welded again at a pole cutter's camp where the Blue River blacksmith had a forge.

Bob left the baby and me with the camp's cook while he drove the blacksmith across the field to his shop. I found myself alone with some woodcutters and drinking coffee with them. They asked polite questions but were stiff and strange with me, which made me stiff and strange with them. I still had to learn the art of jollying along. When Bob and the blacksmith came back we were pressed to join the crew for lunch, which seemed to put the little cook into a panic; however many bowls of amazing mixtures were put in front of us all at once and nobody spoke a word as we ate.

"He wouldn't take any pay," Bob told me, once we were alone and bumping back across the field. The hitch was superbly welded. "I gave him ten bucks anyway. Where would we be without people like that? I ask you, where would we be?"

Blue River had a bus terminal of sorts, with gas stations, stores and houses spread along the jack pine flats. The road south out of it was graded gravel, wide enough for cars to pass most of the time, but sometimes not. Used as the North Thompson Highway, it was very narrow for trucks and buses and sometimes dangerous.

All the little names went flying by: Angushorn, Wolfenden, Messiter, Cottonwood Flats, Avola, Vavenby, and Birch Island. Some have survived and some have not. There was once a Porte d'Enfer Canyon, reported by the Overlanders.

We were cruising happily along the home stretch for Kamloops, passing well-known sportsmen's meccas like Clearwater and the country around Wells Gray Park. It was outside Clearwater that a piece of the engine dropped through onto the road and Bob simply shored it back into place by putting a roadside board under it.

The North Thompson was flowing smoothly now with islands in it and sand bars. Gold leaves were fluttering off the poplars that lined the banks or grew on its islands. Their white trunks gleamed for miles. Further down the poplars were overridden by birch, alder and cottonwoods. The rest of the trees were jack pine, but among the scrubby pines there began to appear a newcomer, to me at least—the ponderosa. This is a pine among pines, with huge cones.

It would become my next favourite tree to the madrona or arbutus on the coast. An arbutus trunk was something you could walk up to and put your arms around with its smooth red-brown warmth. I used to play with the silver curling bark, revealing its bright green undersides and pretend to be writing on parchment—not the first child to think of it. Now the ponderosa woods could fascinate with their open sweeps of land among the trees, the ground laden with those enormous cones to crow over, with a heavenly warm scent everywhere. The ponderosa has majesty and generosity.

Cottonwood prevailed near the river. They made a vista of gleaming white trunks with black knotholes and leaves with silver undersides stirred by the river's breezes. This was cattle country and in some places it looked like Kentucky Blue Grass Country. There were miles and miles of paddocks with white fences and green, green grass across which shiny black stallions paced leisurely or nosed over the rails.

There was no suitable camping spot near Clearwater. We tried the ranger station on Birch Island, approached by a bridge, but there was no one around to sanction camping nearby. The closer to civilization, the stricter the rules.

"Better keep going," Bob decided. There's bound to be some spot by the river sooner or later." It was not on the North Thompson when we found it. Backtracking north we returned to a road we had seen going up beside the Raft River, which was quite wide and full of spawning salmon. The red of their backs was visible from the highway. "This is it!" we agreed, turning into the bush and spurning organized campgrounds.

On a sheltered flat greensward beside the river we stretched the tarp out fully and made a fine home of it. With a one-day stopover there was plenty of time to wash clothes, wash the carryall, repack shifted belongings and eat our heads off. The main goal of course was to get salmon. There were quite a few edible ones hiding their long olive-green shapes behind boulders before the next dart upstream.

Since they would not take the bait the plan was for me to grab one by the tail, my own idea, while Bob, standing up close, bashed it with a club. At first he thought of shooting one as he had on the Telegraph Trail, where the streams were so full of fish you could almost flip them out. He had simply put a bullet into a fish's head. We discarded this idea because of swift water and ricochet. The fish were so big and represented such a feast after cans and cans of this and that; the whole prospect was such a lark.

I rolled up my slacks and soaked my sneakers as I stepped into the icy water onto slimy round rocks. We looked for edible ones turning from silver to green, as anything darker would be mushy. Then I saw a long green form of qualifying

213

hue in front of me, barely visible, fanning its fins in slow lazy fashion as it rested in the lee of a rock. It didn't seem to see me as I got closer.

"Get set. I'm ready." Bob had positioned himself in the water with club poised, prepared to move closer. We held our breath as I got right behind the salmon, which still did not notice me. Slowly, slowly my hands reached out towards that tail fin and, aiming at a double sure-fire grip, I clamped it suddenly with both hands as tightly as I could.

It shook me like a rat. I was hanging on to a fully charged power station. There was no holding on to so much strength and force unless I wanted a wet ride up the Raft. I had not really expected success and felt grudging admiration. I let go. It shot up the river, dodging and darting with indignation.

Bob was more convulsed than concerned over a lost dinner. "That's that. Guess it's just as well we didn't try to shoot it. There's no way we are going to eat salmon now." It is too bad spawning fish don't take a lure. We ate fried Spam and watched the fish fly by.

Our next stop was at a little round deep mirror called Dutch Lake, where a couple of old ladies presided over a lonely little resort with a charming old main house. It had a veranda, where you could take tea. There were one or two cabins for rent. It all appealed to Bob who was sweetness and light to the old girls, finding out their cabin rates and dallying by the dock. He declined their kind offer of tea politely while secretly raising his little pinkie at me. I would have loved an old-fashioned tea, but Bob wanted a steak.

Over the years we never knew what it was about Dutch Lake that was to draw us back on North Thompson family outings. Perhaps it was the old world aspect. Any deep round little lake is fetching, fringed with trees and sporting busy fish, flitting swallows and dragonflies, a good stop off for a break or having a picnic.

"Good Lord, look at all the fish!" I called from the dock.

"Ugh!" shivered Bob. "Those are just big fat suckers. The other fish won't stand a chance. Any lake this size with those in it has had it." Always some new dampener to learn about.

Suckers were presentably sized silver fish, looking edible but for their horrible gaping mouths. They ate everything in any lake they controlled.

With steak calling we were finally, towards dusk, at the end of our journey and over the little red bridge into Kamloops. After that would come the coastal firing squad.

Home Fires

Both grandmothers made idiots of themselves over Mark.

Bob's mother was a very pretty woman with a plump bosom, a very direct and cheerful manner, and an agreeable approach when faced with me. His parents were in an apartment in Kitsilano and had no penchant for the bush life any more. This was my first meeting with them.

Bob's father took Mark upon his knee and said, "We're keeping this one." He referred to Tom's son Larry, totally lost by divorce. I told him he could keep Mark with bells on. No danger of history repeating.

Bob's father was fair and balding. He was the same height as Tom and me—five foot eight—and had been very stocky. He was a Yorkshire man through and through, well spoken and gentle of speech but very firm. He was a retired bank manager, self-educated after the age of thirteen and very erudite.

Then the little monkey was laid upon Granny's bosom where he sprawled himself and wriggled and wriggled in, just loving this warm soft spot. That will be enough of that, I thought. Was she encouraging him?

In Victoria, my mother was not much better. Definitely not the type to encourage sensuousness, she yet cooed over my baby to a nauseating degree. Any baby completely unbuttoned her.

Reception of us was a little different.

Bob's mother had received me with a sort of fifty-fifty attitude and would, he told me, "meet anyone half way." Bob had been right. She would meet anyone halfway as a conscious policy, but if you didn't do the same, look out! She was as direct as my mother (both Englishwomen).

"Well, Stella? What shall it be? I can't stand the idea of 'Mrs. Smith,' and you won't want to call me 'Mother' (as she sized me up), so I guess it would have to be 'Dorothy.'" I didn't call her anything for years if I could avoid it, but referred to her as Mrs. Smith.

My mother was immensely shy and reserved, but if she didn't approve she could be formidable.

"Well Bob, we meet at last." They shook hands and she took the baby to cover her lack of composure under his friendly stare, which was on a level with her own.

This marriage of mine had taken a lot of swallowing. I was supposed to have had the sense to pick, the second time around, some tall lean Englishman with private means who would escort me all over the place socially. Though not in the least averse to tall, lean Englishmen, I had for years turned my back on the vapourings and inanities of the then existing "Four Hundred," the supposed cream of Victoria society. They filled me with disgust. I was not alone in this if one considers Winifred and the other rebels living incognito in the BC interior. They must all have gone into the bush to prove something.

In any case Grandma was now cheek by jowl with our bundle and I could see thawing going on. As the old prospector had said, there couldn't be too much wrong with a relationship that could produce Mark. He was a big, fat, bonny, handsome little lump, full of smiles.

I had assured Bob that my dad was a pussycat, as friendly as his mother, and just as ready to meet anyone half way. Thus it turned out that the two men were getting along very well as my mother bore Mark into the house, to place him on a blanket to kick by the fire. My sister Faith's outlook was the next gamut to run. She was fair, fashionable, popular, and went with the trend.

A few minutes later I was on the phone connecting with some old friends, sitting with my back to the room, when someone came in behind me. She squealed, "My God! She's fat!"

Typical. I had put a few pounds onto my usually skinny

frame, as cooks did among mountains, but fat I was not. I went down into the basement to see how the men were making out, leaving my mother and sister to glue over the baby.

The men were conversing amiably beside the tool bench, but soon a pair of feet in dainty spiked heels came picking carefully down the stairs. Even without her face in view I knew by her step that she was bracing herself to meet This Man.

Bob came forward with good intent, doing his halfway bit to the hilt. She leaned towards him, extending her hand to her new brother-in-law, cooing "Hello Bob" with dovelike grace. I could see she was rallying from shock, but she should have known I couldn't stand her type of fop. Bob's very short height, the same as our mother's—from which vantage point he would learn to couch bold brown stares against Mother's blue flint—his bright red hair and freckles, his shy but cocky stance, all hit Faith like a bomb. She had known in advance what to expect but was not prepared for reality.

"The minute I saw him," she admitted to me years later and when she was in no danger of bodily assault, "I said to myself, 'It won't last five minutes.'" She had quite thought he would desert me within a few months. Our father had not been too happy about my prospects, but was decent and hoped for the best now it was done.

The attitude of Bob's people was not as bad but justifiable. It came to light when the two grandmothers got together on the phone. God knew why. Probably to establish our whereabouts or perhaps to be civilized. They were both brutally direct about things.

"Well, what do you think about it all?" began my mother.

"She's a nice girl. We like her," replied my mother-in-law, being half way again. "But," she snapped, "he'd no business marrying someone with four children." Mother didn't repeat to me her reply.

Quite. It was the only recrimination I got for carrying off her dear son, the apple of her eye. I knew she hated him marrying anyone, her pet who was so much like her—in other words kind, wilful, lovable, and sometimes very selfish.

With the home ordeal surmounted in the main, but with

the resultant tension and inner disappointment occasioned by it, we could not wait to hit the road again.

Indeed, after we had gathered our gear from a garage in Kitsilano, after we had braved Jackass Mountain and the North Thompson again looking for work, after we had gone into village after village looking for it and accommodation, once even filling Mark's bottle from an irrigation ditch, after we had found work and shelter, then my back packed in and Bob had to take me into Kamloops for an anaesthetic needle into my spine. Otherwise we had survived.

CHAPTER ▪ X

Nanny Tatty

Barriere, BC

We had come up the North Thompson River, out of Kamloops, as far as a little settlement called Barriere; we'd been inquiring about rental possibilities in the area at the general store, and the manager had suggested an apparently abandoned small homestead on the Barriere River flats, just up the road. He'd told us we would find the owner, Mrs. Davis, at a nearby crossroads and told us how to locate her. We had decided to find work first and then trust to luck for accommodation. There was the usual bush sawmill outside the village and Bob had been taken on. Now we stood on a bridge over the Barriere and looked down at the winding river flats and a pasture with its small home below, then went to seek its owner.

Together we went up the path to a little house, as directed, and knocked on the door. Knocked again. Eventually it opened and a huge old woman looked out at us.

"Good afternoon," I began. "We've been sent by the storekeeper to see you because he says you own the house on the flats below and it's empty. We were wondering if you would consider renting it. We have to find somewhere to live right away I'm afraid, as my husband has just got a job here."

"It's not for rent to anybody," said Mrs. Davis. "Anyways I don't take children." She slammed the door in our faces.

"Christ!" said Bob.

We saw, besides Mrs. Davis's place, a string of tarpaper cabins stretching from her fence eastward along the bank of the Barriere River just below. The river ran due east and west, and a road accompanying it in front of the cabins ran east and west also. We had come up from Kamloops by the north–south road that intersected the junction.

Disconsolately we returned to the general store. We bought some canned milk and asked who owned the cabins by Mrs. Davis. Anything else around there seemed solidly occupied, judging by flower beds, cars and tricycles in front of houses near the general store. These were few. A little red schoolhouse among the trees and a gas station with a garage seemed to complete the picture.

Our picture, so far, was this: north of the general store the highway went up a hill, bridged the Barriere tributary to the North Thompson, and rose again slightly to intersect that dusty crossroad. At the crossroad was a little group of houses. The small house, which was Mrs. Davis's, was kitty-cornered across the intersection from a house with a white picket fence, sited at the crossing also. Mrs. Davis's house sat in a sort of triangle fenced with wood and wire, with the garden tip at the crossroads and the broad base of her property triangle spreading along the tributary's bank.

The remaining two crossroad corners were occupied by a forest and a big school. The forest faced painted houses on the northbound road's continuing dirt track on one side, while its other dark front faced the string of cabins stretching along the smaller river. Down the bank below these cabins the tributary raced westward to the bigger river, with rapids boiling over its boulders. The northbound road from Kamloops meanwhile turned left and west at the crossroads to cross a bridge over the North Thompson and then turned north up the Blue River Road, down which we had lately come.

After crossing the intersection, the northbound road, as previously indicated, petered out into a dirt road when the main traffic turned left to Blue River. The little box houses along this dirt road were nicely painted. Also, in full view of the riverbank cabins on the east–west road, glimmering through a forest of jack pines, was the white-painted house of the forest ranger. Jack pines were widely spaced, giving way to ponderosa. Distant views were possible. Sound carried well also.

The large old school, the senior one, which filled the fourth corner, was big enough to have a broad flight of steps and its own football field.

"Shacksville is what this place is," exploded Bob, who by this time was shivering with nerves and worry after the Davis encounter. We were waiting in the dust beside the store. The storekeeper had smiled grimly at our report on Hattie Davis.

"I didn't think she'd rent it. But the cabins near her are always changing. It's worth a try. Wait a minute." Obligingly he telephoned somebody and spoke to him a little convincingly about one cabin he knew of.

"The owner's coming right over," said our new friend. "He'll be driving a yellow truck if you want to go out and wait for him."

Fairly soon a man got out of a mustard coloured pickup and stood surveying our forlorn little party of three and our travel-worn rig. We were weighed thoroughly.

"Four of those cabins are mine," he said, "and a girl in one of them has gone down to the coast and I don't know if she is coming back. I'm supposed to be painting it out. It isn't earning me anything at this rate so you'd better have a look at it."

We drove after the little yellow ray of hope ahead, turned right onto the tributary's road and pulled up in front of a cabin right next to Mrs. Davis's home. Thus began the war with Hattie Davis. We were to know her later as Nanny Tatty, thanks to a little nephew.

Fathering

At first we had no time to notice Hattie. My just reward came finally and my two youngest children were returned. One school year in their father's establishment, with two babies, had been enough for their stepmother. Rightly so. This was a time when Joan got off the train with a flowing head scarf and the independent ideas of a thirteen year-old, though Robby, at seven, was his cute little self but a bit more leggy. And with them was Snoose, the dog they had acquired in Smithers.

Disappointment at their new quarters was soon overrun by the children's desire to explore their new surroundings. They had arrived just before the first day of hunting and were in time to accompany their stepfather on an illegal chase after a flight of geese.

He had taken their return and their first sortie into his married life with his meet-'em-halfway philosophy and a strong determination to break them in and see what they could stand up to, right now. He imagined the creature comforts they had left behind, whereas I knew the background to be pretty Spartan but didn't say so. There were areas we left alone. Avoiding unnecessary discussion was safer.

The three children sat with me in the power wagon where we were posted as sentinels to warn Bob if the game warden's car was approaching, as we jumped the hunting season by a day or two. An RCMP patrol car came instead. It went back and forth several times without paying attention to a vehicle full of children or seeing what went on in the field. Birds were veering and vee-ing crazily over Bob's "firestick" (12-gauge shotgun) and looking for a swampy pond to settle in. The children shouted and yelled each time the police approached but he had ears only for the honking of the geese. He fired and got one, picked it up, and carried it before him triumphantly. It was a huge Canada goose about as big as Robert. We had all been waving our arms and wig-wagging at him.

"We now have our Thanksgiving dinner," he beamed. "What's the matter with you?"

The children covered the bird with a jacket as we gunned up a dust trail just before the patrol car flew by again. The police were on a different mission than catching poachers for the warden; in any case they were used to locals jumping the gun on the season and even the game department looked away as locals helped themselves for the larder, as long as they didn't let themselves be caught. Bag hunters were the quarry, the kind of people who chopped off a trophy head and left good meat to rot.

It was a nice beginning for the kids while the weather held. My spirits lifted, especially as we heard that David, my oldest, would pay us a visit when feasible.

Our quarters were cramped. It was the usual blend of two cabins stuck together: one longish one for the main room and one box-shaped and divided into two rooms. The place had all the rented fixings of stove, table and chairs, with bare light bulbs hanging down from the ceilings.

Outside, the shack had long thin shingles over tar paper. An overhang sheltered the doorstep. In front was a wide clear dirt foreground with an oasis of pines near the road. Behind the shack was a long deep bank going down to the river.

Inside, the walls were lined with building paper. It was not that private. A couch lay along the kitchen wall near the only outside door. At the foot of the couch was an archway. It curtained off a six-foot square vestibule with a window, beneath which was Joan's rollaway. Across from her was a small tin heater. The main bedroom door opened off this space to reveal a double bed for which there was scarcely any room. Beside the bed another door opened into a still tinier room which was Mark's. It should have been Joan's room but we all saw that Bob and I could not retire early without her passing through our room and that if she wanted to go outside the same thing would apply. We managed. Robert took the couch in the kitchen, which meant he'd stay warm without supervision. In no time at all Mark had his own attractive rustic crib made from saplings.

Joan took everything meekly enough until it was time for her to go to her new school. She was in denims again, rather more conscious of her looks on meeting another sea of young faces; she was stiff with doubts. I walked with her slowly to the few steps going up into the schoolhouse. Suddenly she balked and refused to go in.

"You've got to!" I shouted, when reasoning failed.

The teacher came out and took in the situation. I had intended to speak to her in any case. Stalling for time, she asked Joan her name and other particulars, and then taking her gently by the elbow said, "It's time now. Let's go in."

Politely Joan let the teacher step through first then placed both hands on the door jambs, stuck her denimed butt out at me and braced her feet. It was like moving a rock. I shoved hard and in she went, red-faced and with tears in her eyes.

The other children, big and little, had by now turned around to watch. I left the teacher to handle it. It seemed impossible that my decent, sensible little girl should turn into such a wimp. I knew the changing of schools was taking its toll, but what I did not know was that at first glance she saw she was the most senior student there and she didn't want the boys to see her tears over that. It was a typical one-room grade school with varied classes and ages, and she was almost ready for high school.

Within a week she was playing softball with them, the only girl on the field, pitching the ball straight up out of sight. By next spring that same denimed bottom was sashaying from side to side in insolent defiance of mothers as she stood on the pedals of her bike and ground up the hill. I had caught her bandying quips with the boys around the gas pumps and sent her home. I knew my work had begun.

Besides making the crib, Bob had one other thing on his mind for the children before snow flew. He decided that if he was going to raise them they must learn to ski. And Robert was to learn how to handle a gun. Robert was attending a tiny primary school a little further into the trees. It housed a total of thirteen kids from grades one to six. Joan could see him from her schoolhouse window coming and going. One day she saw him carrying home a rabbit. They were wild in the woods and hosted ticks, but what of it?

There were wild pastures not far from our cabin with sloping hills and rises that looked just dandy for snow. We planned secretly to give the kids skis for Christmas. Bob surveyed a suitable hill thoughtfully.

"If that irrigation ditch wasn't there we'd have a wonderful run," he pondered. "Hmm." Going over to the power wagon he got out a shovel and started walking up a grassy hill.

I ran after him. "You wouldn't! What if the farmer catches you? Besides you can't stop his water from running."

"Just watch me. There isn't any water at this time of year, dummy. And by the time there is the snow will be gone and I can come back and open up the ditch again. He'll never even notice."

Setting to, he filled in the ditch across the rise for about eight feet, just wide enough to aim for from the top of the hill. When they got their skis the children did go up there to ski their heads off, at least they and Bob did. My skiing was no better than my weak-ankle skating and I'd wind up at the end of the run on my bottom. I thanked God the children did not disgrace me; Bob's profoundly disgusted look at the progress of his mate simply devastated me. We did go cross- country skiing and at that, since walking was my strong point, I was pretty good. I think he was proud of that.

Once, I had to be very good. Bob had poled across a field and had climbed a snake fence with me following. Neither of us had noticed a big bull in another corner of the field, which saw us. Letting out an annoyed bellow it started trotting to- wards us, gradually picking up pace.

"Ski! Ski!" shouted Bob, wreathed in glee from behind the fence. "Faster! Faster!" They were the longest, fastest strides I had ever achieved as I landed in a tangle at the fence with skis, poles and rails all mixed as somehow I scrambled over.

Another time, when we were visiting some farmer, he dropped me with Mark in my arms at the front door right into the midst of a herd of cows. The lady came out and rescued me, seeming not to see any problem. Later he mused, "I've heard cows can get sometimes worse than bulls."

Such situations helped break up winter tensions.

When the snow was chest high beside the ploughed road and a deer carcass hung board stiff under our eaves, and Baby Bunting stood up in his snow sled to watch the children build- ing snow forts, then Mrs. Davis—Nanny Tatty—began mak- ing overtures.

The Dear Dead Days

By winter our dog Snoose learned to lie behind the shack in a small kennel that had been asking for an occupant. It seemed nothing but a high mound of snow with a black hole in it, into which he crawled quite happily to sleep. His black coat was silky with a beautiful gloss and he stayed healthy. Hattie had begun to lure him with scraps. That she was lonely there was no doubt. Then she began passing out cookies to the children. Finally she came to call.

After our initial reception Bob did not care if he ever saw her again. He did not waste time on people who were not amenable, nor did he give them a second chance; he simply went on from there. My own attitude was semi-friendly, a nod or two but no hobnobbing. I still did not like old ladies who did not like children and wondered what this one's game was with mine.

One day before snowfall, in the late fall sunshine, while Bob was at work, I saw Mrs. Davis's bulk filling our doorway hesitantly. I pulled up a chair and offered her tea. She declined the tea saying that her fingers were too gnarled with the "rheumatiz" to hold a cup; it was apt to slip and spill. But she sat on and on and told me her story.

Her name, she said, was Hattie. "The little feller here" reminded her of a little nephew who called her Tatty. Nanny Tatty. For us she remained formally Mrs. Davis. You didn't take liberties with an independent old bird like that who knew her manners and expected you to know yours.

She had a huge bony frame, bent over, and a seamed and withered face. She had acquired a husband, obviously, but her father featured mostly in her reminiscences of the "dear dead days." Her parents with their effects had come around the Horn and had started ranching somewhere in BC. Of this she never tired of talking as she visited us subsequently, or showed me her garden or met me in the road.

I heard about juicy operations, damaged virtue in the village, and buggy and bobsled days with the dear departed. I heard how Hattie had driven her father's team as the hired man could never do, with her gold locket hanging and her yellow hair flying in the wind.

"And I'd drive like that in the buggy or drive the team with my father yelling after me and my hair flying out. He was so proud of me. He wouldn't let the hired men or anybody touch the team other than he or me." From there we went on to undulant fever, the "Bad Disorder" of cattle, and the flood that had chased her out of her widow's home down on the pastures.

We soon found out what her game was: Hattie wanted errand boys and a handy man and a woman to gossip with. Whenever she had tried to get her roof mended or her wood cut she found the men in the settlement all in league. One by one she tried them with her small offers of payment and her heavy tactics as if with former ranch hands. She found the ranger needed every man for fire fighting, the roofer had jobs piled ahead and refused to take less than he charged others. The village handy man was always strangely busy. She turned to her young neighbours.

She was not too successful. Silver quarters and apples did not compensate the kids for hours spent on her woodpile and toting heavy groceries and mail up the hill. Nor would Bob let her hire him. He did get up on her roof once with rare philanthropy but her bossiness soon put him off. She got his back up so much with niggling and orders that he came in and blew to me.

"That's it. If she can't look after herself and pay proper wages then she ought to go where she can be looked after. And if this keeps up I'll see that she does!"

Although I told the children that they did not have to work for peanuts, I said they should still have compassion and help once in awhile. They continued to work on her woodpile when they felt like it but her tongue was ungratefully critical and her pay so low that their pity had worn thin. As an unwilling conscript Bob had been expected to mend her axe, remodel her table as well as repair the roof. She had spoken airily of "hiring" him as a prelude to a haggling spree, forever cooking her own goose. In the meantime, Hattie was now keeping me vastly entertained.

Soon other things claimed our attention.

Adapting

The carryall ate too much gas and kept us from venturing across the country. All we did with it was go for water over the North Thompson bridge to a landing place and fill a tank on our trailer, bucket by bucket. Our rent and overhead were very cheap and an allowance came for the children, so that Bob put by most of his wages for a trade-in. The carryall was exchanged for a secondhand jeep just before snow fell, and now the trailer, to keep Bob's hands busy, was to become a sort of travel trailer with removable housing when needed for hauling.

It was pathetic. I felt the whole performance was for him to have ready a personal escape hatch from the close quarters in the shack and to be able to get away if circumstances warranted.

The trailer conversion went on until zero temperatures prevented it. Then my scepticism was confirmed. Into the trailer went Bob's personal belongings, his own pictures and yearnings. It was a typical male doghouse. It hurt me, though I had the sense to say nothing. It was too tall and top heavy, and a trial run next spring did little to endear it to its owner. Again I said nothing.

Joan was on my mind also. She would be fourteen in midsummer but was still very much a tomboy. Except for her paintbox and some tiny porcelain pieces inherited from her grandmother, she showed no interest in girlie ways. She was like a sister to the village boys, but that could not last. Everything began one night when a school party was rife and a skimpy young male downed his timidity enough to ask her to go with him. This was her first real date and we were horrible to her.

First of all everyone had to remain in the kitchen while she had her bath in the middle room in a tin tub beside the heater. She endured our jibes through the curtain and came out in her dressing gown. Her party clothes were laid out in the kitchen on Robert's bed and we were making much of these, holding them up and fingering them daintily and otherwise depicting the finished product. I could not resist teasing after all the baseball bats and jeans, and besides, I didn't want her to think of dating as a social function, at least for several years.

We sat around the kitchen with her, waiting for the knock that did not come. She sulked and surveyed our mirth with hate. My heart began to sink for her when at last there came a manly bang. Joan opened the door only to find Dipsy-Do standing there, her rather lanky hillbilly girlfriend from next door.

"Are you ready?" asked Dipsy-Do. There was a flashlight circling beams away out in the road behind her. "Don sent me to get you because he's afraid of Snoose."

He wasn't the only one to be afraid. Joan had her turn at a fear of something else one night in late fall, when the mud was crackling with frost as she was coming home from a near-by friend's house, where she had been doing homework. The road was deserted. She got as far as the bridge near us, over the Barriere below our cabin, when she heard hoofbeats behind her. Thudding hoofbeats. She leaped behind the bridge abutment and hung on to it, with the river racing below, and turned to look.

A pack of ghostly grey horses was streaming towards her and over the ghostly bridge in the moonlight, galloping and thundering over the planks above her. Their joyful neighing and heavy breathing drowned out her thoughts. Eventually she got up nerve to emerge and cross the bridge herself, only a block or two from home.

Just off the bridge two yelping curs ran out and snapped at her heels and in backing away from them, kicking out and yell-ing at them, she sensed a presence behind her. Turning sharply she found herself nose to nose with a great moonlit cow. Her feet couldn't carry her fast enough. All the while, through the bellowings of horses, dogs and cow there had been a chorus of coyotes.

Years later she said, "I liked coyotes but not then. It was the first time in my life that my hair really stood on end." As for cattle on the loose, it was free range country.

Her story shook me. I went to investigate where she had hung above the river and didn't like what I saw. Cattle were often loose in this country and it was nothing to open our door and find some old horse grazing in the little oasis of trees that formed the centre of our driveway. Hattie had something to say about free range country.

"They shouldn't let The Animal loose. I see some people don't keep him fenced in." Any bull to her was "The Animal." We did not encounter any bulls on the roads thereabouts, only when trespassing.

The children did well in their rural school life. Joan was made editor of the senior school magazine, called the *Monthly Monarch*. This title she pronounced as the Monthly MonARK. I corrected her crossly and said "It's not MonARK, it's MONark." Consequently she avoided naming it before me and went on calling it MonARK before her friends. It was the battle of "Do I follow my peers or listen to Mum?"

The jellied inkpad for its production was contained in a shallow rectangular Christie's biscuit tin, off which came purple drawings and probably purple prose.

It was not hard for her to shine because she was the most senior girl in grade eight, with three classmates all told. There were two other grades with as many members in each but when party time came they used the high school across from Hattie. Here Joan went to her first dance and was made much of by all the fool fathers who told her she was a good dancer. She was. My hands looked likely to become full with an adolescent. She would never be like her old friend Lucille of Skeena River days, she'd be far more subtle and real prematurely, if innocently aroused; a danger to herself, I thought.

On the other hand, Robert was doing well. Bob had already shown him how to take a .22 apart, with long warning lectures. He was given a role in the school play at Christmas. This was put on in one of the several villages down the highway, in a hall. On its stage we perceived a semi-naked little Indian, with headband, feathers and beads, sitting cross-legged before the footlights and banging away confidently on a pair of bongo drums, grinning ferociously. Why are mothers surprised?

The next thing we knew it was Christmas Day.

The Indignant

The smoke from her chimney went straight up. I tiptoed out to see how Hattie was faring. We had summoned courage and had asked her to join us for Christmas dinner.

"No thank you. I don't partake. Folk make me nervous and I drop things. And it brings back too many memories." I'd decided to try her once more.

Snow was piled three feet deep around Hattie's house, with no footprints going in or out. Alarmed for some reason, I crept up to her window and looked in, in case she might be flat on the floor.

She was sitting in her kitchen with her back to the window on a chair drawn up to a shelf, which served as a table, with an oil lamp beside her. It was Christmas dinner time and before her was a plate of cold meat and bread with a big mug of tea. I made a little noise in my consternation but Hattie didn't turn; probably thought I was a porcupine chewing her outhouse wall. In the morning she'd see the footprints from gate to window and back and guess our anxiety. Let them worry, she'd think. Didn't they know Christmas was just another day?

Winter passed in the usual solitude.

One spring thaw morning, returning from the store, I saw bright sun warming the great bent shoulders of Hattie's rawboned figure as it picked its way up the hill from the village. If it were not for her bigness and decayed strength she would have been the regular rag, bone and hank of hair, with her purpling coat exposed to the day's brilliance. Coming along behind her I gained rapidly.

"Let me have your parcels." Hattie turned and said "Good morning" with dignity. I extracted the parcels gently and she took my proffered arm. Hattie was still fuming over the storekeeper's attitude.

"That man had no right to look at me like that! All I asked for was six brown eggs and you'd think I asked for gold. He fished and fished around out back for ages and I'll bet they are all cracked, the way he put the bag down."

"He has to pick each one out of the crate, you know. They aren't sorted."

His attitude had been, "If only she'd order everything at once I'd be glad to send it up. Six eggs only and she says they must be brown. She says the white ones make her sick and she thinks they give you cancer. You can't help wishing someone would do something about her. See there she goes, up the hill. Can hardly make it on her poor old pins."

My remark had made no dint on Hattie. She knew what the villagers wanted—her removal—and they'd bring it about if they could.

We stopped on the rise. She was winded, even without the parcels. The road continued some hundreds of yards to the crossroads. The cottages and shacks were up there with the high school on one side and Hattie's triangle property on the other. The bridge over the smaller river was just ahead of us and to the left beneath it the river foamed out and curled around its banks, where tufts of green showed already in the brown drowned grass. Patches of snow still lay about and bits of ice hung from the sandbars, but the Lombardy poplars standing sentinel over the flats and pasture below were just coming into bud. Under the trees' shelter, safe from winter blasts and blazing sun, stood Hattie's neat white ranch home.

"I could manage just as well down there as where I am. It isn't even far from the store. And it won't flood no more because they changed the banks after last time."

She began to tremble as though the walk had been too much.

"Do you know what they say?" She turned to me. "They say I ought to be in one of these homes for indignants." I looked blank. "People with no money. Old people who go into a home because nobody wants 'em. They take everything you got and boss you around." Indigents! Of course. Her brown seamed face screwed up. "I dream about it, I'm that frightened."

We talked about it for awhile and I promised to investigate the truth if we were in Kamloops.

"Oh, would you? Would you do that for me?" It was going to be a must.

Home we went with our parcels, going through her front gate and around to the back. Here was where she stooped in her war with the cutworms. Pansies and herbs abounded, dead iris leaves trailed down the bank, and little rows of cans with their ends cut out were inverted over her early seedlings. Snoose bounded at Hattie through the side gate of our mutual fence.

"Here's my glassy friend," she cried. Glossy indeed.

The Dugout

Spring released us. By now Robert had an old bike and joined his sister on woodland forays. Far off, Joan espied a flash flood that suddenly disappeared, leaving its course full of flapping fish. She couldn't believe their luck and filled the carrier of her bike with them. They were big and silvery but I didn't like the look of their mouths, (which stirred a memory.) Bob took one look and went for his shovel again. He laughed and laughed at Joan who was amazed at his lack of praise and gratitude.

"Those are suckers. Fit only for fertilizer. You don't eat them. Besides they take the food needed for other fish." He'd explained to her as he had to me at Dutch Lake how fishing vanishes because of them. Suckers and leeches were two things that made my skin crawl. Many small interior lakes were full of leeches, preventing any swimming.

Testy about being teased, Joan soon had revenge for her letdown because Bob was the next one to strike out. A beautiful stand of cottonwoods grew up the river from us and close to the water. Bob decided to make a dugout canoe, Indian style. In no time at all he had felled a nice fat tree. He stripped off all the green-lined whitish bark which exposed the cambium to flies. If I had not seen it I would never have believed that flies would be interested in bark. A sweetish odour possibly accounted for it. Flies swarmed for several days over the wet strips on either side of the log while Bob ignored them and hacked away. It was a long job and I left him to it.

Eventually it was launching time and I went to inspect the new canoe. It looked expert. It seemed to be hollowed out evenly and a single seat stretched across the beam. As it was too heavy to lift, and he didn't want us to bother the men around, he decided to lever it into the river and ride the rapids to a spot below Hattie's place and ours.

"You'll do no such thing. You must be mad."

"A mere nothing. You don't know what rapids are."

Visions of widowhood haunted me but he did it. I did not watch and stayed home. Eventually, about an hour later, the door opened and a dripping figure surveyed me saying, "Brrr! Got any coffee? You have to part your hair in the middle to ride the damn thing and it dumped me in the river."

Man and canoe had spun separately to fetch up at the bend below. He was a very strong swimmer, luckily, and had managed to save his craft and get someone to help him get it up the bank below our cabin.

He was really cussed in other ways as well. While splitting wood he had swung the axe blade into his leg beside the shin bone. It was a nasty cut and deep.

"That needs stitches. We'll have to go into Kamloops."

"No fear. I'm not wasting all that gas for a cut. Just gimme some disinfectant and I'll pull it together with some adhesive. That's what my mother used to do." I demurred about adhesive over a raw wound.

"Ah don't be so silly. It will heal underneath it."

By about the third day a long red weal crept from the injury right up inside his thigh and I knew it was blood poisoning. Then we did go to Kamloops for antibiotics.

While we had our drama Hattie had hers. She hoed and hoed her garden. Then one day she came to knock on our door in great agitation.

"I want you to come and see. There's a terrible smell. I think somebody's been murdered around here and they've buried the body in the bank."

"Don't ask me," I said, appalled. "If it's true you'll need a man to look. Why don't you ask Mr. van de Kamp over there. He'll help you." I had my doubts about the smell, but you never knew.

Van de Kamp lived in the immaculate little house with the white picket fence opposite Hattie's place. He was not at all partial to helping Hattie but was in a vulnerable position, living across from her where she could see his movements. In order to maintain his distance he was often rude. Still, an emergency is an emergency and he was looked to by others at times. He came with several men who probed the bank below, picked up the horrible smell and traced it back to Hattie's own outdoor convenience. The Dutchman had a wonderful time in the village regaling people with the story. "And all the time it was her own outhouse!"

Swimming Holes

The summer of 1951was idyllic. At this point Mark was walking chubbily and spending his days in a sandbox made for him in the pine oasis outside the front door, or being placed in his stroller or highchair. More out of the way than making waves so far.

Joan was occupied with her girlfriends, making daisy chains as they walked through fields exchanging confidences, or in visiting other friends' homes up the railway line for parties that meant staying the night.

Robert could break down the .22 and handle it, without ammunition, and was happy in the woods.

For Bob and me there were no friends, except the ranger's wife with whom I took tea while Mark played with her baby girl, or who took tea with me while her baby played in Mark's sandbox—unless as a friend you counted Hattie. Bob simply worked and tinkered, or sometimes explored.

We had discovered two paradisiacal places to swim and picnic; a small lake accessible only by four-wheel drive and a lagoon in the river below, sheltered by a bar of fine sand.

The two Genier Lakes were on high ground, and the jeep had to crawl up a washed out track with difficulty. The smaller lake was a round jewel set in grasses, surrounded by shrubs with a background of pines. It was full of enormous rainbow trout that came into the shallows, refusing all lures. The water was alive with feed and the fish went up to twenty pounds like great salmon—a well kept local secret. Turtles were in there too, and beavers had lodges each side of the lake.

Flowers abounded in spring and dragonflies were all over the water like blue fire.

Here we brought the dugout by trailer with its unaligned keel, which Bob and Robert managed to unload and paddle, taking turns, each sitting in the bottom at an angle to keep balance. The whole place was so encircled, green and untouched, that after a swim and sunbathe without a soul around we hated to leave it. Mark ran around naked with a little white sun hat on his head.

When the temperature was at 100° Fahrenheit in the shade we all needed something more immediate and would climb down the bank to the river. Our bridge to the sandbar was a fallen log across the lagoon, over which Bob would run saying, "Come on."

I couldn't. Vertigo was one of my failings and his sang-froid in stepping casually to the edge of cliffs and looking down made me turn my head away. I was not the only family member in disgrace; Tom suffered badly from vertigo and had once been marooned up on the roof of their hotel. The children were far braver.

"Chicken!" Bob would call, when everyone but me had crossed over. I sat astride the tree in bathing suit and cap, inching my way across. He didn't really mind.

The water was divine, even if the lagoon did not permit a decent swim. Outside in the river it was all boulders and riffles in summer with swift depths and rapids in spring.

Bob's chilling nerve with regard to cliffs, swimming in turbulence, and in particular his disregard for safety with a power saw, was always a worry. We often went for wood with the trailer, where I was a witness to his logging methods. In logging boots, he would leap from fallen log to fallen log to limb them, running the slippery length of each with the power saw going full blast. It was too time-consuming to shut the thing off between trees; safety catches were for fools that didn't know what they were doing. The axe cut had been a prime example of his carelessness, and yet he was extremely careful with guns and scornful of anyone who went log-stepping without his gun cracked open. I did trust him with

Robert in that respect. He didn't expose us to danger, only his foolhardy self.

Sometimes on a Sunday we would go on an expedition. The kids bounced primly in the rear of the jeep and Mark sat on my knee. We would start very early with a basket of food and perhaps drive past the houses lining the river and CNR northwards, follow the tracks through abandoned settlements then turn off to Dunn Lake. Then we'd launch our Whitehorse boat with its newly acquired outboard: a secondhand, two-horsepower Seagull, the result of a swap. Bob would go out on that lake and fish, maybe take Robert. I stayed on the beach as a rule because I did not like that lake. It seemed sinister, gloomy, surrounded by beetling hills, and the water was very black. I did not like what might be in it. Being on its beach was plenty. The place had an aura and if I'd been an Indian I would have said that spirits dwelt there and I would have avoided it like the plague. My children thought I was crazy. Fishing was poor too.

It was satisfying when we could afford gas enough to go up to Clearwater, or show the kids Dutch Lake, or go towards Wells Gray Park.

Before the summer was over David came up. The visit was a comfort to me but was not an unqualified success; at eighteen he was now six foot three, looking older than his years, and Bob had to look up to him a long way. Gradually my boys would develop a manly camaraderie with Bob, which usually started by their placing a twenty-six of rye in front of him. That language they all understood. In David's case the rapport was instant because anyone who knew the bush backwards was a pal of his. An accomplished fisherman from the age of twelve, when last I trudged after him, he was now a constant hunter in his home hills.

He stayed a week, using Robby's cot while the boy used a rollaway. The children were out of school and while Bob was at work we all walked through the village pushing the stroller to where the river carved out a nice bend full of log jams. David liked to fish log jams. We went through an airfield where farmers would bring down their tiny Piper Cubs, smaller than cars. I discovered with a shiver that David was licensed to fly them. He was a boy who chested his cards, especially around mothers.

In the summer evenings we took him to our secret lake and to our swim hole but not to the gloomy lake. Bob, who now had in David another man along, arranged a much grander goal. We were to take a boat up the length of Adams Lake which he had not yet seen himself.

On a Sunday, after driving south down the highway and taking a dirt road inland to the public landing, we hired a clinker-built boat with an inboard motor and all of us got into it. Bob sat at the stern with the tiller, Robert and Joan sat amidships, and David and I sat with Mark in the bow. With this load the waterline was quite passable, about six inches below the gunwales. The sun was shining and the lake was placid, with mirror-like sweeps along the shores.

Adams Lake is a long slot, like lakes in the Okanagan. We hummed merrily along with a line out, cruising about a mile or two north from the landing, then decided to put in on the opposite shore, have a swim and eat lunch. This we did with the usual gusto and I was just getting out of a wet suit behind a rock when Bob noticed the skies were becoming overcast. For some reason I couldn't understand he looked tight and nervous.

"All right !" he ordered. "Everybody into the boat. We've got to git. Right now!"

The kids hopped into it in lively fashion as he started to push off and I leaped into the bow crying that I'd forgotten some underwear. "No time! Forget it!" We were half way into the middle of the lake before we knew what was happening. What he knew full well and didn't want to tell us was that squalls can come up narrow lakes with sudden fury and rip right down the centre. We were half way between two shores when the water became choppy. Bob was looking pale. Then a wind came up and the water got a black look with little flips of foam. Being half way across, it was senseless to go back and just as crazy to continue to our boat ramp.

The children were still unaware of danger, but David, who was, began to sing. Bob kept the throttle full out and looked greyer in the face each minute as the wind got worse and the lake much rougher. It was licking the gunwales but not yet spilling inside, though the children, by this time aware and peeping out from under a tarp, had the bail can at the ready. They were scared too, but determined not to show it. We did not have life jackets. Nobody but sissies carried life jackets in those days. It was the sign of an amateur.

Looking at my kids I wondered how I could save the young ones and keep them afloat. Joan was thinking the same thing while keeping her brothers preoccupied. She could swim, but Robert could dog paddle only a few yards and David was not much good for long distances.

Somebody up there liked us. We should have been swamped. It seemed hours in the squall, all of us riding along by now in deep silence. I prayed like mad. We were still head-ed upwind in the centre of the lake. Finally the landing be-came visible. Until then Bob had not put into shore anywhere because he didn't want to run parallel to the big waves coming down the lake until he had to and possibly, if the storm did not let up, he thought we'd be marooned overnight and he'd be missing from work and get fired.

We made it. David made a joke or two. I had been watching his face during the ordeal and it told me nothing. He had been moving heaven and earth to keep the kids and myself from being afraid. Fortunately the children had had their backs to Bob's ashen face in the stern. My fury at what my dear ones had been through was gradually eroded by contrition towards Bob's guilt over his own poor judgment and his intention of giving my family an interesting adventure. Nobody spoke much on the way home.

Though balm to his mother for awhile, David's visit was a mixed blessing to his very young stepfather. They became good friends bush fashion but were too close in age for Bob to carry any weight, polite though my young man was and the soul of tact. Bob began to look sulky and when we were alone I asked him why he looked so glum.

"Wouldn't you? You bring me this great big love child twice my size."

His forked tongue and uncalled-for remark made me realize that David should not be exposed to the reality of being out of place or downright unwelcome, but he had decided to take the train home in any case.

There was an errand to do in Kamloops and I resolved to ride down with him. I was going to get Mark a silver mug and have it engraved, my only child without one. Bob agreed and left us at the station.

As we boarded David collapsed the stroller and put it somewhere while I went with Mark into the coach to find a seat. The conductor came along to take our tickets and said, "By the way, your husband has put the baby's cart in the vestibule ready for when you get off."

"My WHAT?"

David approached and the conductor turned and looked at him.

"Your whatever he is then," snorted the man disgustedly.

With great guffaws and a certain amount of pride in my own looks in my mid-thirties, I told David what the man had said. At eighteen David looked twenty-eight, so you couldn't blame the conductor. David's reaction was quite unnecessary. He gave me a filthy look and shuddered all over. One thing though. The train episode showed me exactly what Bob was up against and I returned home much wiser.

The Welfare Woman

Back at the crossroads the summer went on.

Hattie came over gingerly at correct intervals and I would see her home through the gate to look at her garden. She taught me what flowers survive below zero temperature and of course how to defeat cutworms using bottomless tin cans. I learned that during the heyday of Hattie's great strength she had got in her own firewood the lazy way, by hauling a tree length indoors into her scullery and sawing it up as she needed it, rather than bucking it up outside.

One day I received a different sort of visitor who reminded me of Effie's former plight when she had been investigated as a possibly unfit mother. Had someone in the village been gossiping about us? It was the local welfare woman, very English, very professional and very stiff. Again the door was open to let sunshine in and this time Mark was on his "pot." It was under the lid on his highchair as he was too small for the outhouse. He was sitting there having just completed a very good effort. The woman simply appeared in the doorway and stood, smiling feebly, and saying, "Knock, knock." I have no idea why she picked us to call on.

I met her right at the doorway hoping to head her off and get at my baby but in she came, as one with authority, sure of her welcome. There was nothing for it but to ask her to sit down. After that I could not bring myself to dethrone Mark in front of so much starch. If I lifted him down the room would be permeated—which is what she deserved. I opted to leave him there, thinking she might leave soon. She did not and continued to talk. As the kettle was boiling its head off I had to offer her tea, gulping with embarrassment. Still the visitor did not catch on. She was too busy sizing up our affairs and being terribly, terribly kind.

It was now far too late to disclose Mark's position for she'd think me a fool not to have removed him in the first place, whereas nothing short of a shove and shutting the door at the outset would have done any good. Or perhaps she guessed about Mark and just thought me a careless hillbilly. Acute embarrassment grew to the pitch where I didn't know what she asked me or what I replied. Eventually she left.

Bob was furious. "Nosey old bitches! What did she want coming here?" It was all part of village existence.

CHAPTER · XI

Mother Goose

The Intruder

From late summer and through that first winter several neighbours left the crossroads, the first of whom were the van de Kamps. Their immaculate little house across from Hattie's was vacant. The Dutchman had left most suddenly. A big forest fire in late summer had broken out along the main river further up and the ranger gave notice that he'd be rounding up volunteers at the crack of dawn. Before the first glow of light the Dutchman had rammed his wife and possessions into their trailer and had driven off into the night, never to return. Hattie was overjoyed. Her gossipy detractor had flown. Their house was sniffed at by one or two comers and then it stood empty all winter into spring.

One morning Hattie was disturbed in her weeding by a high metallic screech that cut the still pine air. Another screech followed and then another. I came out and stood on our step. Hattie stood leaning on her hoe. Our heads were cocked simultaneously until we saw the cause of the noise.

Yonder, across the street and behind the white pickets of the deserted place, stepping briskly among a pile of packing cases, was a tall and ancient figure in a flowered black coverall, wielding a claw hammer. A white bush of hair and a long aquiline nose stuck out beneath a huge black straw sun hat with a plate-like brim and a crown that came to a point.

"Why," I breathed. "She looks exactly like Mother Goose."

Electrified, Hattie all but pawed the ground.

"Doesn't look as if she's done a tap of work in her life."

"She wasn't there yesterday."

Hattie wasn't listening. She had thrown down her hoe and gone indoors to think. Fortified by tea she emerged later bearing a crowbar and saw. This was her territory and by heaven she was going to get to the newcomer first. Arriving at the picket fence she opened fire.

"Good morning. Do you need any help?" was what floated across to me. I wasn't going to miss any of this.

A surprised white face regarded Hattie from under the hat's shelter—my long distance peripheral vision was very keen, which made everything obliquely clear. The hammer suspended in mid-air.

"Hattie Davis's the name," Hattie continued. "I can use tools without the help of anyone and that claw hammer of yours will take all day."

The hammer was lowered and transferred over as the lady quickly opened the gate. Hattie's thick gnarled fist found itself enclosing a long blue-veined hand that bore an opal.

Fascinated, I began to clean up Mark's sandbox and eavesdropped shamelessly. All sound carried in these parts.

"Violet Travers. Please come and see what I'm trying to do. So good of you. As a matter of fact," Mother Goose went on chirpily, "everyone has been so kind. The milkman brought my things down from the station. I'd been wondering what on earth to do. The forest ranger stopped by on the way to his office and heaved these cases nearer the front door. He says he'll be back later. Then a lady with a truckload of cabbages…"

"D'you want help or not?" Hattie waved the crowbar. The white bush and pointed hat nodded vigorously.

"Then grab that end and hang on hard." Two pries and the side of one packing case came off.

Ostensibly I was going in and out of our house about my

business. Village children watched through the fence as the old women got loose the sides of crates and the milk van idled while the driver inquired how were they coming? Then the ranger returned and Hattie took off.

It was clear that here were forces beyond her control. In addition to having a popular person at the crossroads with a winning way, the boxes had revealed appliances, a curiously carved Chinese chest, and a glimpse of shawls and vases. Maybe even jade. The news would be around in minutes. One trunk was labelled Hong Kong.

As the days went by Hattie tended her own knitting. She did not know how to tackle Mrs. Travers or what to think. Clearly the creature was no softie or what would she be doing in a place like this at her age, and by choice? Hattie tried hard to think how she could use this development without winding up looking like a fool. I could see the wheels going around. All that help for a stranger. It would not improve Hattie's own cause if she showed annoyance. There was always somebody loitering on Mrs. Travers' doorstep. They came at first with pie and pickle offerings and flimsy excuses to gape and admire. Until something happened concerning this new arrival Hattie decided to stay aloof. When the two women met she was grumpily civil. And it was galling for her down in the village.

"I'll take that up to Mrs. Travers," she heard. "I'm going that way."

"Thank you," grinned the storekeeper. "Did you know she's got her house open and is asking people in? The wife says it's a rare treat the way she's got that little place fixed up. Sure is artistic."

Mrs. Travers astonished me and I made myself known partly because she reminded me of my mother's eccentric friends. I was invited inside but didn't tell Hattie.

One sunny afternoon I observed her heading for the bridge and groceries. Mrs. Travers waved her pruning shears as Hattie passed.

"Come in and have tea on your way back."

"Thank you, I'm sure." Hattie was greatly relieved. You had to know where you were if you wanted to come to grips with things. Know the enemy. How would her position in the village be affected?

"You look puffed out," the lady welcomed her later. There was always a mark under Mrs. Travers' chin left by the elastic on her black sun hat and the black smock seen up close had roses all over it. Her tiny living room was furnished by up-ended crates concealed by the most extraordinary array of rich stuffs. Small oriental carpets and long fringed shawls covered boxes, floors and walls. Silk cushions turned two crates into a divan. Hattie, who never bothered with her parlour, was over-whelmed. By the heater stood a small armchair before which was a leather hassock with designs inlaid. Watery prints hung between gilded mirrors, a long vase on the floor was full of lilacs and a gilded pot thing with a long pipe running out of it stood by Mrs. Travers' chair.

As soon as Hattie got home I was the recipient of a torrent of information which could be thusly reconstructed.

"Ah that," Mrs. Travers explained about the pot thing with the pipe. "That's my hookah."

While she busied herself behind a curtained archway with the tea, Hattie had taken stock. She was seated on the sturdiest box and was looking directly through a bead curtain into the kitchen alcove at strange electrical equipment.

"How long have you been here?" Violet Travers asked, setting down the tray. A folding card table served for dining.

"Before the Depression. We had a ranch below with a hundred head of cattle until my husband dropped dead in the bull's corral. The Animal never touched him. I sold the herd and some acres and they pay me to graze on the rest. I could rent the house but I plan to move back some day, now that they've rerouted the river."

"Does it flood then?"

"Not since they banked the bend. The bridge is safe, don't you worry. How about you?"

"Bank manager. He died in Hong Kong. We moved around a lot, especially India and Persia. Everything I have is every-thing you see. I travel light. But you have to come to roost eventually.

"Frankly, I have to be unwatched by certain sorts of people and I'm staying where they can't supervise my end. And I love the feel of this river place. What you've done and what I've done make no difference. East or West makes no difference."

"You certainly got some lovely stuff here. Minds me of what's in my sea chests. All my family's things came around the Horn. Every good thing I got."

Violet looked up with interest. She had been busy inserting a cigarette into a long holder which was poked into the area of her navel to steady the operation. Her facial lines were long to match her nose and her chin came to a point. As she lit up she surveyed her guest with a calculating blue glimmer behind the crinkles and smoke.

"Come over and see sometime," offered Hattie.

"Glad to. Some day you must sit down and try this thing" indicating the hookah. "The smoke is drawn through the water and cooled. It's very…"

"Not on your life. Thanks for the tea."

Gone was the "rheumatiz" that couldn't support a teacup. Thereafter Hattie was seen bustling back and forth to Mrs. Travers' house with help and advice. The neighbours gave Mother Goose one week in which to get fed up.

They were totally wrong. That distinguished example of charm and grace considered Hattie a powerful ally and friend. Hattie's strength and experience would be buffers against hardships, and the presence of someone Violet's own age, also alone, bred confidence. Very cannily Hattie failed to speak to anyone about her new friend. As she would have said, "It's for me to know and them to find out."

When she was not dispensing tea or planting sweet peas, Mrs. Travers was often seen crossing the fine hot dust of the road, followed by several small fry, and being welcomed at Hattie's by our own faithless dog.

The door to the white cottage was open all summer. The tea was dispensed in eggshell china and accompanied by stories of the Far East by the score. Violet was not a "yarner," but she loved people. Having come impoverished but cheerfully to hide her own lonely finish, she had decided to make these

246

souls her own. She had worked her way up the North Thompson through the settlements, away from telephones, and had found Barriere to her liking. Adventuring was her game and Hattie's tough spirit was the essence of it.

The Green Light

It was soon evident that Hattie was moving, supposedly out of pique to get away from the crossroads. The truth was that apart from the fact she could still hold a teacup, her "rheumatiz" vanished, her own chests were gone into and the two women became fast friends, matching linen for linen and yarn for yarn until the old ranch owner decided that God had given her the sign. If a frail woman of Hattie's own age could set herself up so successfully, then she, Hattie, could take back her rightful heritage and position in the village. At first most of the villagers were still unaware of this next door liaison as the two women had not appeared together in public.

Soon after the friendship began it was discovered that Hattie was back at her old games with different results. Men who had fallen under the spell of the motherly sorceress scrambled all over themselves to help Mrs. Travers, mostly because their wives told them to. They could hardly refuse now to help any old person, herself included, Hattie thought. Violet might hear of their refusal and interpret it as unwillingness to help the aged. Their families would be the losers because she brought colour into their lives. Hattie began to take advantage. She went back to asking heavy favours and undercutting pay when she hired.

When I went down to the riverside ranch to give Hattie some help, taking Snoose and the Little Fellah with me, I found bare floors shining with varnish and the plastered wall board freshly painted. But Hattie was never satisfied.

"The tape doesn't cover the wall joins and that chimney plate doesn't fit. The first big wind this winter and my white paint will be all smoked up."

The dog was loose and so was Mark while I repainted Hattie's kitchen cupboards. On one side of her house was a deep well covered with boards and on the other side cattle were roaming. I was treated to an unnecessary lecture on letting the Little Fellah go near the well, just as if I was not dropping the paint brush every minute to check. Finally I tied him into his stroller with biscuits offered by Hattie.

It was while standing on a countertop to paint inside a cupboard that I got a fully fledged view of a real Hattie event, like driving teams with hair flying. A hullabaloo had arisen outside, and through the window was visible the extraordinary spectacle of a herd of invading shorthorns being put to rout by a snapping dog and an old lady who, with both hands raising a broom aloft, was bringing it crashing to earth repeatedly while emitting wild cries at Snoose.

"Skitch at 'em! Skitch at 'em!" she shrieked, with every bash of the besom. Cattle stood off among the trees and in the river gulley watching as if she were mad. And Snoose was all bark but no bite.

Hattie took out her change purse when I left. I shook my head emphatically but two old fists held the purse tightly and her eyes filled with tears.

"You worked four hours so that's two dollars. I always pay my debts. I don't owe nobody nothing and nobody's going to say I do." I took the money.

Towards the end of summer amid unseasonal rain the handyman's truck came down the greasy hill bearing most of Hattie's furniture. Then with very bad grace he and his boy hooked up the stove and heater, knocked together her bed, and hustled furniture where she wanted it. But another load was still to come. I had dropped by and was there when it did.

As it arrived at the gate the man stopped his truck and cut the engine; from the highway gate to the house on the flats was a long drive. He got out slowly and his son stayed in the cab. Hattie saw war. Pulling on her reliable purpling coat she went out to wage it.

"Yer truck break down?"

"No. I've just heard from my neighbour that you don't pay more than fifty cents an hour. You know my rates."

"Fifty cents an hour for labour and labour is what this is."

"What I'm saying, Mrs. Davis, is that unless I get my rates this stuff gets unloaded in the ditch and we drive on."

In the late Dirty Thirties an unskilled labourer could expect no more than forty dollars a month. That worked out to $1.42 per day or seventeen cents per hour. That was Hattie's training in firing hands. She had raised the ante magnanimously by 1951. But labourers by then were earning at least one dollar an hour.

Coming over the bridge at just this moment was a wondrous figure with snowy aura beneath a big, dark woolly tam. A large umbrella vaunted aloft and the body was clothed in a long navy Burberry, well belted, surmounted by windings of a long white knitted muffler. Gardening gloves grasped a stripped sapling as, walking stick in one hand and the "brolly" in the other, Mrs. Travers slid her way in floppy overshoes through the greasy ruts.

"How's the moving going?" She was breathless, with umbrella aslant one shoulder, as she raised her wand in accolade.

"Our Mr. Jones is so helpful," she went on. "I had to put in a new boiler the other day."

"What did he charge you?" inquired Hattie nastily.

"Oh. The usual. Fifty or sixty cents an hour for the work part, isn't it? I don't pay much attention to these things. Do me a favour Hattie, and come to the store with me. I'm not much good in this mud. Mr. Jones doesn't need us women around, do you? And Jimmy here is so big and strong. Please give your mother my kindest regards, won't you. Mrs. Davis won't be long."

Jones tore down the driveway at top speed as the two old girls picked their way to the store. I was going there anyway and so followed at a respectful distance, overcome with mirth.

The proprietor was behind his counter as usual, but today he had chosen to display some eggs in trays rather than leave them in their crates. The big drum heater was now alight to ward off damp and was glowing centrally, with an occasional glimmer cheering the scene.

Some Americans were talking moose to a local and buying shot against the coming season; they had just pulled two huge trout out of the secret little lake and I could have killed them. On the other side of the store were the welfare woman and the proprietor's wife. Both these women turned to greet Mrs. Travers and stiffened a little when they saw Hattie behind her.

"Hello everybody," quoth Violet. "What are you cooking up today?" They laughed apprehensively.

"How do." Hattie inclined to them with dignity and they murmured back.

"What I would like, Hattie," her friend told her loudly, "are some big brown eggs." Eggs must have been discussed. "Here they are displayed already. How very convenient." She looked across to the man talking moose with the sportsmen. "How are your hens laying in this change of weather, Mr. Hay?" He had no ready answer.

"Oh God for a camera!" muttered one American. He was taking stock of that huge old woman and her prissy mufflered friend.

"How many?" The shopkeeper stood poker faced.

"Just six. They'll last me a week, you know," laughed Hattie's mentor, full of innocence.

"I'll take six of those as well," added Hattie.

On further thought she had more to say. At last she had found out how Violet did things and gave it a try. "They look real nice laid out like that."

The man behind the counter smiled at her for the first time, the other women moved unconsciously closer and in the flicker of flame from the heater the eggs seemed to glow— as if made of pure gold.

Brassy Reality

While Hattie had been having these experiences during the summer, her young neighbours had dealt with different things. Joan had been to stay with friends up the railway, where unknown to me, the girls had attended sock dances at small places like Chu Chua and Little Fort. She was growing up too fast and apparently somebody else was worrying about her too.

One night late in summer, while she was away with friends and Mrs. Davis was having moving problems, I was coming out of our room into the kitchen, which meant passing through the tiny anteroom. This, after a trade with Joan, now held Robby's bed. Above his sleeping head and through the window came the glare of powerful headlights, which were moving right up under the window itself.

We knew nobody who would do that. Inside me, though, I knew somebody who would. My heart nearly stopped when I heard a familiar voice outside. Car doors slammed. He wouldn't. Oh yes he would!

Bob was sitting at his customary place beside the kitchen table, a can of tobacco in front of him and rollings in the making. His usual bedtime potion of cocoa, canned milk and sugar was beside him, as beer was for Friday nights. The heater was stoked, nights were drawing in and a single bulb suspended from the ceiling did little to dispel the gloom.

There was a loud and cheerful thumping on the door and a silvery head appeared. It announced itself to my present husband's astounded glare. I could not manage to squeak, much less speak. But the men seemed to sort things out without declaring war.

In two strides George, my tall, skinny ex, was over at the table saying, "Don't get up. (Who was going to?) We were in Nelson seeing my wife's sister and thought we might as well run up and see how you people are." He'd probably been plotting it all summer. Bob fought for a suitable crushing quip but couldn't find one fast enough.

There was a small flurry behind me where I stood rooted to the floor. My successor, my children's stepmother, had flown in saying "Where's my Robby?" as she poked around the curtain and found him, awake now, in his trundle bed. As he sat up rubbing his eyes, astounded to hear his father's voice, she swooped him into her arms from a squatting position beside his bed. He was too surprised and sleepy to react.

HER Robby? Oh shock upon shock. Meanwhile, Bob had

to be rescued from that overhanging presence. Rescuing and ruining were needed. Snatching up a cigarette lighter from the table I held it in the palm of my hand under my ex's nose.

"See what I have?" It was of solid brass inlaid with black onyx. "Bob got it for me in Juneau." In short, this man gives me presents even if this inspection tour implies nothing of the sort could happen. It was the best I could manage.

Bob had now recovered his poise but remained seated. After all, they had damn well broken in. He regarded my ex with lofty dignity, forcing him to remain on his feet while chattering away about the highway and trying to find our house. The lighter was taken out of my hand, turned over and examined carefully. "Japa-nee?" he asked Bob guilelessly. Bob got up and went outside.

Their errand was to say that both Joan's grandmothers were worried about her. His mother wanted her to be sent to a convent school and when that didn't wash with my mother, changed the suggestion to a private school near her. My mother wanted her to attend my old school. I blew.

"What is this deciding by other people what I'm to do with my daughter?"

"Now don't be like that!" put in my cheeky successor. I gave her a foul look.

Certainly I'd known Joan couldn't stay in this area much longer, but I needed time to make a plan. I knew too well their bossy huddles down on the coast and their arbitrary decisions.

"Well, we gotta go," said my personal monster. "You do some thinking. Your mother's willing to take her. We just wanted to see if everything was okay. No news is bad news in this case." With that they drove off.

I couldn't look at Bob when he came back in. He said nothing because there was nothing left to say. He sat by the table again quietly, looking at me inscrutably. I felt indignantly soiled.

"I think," he said finally, reaching under the table, "that this calls for a beer." We let things ride for awhile.

Joan was not to be influenced by other family members if

I could help it, but to deprive her of chances such as I'd had would be cruel. In the end, after corresponding with my mother a few times, it was decided that Joan should go down and live with her while she attended my school as a day girl. Food and fees would be covered by allowances, paid to Mother instead of to me, with Joan's father footing a few extras. He had another family and obligations, and for my part financial heroics were not expected as long as he helped out with his children's board. Anything else they had came out of their stepfather's lunch bucket from day to day. It was a tight situation.

On the Move

By now Bob was restless again. There was little wonder at it. Nothing but shakes and bush sawmills. What he did was to place the top-heavy housing back on the trailer, hitch the whole to the jeep and take off on an exploration junket, leaving us stranded in the cabin. He was gone several days over the Labour Day weekend but came back glowing.

"I've found it! I've found where we're going to live, I think. You must come and see what you think too."

It was the end of our little ménage for awhile. Once again Joan was put on a train in time for the new fall term, a week after Labour Day, the beginning of a series of endless goodbyes and hellos as she grew up, graduated and went to work. This time she would be with my mother, my poor mother, over seventy. And at the same time it was decided to send Robert down with her until we were settled and I could fetch him back around Christmas time. It was common sense and Bob seemed to think it safer. Another parting, another school.

"You'll have to get rid of the dog as well," pronounced our doom-maker. "You don't know what we're going to run into and he's another mouth to feed. The old girl will take him, you will see. She's always trying to take him over."

Hattie was delighted and agreed to have him for a weekend while we searched for a new home.

Again it was hunting season. And I would soon have to find yet another school for Robert when we settled. That put spurs to me. The next Saturday saw us three family remainders setting out at dawn on the Bridge Lake Road towards the other north–south highway.

"What I'm going to do is build a house," said Bob with decision. "A log house. There's a lot of lodgepole over there.

"Around here is all very pretty but it's too far from anything unless you're a rancher. I want you somewhere settled so I don't have to worry about you."

We had left Barriere at dawn and now we drove on in silence, coming out at 100-Mile, then down past 70-Mile and I wondered why he was heading south. In no time we came to a valley in which was nestled the tiny town of Clinton and as we came down the long hill towards it Bob pointed a far-flung finger out the jeep door.

"See that? Dogpatch. And down there? Boot Hill. That's it. This is where we stay and that," indicating a grassy hummock, "is where I'll rest my bones."

He was right. We settled on The Chasm, several miles out of town on a school bus route, renting a two-bedroom cabin from a rancher who owned surrounding land, then ascertained that there was no dearth of employment at the usual, ever-present sawmill.

Hurrying back to the North Thompson, we packed our bags and said our farewells. It would be bleak at first without the other kids, but we were all used to these comings and goings. Snoose was busy skittering around his new ranch home and in a way we were glad. Hattie's need was greater than ours. We were never to see her again, but my friend, the ranger's wife with whom I'd taken tea in the house among the jack pines, promised to write and give me all news and report on our pet.

As soon as we'd moved Bob went down into his Dogpatch and began negotiations immediately at the government agency about buying a lot in town. Sure enough, there was a piece of unwanted crown land right opposite a big new school, and on the edge of what was earmarked as a park but was in fact a willow swamp.

Before long, somewhere between our temporary cabin and

100 Mile House, a log deck grew, beside a gravel road off the highway, of thirty-five- to forty-foot lodgepole pines for which Bob may or may not have paid stumpage. These logs were to lie and season all winter for building next spring.

Meanwhile we had a larder to fill and there was somebody new to meet.

CHAPTER · XII

|||||||||||||||||||||||||||||||||||||||||||||||||||||||||||||||||||||||||||||||||||||||||||||||||||||||||||||||||||||||||||||

Around the Dam

Briar in the Willows

At the first opportunity we began to explore the terrain around our cabin, which sat on a small rise overlooking a gravel road and a valley full of ranch lands. In a far meadow, running along the trees edge, were railway tracks. Over to the left of our view, where our road met the tracks, were some white-washed stockyards.

On the first day at Chasm we heard a horrible noise that turned out to be a train approaching the stockyard crossing. The new train was a diesel and its shrill whistle made the wail of the BYN's Cannonball a thing of nostalgic beauty.

"Cats on the keyboard," I remarked bitterly.

Beside the cabin and running down from the hill behind us and under the road to the ranches, was a gurgling stream. It emerged from a small forest, also behind us. Where there are streams there are often lakes and we took our fish poles to follow the water course back into the bush. We were not far wrong.

A small square lake, or reservoir, had been formed by bull-dozing up four earthen walls in a marshy field into which the stream ran at the top end to emerge at our end over a weir. It was quite a size, and no pond, and very obviously supplied the ranches below with water for drinking and cattle. The dam was surrounded on all sides by scrub brush, and lily pads crowded the far end, among which were paddling some good, fat wild ducks. A small pier of one plank on supports was at one side of the reservoir and around its rim the uneven clumps of earth that contained the water were grown over with willows.

We followed a thin path behind the willows right around the small lake, heading for the plank pier on the other side, thinking to use it. Just ahead the trail curved around a tree and, too late, we realized we were not alone. We were trespassing. The strong scent of bitter pipe tobacco reached us, simultaneously followed by puffs of smoke curling out from behind the tree into still air. Unable to back up without looking stupid, we became aware of a black figure, tall and old, watching us calmly. Black pants, black shirt, and this time a corncob pipe. The figure did not move or blink. Rallying silent excuses for being there, we looked to right and left, uncertain what to do.

"Did you catch anything?"

Quick to seize an opportunity, Bob emitted an embarrassed fox bark and started to summon his bush wits for an angle.

"You'd be van Horlick's tenants," continued the apparition, wisely giving us time. "I see you aren't lucky. Well, the best place to get 'em is over by my dock. Rainbows are small in here and a mite lazy and they've probably finished feeding this time of day. Well, I'll be getting back." With that the tall dark form with its white crew-cut disappeared into the bush.

"What about that!" erupted Bob. "Didn't I tell you what the folks around here would be like?" Too rattled to fish, we headed for home. "But not all of them, mind you. Am not sure how it will be with van Horlick after some incidents I've heard about, but I bet I can get on with the guy. I'm sure going to look up that old boy. He'll be interesting."

Our cabin, though new, was a typical sawmill shack with which the woods were sprinkled. Local landowners would throw them up for revenue to rent to mill hands who would otherwise have a long way to go to work. The sawmill itself was deep in the woods down its own road, which branched off ours.

The cabin site was unfenced in open range land, which left our toddler unprotected from roving shorthorns and caused me to tether him on a long rope; this after a battle. He was old enough to talk a little and assert himself and when I told him a definite no to setting off down the road, and had brought him back several times, I saw that words were useless with this venturesome kid. I tied a cord around his waist, drove a stake into the ground near the back door and gave him plenty of slack. Not only were cattle loose but the place was haunted by roving dogs.

At such times I could see him a few feet away from a window. Cattle never came near the cabin, which was on a rise, but he would have wandered far afield among them. Buster van Horlick's dogs were not interested at all, unless they came with him, or were interfered with.

In any case, tying Mark up didn't work.

Bob told me once that I would try to mould Mark to be like my other children and that I wouldn't succeed. When he discovered his walking limits Mark was so furious he threw himself to the ground, stomach down, pounding toes and biting dirt. I had never seen such a display or such a baby. Later, in the banked snow paths of winter when he still ran off, I would have to lay him over the chopping block and paddle him through thick layers of clothes with a stick from the woodpile. It did not hurt his spirits one bit, or cure him either.

Across the road from us was our landlord's, Buster van Horlick's ranch, though "ranch" was a slight exaggeration. His snake fences were falling down except where his cattle had to be penned, and his sun-blackened barn with its hayloft and his house were in disrepair; old machinery rusted near the back of the ranch house and behind the outhouse in the rear of their property was their dump. Haystacks lined the fence inside the front yard. It wasn't so bad, probably typical of a lot of ranches, but we were shocked after seeing the neatness of North Thompson ranges. Inside the house the centre of activity was the kitchen, full of steam and shouts, where the coffee pot boiled endlessly and you got a mug rinsed out in a bubbling boiler full of clothes.

Everyone around the Chasm made a hit-and-miss living at the sawmill, including Buster. His wife Una and her two impish girls ran the farm. She was a yelling fury and her girls were teenage queens in Stetsons, riding bare back, flailing their horses with riding crops all over the country to see what they could see. There was also a little boy called Bobby who liked to tease kittens. To round out the establishment there were those two bloodhounds that meant business.

The noisy rows that took place between Una and Buster were so curdling that children in the area played a game called "Una and Buster" to imitate them. Bob had no intention of being drawn into neighbours' quarrels or of listening to gossip about them; we were determined to get along with our landlord. After all we were experienced in that sort of thing.

Being very lonely, as I surmised, Una came one day to call on me about the milk we bought from them, appearing at our door with the two hounds.

"They won't hurt you," she said, as the dogs coursed around making Baskerville noises and growling through the screen.

Inevitably the chatting turned into frank conversation about Buster's temper, for his was the worst. After enough of this and thinking to smooth things down I delivered a favourite maxim.

"There's nothing like a jolly good fight to clear the air. A good argument is the spice of life. I bet you enjoy it. You wouldn't do without him if you could."

"Me!" she shrieked. "I'd as soon live with a rattlesnake!"

More was to come of that later in the summer. Meanwhile, at the first opportunity Bob set off to follow the trail of the old man we met by the dam until he found his lair. He entered the stretch of jack pine between our cabin and the reservoir where the drumming of grouse was almost constant. A small trail came up through the willows to that tree by the pier and following down it Bob found himself in a clearing the size of half a city lot, full of vegetables. Working around the patch he came upon a venerable log barn, facing the dam and silver with weathering, beyond which was a small log house. Trees pressed against the house and barn site on each side, but the view was open at the back towards the lake and open in front of the house where fields stretched away.

Following a single line of balm of Gilead trees that served as fencing, Bob came circuitously and politely to the front approach. These trees were deciduous young saplings whose roots propagated sideways like a fence. The incense from the trees was heavy. A private road wound up from the main gate to the house which, seen from the front, looked like a small gray sentinel between the forests, facing down the fields before it. A single gable graced it, like that of a wildwoods church. There was a wing built to one side with a white-curtained window; a door and another window were under the gable and that was it. The door opened straight onto all weathers over a four-by-four that passed as a step. Someone moved near the window by the door, which soon opened silently. No dog barked.

The face confronting Bob was long and weathered but with few wrinkles. The stiff white bottlebrush hair stood above screwed up eyes of penetrating Norwegian blue and the ears were long.

"I've been expecting you one of these times." Curiosity in the country worked both ways. "Name's Bolstad." He led the way into what looked like the main and only room, the kitchen. "Have a chair over there."

In the middle of the room stood an old kitchen table, scrubbed clean, beside a good old cook stove attached to the windowless wall with its chimney. On the table were tobacco cans, a crib board and some old letters; under a side window was the eating table with a radio on a shelf overhead. Against the rest of the radio wall was an old black leather couch and two chairs.

The chief feature of this room was a tall rocking chair drawn up by the central table, high-backed enough to support a tall man's head and lined with a goatskin hide, and painted a thick clean grey like the rest of the house inside. Visible through two greying cotton curtains that barely met was the bedroom and the old man's cot with army blankets on it. I took in these details eventually, as Bob didn't notice them.

"How are you coming along with Buster?" began Chris Bolstad, settling into his rocker. He never seemed to sit anywhere else.

"I make a point of getting along with everyone." From Bob's report of this visit it was easy enough for me to reconstruct the conversation.

"He's not so bad. Pretty cruel to that wife of his, which I don't like. About the dam..." Chris went on to describe Buster getting a gang together to dam the creek on Chris's land in return for rights on the weir.

"If he don't like anyone he can fill up his tanks then shut the water off for awhile on any excuse. But he don't bother me. Una comes over with the kid sometimes and brings me a pie. Maybe harum scarum but she's pretty good to me. I don't know nobody now. They're all dead."

"How long've you been here?" Bob would be making a rolling from the tobacco can pushed in front of him.

"Nineteen hundred. Came by on the Trail of '98 and homesteaded here on the way back. The Cariboo Road used to go right by the door and later it was mail coaches. Come on out and see my barn. Got my forge out there."

The barn was full to the loft with hay; embedded in the centre of it were great blocks of ice, years old. He used the barn as a silo for his products and all his farm implements were there. At one time he had kept horses but now, at seventy-five, he did nothing more than dig his vegetable patch and feed the moose who came to nibble at his balm tree boundaries.

Chris's acreage was the maximum allowed to preemptors in early days: about one hundred sixty acres cultivated and more if you wanted to own forestland. No one knew if he'd paid for his preemption or if he was still squatting. He never discussed his business with a soul. Rumour had it that Buster was jealous of Chris's fertile property and had an eye on it, but there was no proof of that either.

Bob arrived home with a skinned rabbit wrapped in a

huge rhubarb leaf, one of many such gifts we would receive through the warm season. One thing Chris grew was his own tobacco and the strong smell of it always announced his presence in the woods.

The Convivial Season

Before long snow was flying again and the two men played many crib games by lamplight beside Chris's black woodstove. Chris's hideaway was less than half a mile down the road between ranches and it was easier to go by road. The winter went quickly and I didn't begrudge such absences because I had a dozen projects going: typing yarns, writing letters and making a plaited rug while I listened to the radio. Besides one was always hopping up and down to fetch firewood and we always went to bed soon after dark.

It had been arranged that Mark and I would go down on the adjacent train to fetch Robert when the Christmas holidays began. When they did, Bob put our toddler and myself on the PGE line for Squamish and thence to Vancouver Island. The train was sooty and old-fashioned and the car vaunted a little coal heater at one end of the kind used by pioneer colonists to cook their meals enroute. The old gas lamps were still hanging up. There was more danger of rockslides on the tracks then, but we had to ignore that.

Robert seemed willing to return, but Joan had settled in and made friends. She and my mother got along well as Joan was trained to help and respect elders. Everything hit the fan, though, when one day Joan brought home a Chinese immigrant girl.

I am afraid to say that Chinese immigrants in Victoria had a hard time with the locals and Mother was no exception. Victoria's provincial, snobby little "Four Hundred" had no space for Orientals, who were mostly Hong Kong labourers seeking the "Gold Mountain" who found themselves working as houseboys, launderers, and truck gardeners. But my old school had no objection to Chinese money and so I had a very interesting classmate called Anna Mae Wong (not the Chinese actress). She was the exception. Nowadays that school has gone "international" and welcomes girls from various Asiatic countries around the Pacific Rim.

However, apart from Joan's fury at her grandmother's attitude, all went well, and she stayed behind while Robby came home to us to the second room of our cabin, a lean-to, approached from the outside, out the back door and around the corner.

We were making friends also. The mill owners were very affable, and Bob also chummed with a tall, dark truly Canadian man called Howard, and his jolly plump wife, the union of a long-standing bachelor and a widow with two grown sons. Howard Lyons was Canadian because he was neither English, American or anything else. A prairie type perhaps. They were an older couple but we had something in common. I was aware that Bob thought a remarried widow with sons might be a good influence on me, and in fact they would become Mark's godparents. We would go into town for supplies on a Saturday afternoon and meet them for beer. Dottie did not seem too bothered about her sons and this was held up as an example to me. Also her view of Bob was full of kindliness and mirth and at one time, after I had finished shopping and had joined the three of them at an overflowing table, she had observed my face as I came in on one of Bob's worthier Baron Munchhausen lying yarns and she patted my arm.

"He's not as bad as you think he is, you know."

Impishness in Bob always bubbled up. His strong sense of humour backed up his desire to keep life on an even keel.

While this sport was going on I would be watching through the cafe curtains the boys outside in the jeep. Robert had his work cut out in reading his comic book and supervising Mark's clamberings around. Sometimes I'd excuse myself and join the gang later. We had to bring the boys into town unless Mark was dead asleep and Robert at nine years old could watch him for awhile. In those days bush children were sensible and responsible because they had to be. Robert was no exception.

Bob's bent for teasing struck a chord in the ample bosom of the mill owner's wife Della Ruckle, a very hospitable come-allye hostess who was a cross between Mae West and her predecessor of the 1920s, Sophie Tucker, but was much more like the latter. They were the fun-loving sex symbols of the 20s and 30s, naughty but nice. Della was a very warm woman who fitted that description down to her ski socks. Her husband, a most unlikely mill type, was tall, gentle and looked quite scholarly, a most deceiving mien when it came to work ethics. He came from Saltspring Island where his father had bequeathed property now known as Ruckle Provincial Park.

There were two other males as well, both single, who ran a small logging operation not far from the sawmill, who would show up at Della's gatherings. One was the owner of the smaller mill, Harold Schiefke, who was well educated, while his sidekick and assistant, Amos Fowler, was a simpler man but stocky, fair and of few words. Bob took to the latter who was friendly enough, but who went mostly everywhere on business or pleasure with his boss. They were a team.

There was a tall, skinny cowboy-turned-rancher with a family and a spread near the highway. All these people were good for a laugh when we met in town and they were the folk that we knew. Two of them at least, with university degrees, were an example of how to adapt to the bush and live there with the proper attitude which was: when in Rome do as Rome does and get on with it. That applied to clothes, speech, work habits and outlook, though always with that little edge which less complicated locals respected.

Christmas passed happily enough in our own little shack with the boys. During the winter Robert caught the school bus and was gone all day. He seemed too busy to show evidence of missing his sister, and in any case Bob was treating him like a man and showing him men's things to do with guns and woodpiles. Respect between them was mutual. They believed in getting on.

We trusted Robert enough one evening to guard Mark while we attended a nearby Christmas party put on by Della, where punch bowls and beer overflowed and food and wine aplenty met our eager gaze as we stamped off snow and left our boots in the great heap of overshoes by the door. We needed the break badly and if Robert had not been careful about fire and other contingencies we could not have left them.

The place was full of a rosy glow caused by candles and tree lights, a fire and red decorations. The mill had its own generator and the house was fully lit. The oldest son sat tinkling at an old piano, of harpsichord tone, and his forte seemed to be "We were sailing along on Moonlight Bay," which his mother sang robustly while beckoning in new guests.

Chris was much more connected with the van Horlicks than we knew and had taken his Christmas with them. And with these things time passed rapidly until about February when it was still impossible in the snow to start on cement footings for the house in town.

Labours of Love

More for something to do than anything, Bob decided to take the jeep apart. Near us was an abandoned chicken shed turned garage, made of logs and very snug. It had been built for some other purpose and eventually a woman showed up with a camera saying it had been her schoolhouse. In early summer swallows would nest in its eaves, making dozens of mud nests and becoming a plague. After supper every night Bob took the gas lamp out there and worked over the engine, gradually dismantling it. It had been a little cranky. If he failed to get it back again in the order in which he took it apart we'd be isolated, not to mention being unable to get on with our building.

"You always said I'm no mechanic. Well now I'm going to teach myself." He was successful and we had no more trouble.

Spring came and those swallows, swooping out at us. Horse trading began. We had a deck of logs to transport into town and nothing on which to haul them. Across the way Buster had a long flat trailer.

Bob's caravan contraption had been dismantled for its lumber and the planks put toward building a better boat, partly started the previous fall. Buster envied us our little Whitehorse skiff as much as Bob coveted Buster's long trailer. Before I could stop them a smooth exchange took place.

The next valued item to disappear was Bob's typewriter. He had kept thinking he would write some fine trapping stories and he did knock off a few, lurid though they were. He now picked up the machine saying, "That's that. It was only a phase anyway." Buster's girls got the lovely little thing in exchange for building gear from his stockpile. The box trailer had been sold at the mill.

Not wasting a second during spring thaw, Bob finished the new boat outside, a bigger flat-bottomed craft that sat across two sawhorses and was painted green like the first. He was waiting for the side road where our logs were decked to become accessible.

As soon as we could get at the logs we started hauling and I found myself at the building site astride one log at a time, perched across the same sawhorses, while I became adept at using a draw knife for skinning the pines as a long green-backed curl came towards me. It became a challenge to see how long a strip I could peel without making a gouge. That was all I was allowed to do. When I hovered around trying to look useful I was told, "Stand back." Bob had his father's idea that women must not be allowed to do heavy dangerous work whereas Tom, with a woman in tow, was apt to say, "Grab the other end," thinking he was being matey.

There was no end to Bob's resourcefulness or scrounging and trading abilities. Except for cement, hardware, duroid roofing, windows and a single pipe for water, everything was free or off the country. The furnace was made from an oil drum set into a pad made of concrete left over from the footings. Over that summer the building gradually turned into a two-storey house with a dugout basement that a car could enter, two bedrooms downstairs and one up, with room for another up there also. The kitchen was L-shaped, with a rustic bar between the dining area and living room; the whole vista from the fireplace to the back of the dinette was thirty-five feet, the exact length of the longest logs. Outside and overlooked through a big bay window, as well as through the dining windows, was a thirty-five-foot porch.

Bob Smith, five foot two and a half, built the whole thing

himself and not another man came near until wiring time. With an A-frame beside the rising structure he hauled the clean shining pines into position, higher and higher, using the notching skills he'd acquired in Alaska to align the corners.

Inspections

In the second week of May, after all the snows had gone and before the mosquitoes came, my father paid us a visit. We got him off the train, took him out to the shack and put him up in the "bull pen." By now that overworked name was used for the lean-to and he loved it.

"But," he warned, "you'd better not let your mother see this." He meant everything.

Mother had never recovered from the trials of my father in coming out to Canada. Formerly a smooth, top-hatted young Londoner, he landed in 1906 with almost empty pockets to escape supervisory relatives and "make a fortune." He was one of the victims of the Canadian land boom advertised so much at the turn of the twentieth century. He had ridden freight, pitched hay, driven a team and himself into an ice-filled Bow River after cutting ice blocks, and had pushed barrow loads of bricks. "How dreadful for a man like him to have to rough it. I don't know how he survived."

She thought muscles and sweat revolting, though she did get kittenish over barrel-chested Mounties. It took her years to understand what Bob was made of and what his dreams were all about.

It was only after his wife Nellie had died (1968) that Laurence Cuming confided to Mark that he had been pursued by the North West Mounted Police for bootlegging to the Natives at Fort Macleod. "They were coming in the front flap of the tent while I was going out the back!" He'd had to leave some of his photography equipment behind.

Around the family my father was known as "Pop." To my sister and me he was Dad, and a kindlier one no girls ever had, though we never dared mess around when he scowled.

He had his seventy-second birthday with us and I made a cake. He accepted his cot in the lean-to with Robert and kidded me about the "bull pen." Then of course he wanted to go into town with Bob and help him build the house. Bob was very good about it.

"I let him hand me tools and bang up a few things but of course he's much too slow." The thought of my father in his viyella plaid working shirt with tie and tie pin, and Bob in his usuals with carpenter's apron and ski cap, working side by side, was too much for my funny bone and I had to disappear for awhile.

Before he left my father delivered himself of some philosophies to me in private.

"If I were to drop dead tomorrow I'd have had a pretty good life. No complaints. But you've got to get yourself straightened out. You've got too many irons in the fire and don't know which to work on." He meant my trying to write, cook, hunt and make rag rugs all at once. He perceived the state of my mind perfectly well, and the cause of its ambivalence.

"Concentrate on one thing at a time and finish it." He had what you call the single eye. "Stop looking back over your shoulder at the past and be thankful for what you have now. Do what I do. Live for each day." Simple. It went down like restorative wine.

Then my mother-in-law came, all by herself. Curiosity about what Bob was up to was too much for her. She couldn't wait to be driven and took the train. She was a good sport, fitting herself into what she found, but experience in camping and mountain climbing had not included shacks.

She loved the log house in its beginning stages and regaled me with plans she had drawn (as I had) for her own home. She did not go into rhapsodies over her son's building feats; she'd expected them. What she did do was cajole Una's bloodhounds. The dogs came over to investigate and I warned her, but in two seconds flat she was outside the screen door with them, patting them and giving them little bits of food.

"Doesn't pay to be afraid. They know, you see."

The Smiths both drove up later, just before we moved into town. His father was overwhelmed by Bob's achievements.

Joan returned to us at the beginning of July. There were no more funds for private school and she needed a mother's eye.

She had shed tears at leaving friends when term was up, but it was too much to expect an elderly mother to raise my daughter. The town school was a new one with grade school and high school in one and had good teachers. Joan moved into the lean-to and hung up a blanket "wall." The log house wouldn't be ready until September, just before school opened.

The weather was blazing when she came and soon she and Robert sat in the stream in bathing suits to cool off. They looked a pretty sight—apart from the ethics of sitting in drinking water—amid the dappled shadows of birches.

News of Joan's arrival must have gone around the dam area within hours, for scarcely had she settled in when a lone biker began to appear. He buzzed up and down the road in front of the shack for several days, then one day when she was just outside the door she saw a slick-haired youth in black leather standing beside the log chicken house some distance away, silently watching her. She watched back puzzled.

"What does he want, do you suppose?" she asked me.

"Just casing the situation. News travels fast." She had just turned fifteen and it would happen often. Clinton youth had spotted her.

The children would push Mark's stroller along the road. They would try to avoid passing a culvert through which the stream ran, but if going that way they would run by very quickly. Returning with them once, I saw why. A great black crowd of bugs rose around them with a hideous whine that could be heard yards away. They ran like the wind, telling Mark to hold on tight, as the black cloud followed them all the way home until they got inside the shack with a horde of deprived mosquitoes winding up on the screen door. There would be other mosquito bouts, but mostly we were too busy helping around the new house to go into the bush.

During a lull in the weekend building, when the weather was sweltering, Chris Bolstad paid a state visit to our cabin. Except for going over to van Horlick's it was not his custom to visit anybody because he really was a hermit.

I had made some home brew previously and the smell of boiling hops had driven the kids outdoors. Bob had provided bottles and a capping machine. He must have passed an invitation after testing it. As soon as I saw Chris Bolstad coming over the brow of the hill I ran down with a bottle or two and placed them to chill among tree roots in the stream bed while Bob greeted him. He came bearing a mess of trout, neatly gutted, strung on a string, and wrapped in another big leaf.

Bob still played crib and soaked up information about the surrounding country in Chris's kitchen on some nights, but mostly he was too tired from wrestling with logs after an early dinner and a day at the mill. He didn't waste a second of the daylight hours. After supper we would go down to the town lot and returning after an evening of building we'd find yet another rhubarb leaf presentation just inside the screen door: two dressed grouse, or fresh vegetable, or more rabbit, or fish. Chris was the only person who could catch trout successfully in his pond; the countryside was full of his little wire rabbit snares. Una van Horlick would make rabbit stew and he'd get some.

He was so good with children. Little as he was, Mark was taken by the hand up to the dam and shown how to fish with an old line on a fresh willow pole, with an unbarbed hook and a little green and yellow float.

"D'you want to see some rabbits? You come over here quietly some time and squat down behind a bush like that one—that's it, down like that—and make a noise like a baby rabbit. They make a funny kissing noise." Chris showed him. "Then the big ones will come looking for you."

The kid so loved him it was once to prove the undoing, in a way, of Buster's much-touted role as a villain mean to family and people in general.

One noon when Bob came home from the mill he found the shack empty and lunch half ready. Then he saw me flying back over the hill behind the cabin in tears. "Mark's missing!"

Using his head, Bob ran straight over to Buster who was also home for lunch and who was soon on the phone, causing the mill alarm to go off and trucks to rev up. In five minutes a group of men, lunchless, with Buster in the van giving orders, were fanning out.

Feeling useless, I set off for Chris's place to see if he knew anything and there was Mark, sitting quietly, eating a chocolate bar. Chris knew nothing of the uproar and thought the siren meant a mill accident. He was just about to bring Mark home.

Rag Mop

There was no holding Buster down for awhile. He basked in sudden popularity. Once his lunchless heroics became known people had to stop sniping at him and say something nice for a change. But only for a while. Soon he was back at his old game of pitch-forking horses, so I heard, hissing at animals or sucking in his breath to deliver a tirade—a blue-jeaned, saddle-bent, beak-nosed bone rack under a black Stetson. He liked trading though. He and Bob kept swapping things in deals where Buster did not always come out on top, but thought he had.

Una was not much better than her spouse. Wild of eye and hair with a vicious temper when crossed, she one day outdid Buster's pitch-forkings with a scene that took place right in front of our shack.

I heard wild yells outside and ran out in time to see Una emerging with a shotgun while several puppies ran cowering from her porch. Shots filled the air as puppies bowled over one by one, full of grape.

"Come on!" she shouted at her girls inside. "Get busy!" They came out and, seeming willing, dragged the pups away. Una called across to me unabashed. "They were all over my kitchen table eating my new batch of cookies. I'm so sick of the bloody animals around here! Throw them on the dung heap!" I was horror-stricken, but wisely I felt, kept my own counsel.

When a horse had to be destroyed it was Una who had to shoot it, not her husband. They deserved each other. The whole prospect kept her weary and hard.

It was actually after this that Una gave up trying and took off with her children for the coast. Buster simply let her get on with it and have a bad time without money. While she was gone a blonde "maid" kept house for him, much to the titillation of the neighbours who were keeping tabs on the van Horlick miseries and enjoying themselves enormously. Buster was much too smart to be trapped by women. He gave out that the girl was a relative and kept it that way. God knows she could have been, as he'd given no indication of being a woman chaser.

When it seemed that Una had had her lesson, he hopped into his truck and went to fetch his woman—dragging her, I adored to think, almost literally by the hair. Quite thankful at being queen of her own domain again, and with Buster's full cooperation, she packed the maid onto one of their horses, with her duffle bag up behind her, and sent them off with a right sharp smack on the horse's rump.

These were the people that Chris turned to when in trouble because he didn't want to turn to anyone else. He was dependent upon them for very many little kindnesses that few knew about.

Una would take pre-school Bobby and herself over the dusty half mile that separated their doors, carrying the usual pie and mail; over this same road by lantern went Chris at night when he wanted medicine or anything fetched from town the next morning. Little Bobby knew Chris was good for chocolate or pop, you never knew what, except that you couldn't fool around. Usually benign, the old guy was suddenly frightening if you did. He wouldn't say anything, just fix the offending child with a chilling Nordic-blue stare. It was most effective.

Neighbours speculated on why seemingly cruel people could be so kind to an old hermit. Their conclusion was obvious; Buster meant to inherit the old boy's land since Chris had no kin. But then again, we thought, if they really looked after him and were kind why shouldn't they? The answer was not forthcoming from Chris. He was smart enough to remain tongue-in-cheek and dodgy if he thought people were nosy or plotting, and he kept his mouth shut. If anyone complained to him about the van Horlicks he would just say, "That's Buster for you," or Una, as the case might be. One knew he knew what he knew and would stay out of frays. And what I do remember about van Horlicks is that they were very kind to us.

More Visitations

There were more visitors. While the children were out of school their big brothers decided to pay a visit to the Cariboo and check out the new house, which still lacked a roof. There had been some hint that the boys would appear during the summer, but no more had been heard. Then one morning, very early when it was barely daybreak, there was a knocking on the shack door.

"What the hell?" Bob sprang out of bed and unshot the bolt.

There in a crack of light were two tall forms, David and Henry, looking both apprehensive and sheepish. They had good reason. It must have been about 5:00 a.m. They had found that the train did have a request stop for Chasm, BC, near the stockyards, but hadn't realized that it went through at four in the morning. They had no recourse but to get off in the dark. They followed the white stockyard fencing but could barely see the road. As it was too early to expect to find beds or welcome they had settled into a dry patch of roadside grass and had tried to sleep. Eventually the discomfort was too much and they wound up at the shack. They had no trouble in finding it. It was the only cabin in sight. All else was ranch property.

To say that Bob was annoyed was an understatement. They came in and had breakfast and their stepfather took off pretty quickly for work. What to do? This was the walking-on-eggs time when I felt like the Virgin Mary with two sons crucified. With our own bed in the main room and only two beds in the lean-to, there was no question of sleeping on floors. I could not really blame Bob's lack of graciousness as the boys had neither written they were actually coming—to give us half a chance of finding them accommodation somewhere and to lay in food— nor had they researched their time tables.

The best thing I could do if I wanted to avoid tension was to find something to keep them busy then put them on the return train that night. Joan came to the rescue with the idea of going exploring and taking a lunch, but it ruled out including me because of Mark. Just seeing them and having them walk across the fields away from me meant crying inside, and for real when the door was shut.

Some miles from where we lived was a deep chasm, from which the settlement got its name. There was a small lake at the bottom, which David, when he heard of it, decided to fish. He always carried fishline and hooks in his pocket. He soon found out how stagnant it was.

They had a wonderful time, slipping and sliding to the bottom of the scenic spot with Joan and Robert tailing after them. And later over dinner everyone had recovered a sense of fitness, especially Bob, who was going to show them the new house before putting them on the train.

And still more visitors.

What we were doing must have attracted friends on the coast. One of my best friends, Sandra, came up with husband, young son and Boston pup. They stayed in Clinton, some ten miles away from our cabin, but I had a good time roaring around in their car and in the course of piloting them through the back roads they saw in the distance what was probably the Pavilion Range. Sandra prodded her husband.

"Look, look. See the cobalt mountains."

Cobalt! How far was my mind from this friend's colours and exclamations. In this country you never, never mentioned scenery. You breathed it into your bones and kept your mouth shut about it. I was getting like the poet Rupert Brooke who wanted to push some girlfriend off a cliff for being banal about the sunset. But that was only half of it. For years Sandra was to chide me about an episode that followed.

We had all finished a meal at our cabin and there was a pause in activities. I thought they might like a grouse or two to take home and said so, reaching for my gun on the wall.

"What are you doing?" cried my friend in horror.

"Going to get a grouse."

"With THAT?"

I gave her a look and went out but was not able to get one. Years later Sandra was still sounding off the same litany.

"I thought you were out of your mind." It was a good thing she didn't know what I pulled off next.

Sometime later, after they had left, thinking to vary our game diet, I went up to the dam with the boys, hoping to get a duck. There were plenty of them cruising around and surely I could manage that.

Keeping the kids well behind me, I aimed at one and missed, reloaded and fired again as it swam away from me in some alarm into the bulrushes at the far end. That second shot got him. To my chagrin I realized I had hit him in the rump and he wouldn't die. Caring no longer about the food part of it we went around the bushes and rushes hoping to find the duck and end its misery. I was full of remorse. Grouse were no problem, dead in a second. We never did find that duck and I'd have to live with the memory, being darned careful never to shoot anything I couldn't get in the heart or head. My own misgivings were as nothing compared with what awaited me next night.

The boys had already reported the duck mishap and I'd had looks over that. Early next evening Bob went over to Chris' place for some reason and came back looking pretty grim.

"I hear ducks aren't the only thing you shoot at."

"What d'you mean?"

"You damn near shot Chris."

"What?"

"You better get over there first thing in the morning and apologise. Don't you know better than to shoot on water? I thought we went into that. Bullet went right by his ear."

I wanted to make a bolt for it. Yet the old man must be faced. Next morning I went over knowing that nothing said would compensate a ricochet accident. He was among his cabbages and I began my outpouring.

He simply looked up and murmured, "Wouldn't have wanted it to come any closer. D'you want some carrots?" Oh, those eyes.

It was all the worse because I was not a careless hunter and was very law-abiding. Everyone up there shot at things and we were over the required three miles from town. There was nothing behind the dam but empty fields stretching away towards 70 Mile, but I hadn't counted on bullets going sideways.

It put quite a damper on me and was possibly the last time, save one, that I hunted alone.

In the past, while we were still in Hattie country, a beautiful buck with a good rack had been standing on a rock outcrop not thirty feet from Bob and myself. We stood still. Then Bob handed me the Winchester.

"This one's yours."

I got him in my sights with an expert head-on focus. But I saw his eyes, those lovely deer eyes, and my finger froze on the trigger. I simply could not pull it. The buck moved off slowly out of sight and Bob said nothing. Not a word of reproach.

Yet I had thought nothing of potting at squirrels near the North Thompson just for their skins. It makes me cringe to think of it now.

CHAPTER · XIII

Dogpatch

Of Bogs and Bulls

Spring and summer had passed pleasantly. In addition to building we often knocked off to go fishing or swimming in surrounding lakes and went woodcutting also. We were all involved in woodcutting and Robert was getting pretty good on the end of a swede saw. Boys in the country became men at fifteen and were often married and in a tarpaper shack by the time they were seventeen or eighteen.

On one of our sorties Bob explored down a ranch road and decided to take a shortcut with the jeep, which could "get out of anything." It was near a small alkali lake. These were often pretty little lakes in which you could not swim or drink from because the water was totally alkaline. Parts of the field beside the lake were boggy from seepage so that three quarters of the way across the acreage we sank to the axles.

Our approach road was untraveled and likely to remain so with night coming on rapidly. Bob worked for a long time with shovel and branches but we simply spun from bog to bog. Finally he gave up.

"There's nothing for it, we'll just have to spend the night here." We looked at each other in dismay, mouths open.

There were trees here and there and chunks of dead branches scattered handily enough, enabling us to build a fire. It was a good glowing one that kept at bay the twilight mosquitoes that were coming at us in hordes. We were inured to them to some extent but not to masses of them. In fact in balmier days upon his own explorations our adventurer had used a mosquito net around his Stetson, which sent his brother into stitches.

Right now Bob was highly amused at us, seeing us hugging ourselves miserably against the coming cold.

"I'll make good pioneer types out of you people yet."

He had brought up to the fire a sort of raft or piece of an old wall that he'd tried to insert under the jeep. The children opted to sit on that.

"At first light I'll go along the road and keep going until I find someone to haul us out."

We enjoyed the experience in a way. By the time it was dark and we'd shared the last leftover sandwiches the fire was a wide bed of coals giving enormous heat and was ringed with logs to push ends on into the core. Nobody had to be reminded to stoke. We had no rugs but simply lay down in our pants and jackets, the kids choosing the wooden platform and their elders preferring cleared off hollows beside the heat. Everyone kept turning and turning as their backs or fronts became cold.

I was diverted by watching Joan and thinking, "This is what it's all about, kid." Not that she wasn't a competent little sport, but she wasn't aligned in some way. She didn't disapprove of pioneering or "roughing it" so much as she always wanted to do it differently and hated being coerced. In fact, forever afterwards when camping, if I wanted her to come exploring or do something splendid she would reach for a mirror and bobby pins or tidy the tent. Although she was tough she seemed to follow a different drummer.

Unknown to me that night she was really suffering. We were in open range country and cattle were loose. Although we paid little attention to sounds, she could not help listening to the weird lowing, trampling and complaining that cows were making all around us. It was the season after summer when the bulls were turned loose among the cattle. Her impression was not helped by waking just before dawn to find her stepfather gone and to hear when he did get back that the reason he was gone so long was that he'd been treed by a bull and had been forced to stay there until rescued. The farmer with him winched us out and we were soon back at work and school as if nothing had happened.

The subject of bulls, which Joan preferred behind fences, reminded her of a scene in late August, the beginning of the mating season for livestock. She had gone about with friends a little after her return to us and found herself stacking hay in a field somewhat beyond Chris' place with a very good-looking nephew of Buster's. The process led to forking hay in Buster's barn and a little friendly innocent horseplay in the hayloft.

Ruffled by this, she was later that day escorting Robert and one or two of his little friends along the roads, when all the children saw a bull being very busy or about to be. Before the bull knew what had happened Joan leaned over the fence and with suitable blessings and gestures repeated what she could remember of the Anglican marriage service over him and his cow. That was the best she could do for the little children who watched fascinated.

School time approached and once again Joan became a large lone figure among the small children who clambered into the school bus on their circuit. Fortunately for her, she would no longer be conspicuous as a big goon among the little ones because the roof was on the new house and the windows were in, rendering a school bus redundant. We deemed it time to settle.

The Good Life

It was now September and the children and I had been chinking logs with moss. Mortar was expensive and messy and could not be hurried. We fetched moss from a perfect place in the woods where it was thick, and filled bags and bags with it each time. The faster we stuffed the open chinks the warmer we would be and the sooner we could move in.

All was excitement. While we insulated, Bob dug a deep ditch in front to bring in the water line and keep it from freezing. One single tap had to do and it came up in Joan's bedroom, which would be the bathroom at some future date. Then he installed his homemade furnace and vents.

Moving day was unreal. We had never had our own home before. We could not stop going in and out and round about instead of unpacking. It was surprising how little furniture we needed as Bob had taken care of everything.

There was a built-in bookcase, there were shelves in the breakfast bar, there was a gun rack made of varnished pine on the living room wall, a rustic dinner table and four pine sapling chairs that he'd made himself. The detachable pieces, along with the new boat, had been made mostly inside the chicken house during the long winter's wait to build. He had not had time to make a rock fireplace with a chimney outside as he'd wanted, but he did lay the concrete hearth to support it. Meanwhile we had an airtight heater installed on the pad that radiated warmth thirty feet around it and up the stairs.

Moving in with us was Dingbat the Singing Cat, a recent snow-white replacement of Snoose. Bob liked cats better. Kids like any pet.

The staircase had no backing behind it, and no risers as yet, so that a stack of records placed there temporarily, were at risk. Mark started to crawl up the stairs and, as my hands were full, Joan made a dive for him. The records were dislodged and many fell through into the basement and some of our most precious ones were lost, the worst loss being *The Wrong Highway* with *Son of a Miner* on the back of it, a second copy obtained with great trouble. The end of our Yukon era.

The children soon made friends at school, the furnace worked well, and Bob drove out to the sawmill every day. On Friday nights we'd open a case of beer and he'd stretch and say, "This is the life." On Saturday afternoons we'd go "uptown" to see what life was good for. No further worry about children left in a jeep or to their own devices several miles away. Bob kept busy tinkering around at night but his dream—our house, his toy—was almost completed and I knew this sweet domesticity wouldn't last.

Everyone in this village knew everyone else and their business; never a day without entertainment.

In 1952, the inhabitants of the valley tended to fall into groups: ranchers, sawmill people, hotel people, government staffs, merchants and Indians—the latter very much in evidence in the pubs on Saturday. We of course had to stick with the sawmill people. Bob never went anywhere on the main street without running into a group of friends. Those he considered fit he ordered me to know and those unfit he enjoyed himself.

When I say "ordered" or "allowed" it was by mutual arrangement. It pleased me to please him. If anything did not please me, he soon heard about it. I was allowed to sit with the older couple, Howard and Dottie, and Della and her family from the mill, as well as merchants if I wanted to. The latter had no time for pubs, so friendships were struck up through the stores. Longstanding ranchers did not bother with mill owners. White-collar workers didn't know us from a hole in the ground, socially. I found the mill bunch too jolly for my bookish ways and the merchants too inaccessible for close friendships; I was happy with family and random chatter around town.

Christmas came again. During the holidays both older boys came up, arriving at separate times as grown brothers will, and David came first. Everything was much to his taste and he settled in as if he had always been there, becoming firm friends with Bob. He spent all his time chinking logs in higher places we could not reach, or in redoing our work. By now we were using a homemade mortar of flour and sawdust slaked with water. It dried like sandy speckled plaster. David stood there and chinked and chinked until every inch was packed smooth and tight while Bob marvelled at his patience.

Then Henry came and it was quite different. He was wearing a navy Burberry and thin shoes in below zero weather and the inexperienced boy had not stayed on the bus right into town but got off too soon, only to find he had miles and miles to go. Rather than wait for another connection he had decided to hitchhike and had succeeded, but not before he had walked several miles and nearly frozen to death.

He stood there in his long thin coat before the fire, holding out his long thin fingers.

"I have never been so cold in all my life!"

He took it as a personal affront. All the poor kid got was derision but we soon had him bundled up. It was not as if he had not brought his Indian sweater. Bob had put up a basketball hoop outside, sent by their father, and they all warmed up around that.

We still thought of Chris Bolstad. We did not see much of him after we moved into town, but sometimes on weekend jaunts we'd drop in and everything would be the same. Affairs across the street were the same also, news of which got perfectly well into town. Unfounded rumour had it that Buster had tried to get Chris to deed over a workable part of his property in return for present and future geriatric care, but Chris would have seen this coming. His independence was likely the same as with Gunnar, Charlie, Hattie and Violet. Nobody could budge the old bachelor with new ideas. Chris said nothing about Buster and we began to realize the whole story originated at the mill.

Growing Pains

During that summer there had been a little discord with Joan. She had been fifteen on arrival and now there was the question of her holding her end up by taking a small job after school. She was also going through the stage where teenagers show their independence by being careless about their rooms. Joan was to become an inveterate tidier, but just then we were getting her adolescent treatment full bore. The boys had not yet discovered this glory. It would take Robert another three years.

One day when she was off somewhere Bob had some work to do in her boudoir. Her bed was unmade and when he went to move it Bob found dust curls, bobby pins and socks. His dander came up at once. He returned to the kitchen for a broom and dustpan and I followed him apprehensively.

"I'll do that," I urged. No answer. His Royal Neatness swept everything into the dustpan without comment until it was loaded, gently pulled back the bed covers, gently poured the dusty pile onto the bottom sheet and carefully replaced the covers with a little pat. He walked past me with his eyes big as usual. He was feeling simply beautiful.

The deed did not endear her stepfather to her one bit. She said nothing and became more determined than ever not to change her attitude towards this new authority, who looked about twenty by then but would never see thirty again. Desperate, he asked her one day to sit down on the couch, depositing himself at the very far end for a friendly chat.

"Joan, what is it you want?" he'd said. His face was bright red.

Now somewhere along the line, back at the last cabin, brother Tom had paid us a visit and softie that he was did not like Bob's treatment of my kids. "He could be more gracious. A lot more gracious. Does he expect them to climb into a hole and pull the lid over?"

Notwithstanding his impatience at times, Bob had seen the whole situation for what it was worth. "You've got the kids pulling you one way and me another and you're walking on eggs right down the middle."

Now he was determined to keep his temper and appear friendly. He asked Joan if she couldn't meet us half way by keeping her room decently and not having to be told what to do.

"Wouldn't it be easier for you?" he concluded. No reply. She stared across the room through the big picture window glumly and, as he thought, with every intention of ignoring his right to talk to her like that. He got up in disgust and walked out. In reality she had seized up and could not speak. Embarrassment held her rigid. It was so difficult for them.

Life for Joan was not all contretemps. She had several girlfriends and the boys were noticing her.

A redhead nearing twenty—who knew better than to date a fifteen year old, yet fully intended to—liked to take her to movies up at the hall. I allowed this with the usual strings about time of return. Then came the annual Clinton Ball in May, which was attended by visitors from all over the Cariboo and was an all-hands-to-the-pump event. The whole village looked forward to it. As all the older girls were going I could not inhibit Joan, and of course the redhead moved in.

This really put the wind up me because traditionally the ball did not end until breakfast time. The evening was always warm and couples moved to parked cars of which the streets were full. In the end I resorted to checking all the parked cars with a flashlight at the ready. I need not have worried. That young man did not need under-sixteen jail bait.

One time Joan did not show up at home when expected and I had to hunt for her. A favourite haunt, the ball park on the hill above, yielded no sign of life. As I was coming out of the nearby woods above the highway a car stopped down below and a face appeared above the roof of the car and addressed me.

"Mrs. Smith, is it all right if Joan comes with us to Ashcroft?"

"Certainly not," I said in panic. A female face, more downcast, joined his. There she was in the car already. If they had not seen me they would have driven on. Mere boys were always killing themselves on the highway.

"Get home this instant!" I shouted, appalled.

She climbed up some distance ahead and made disgusted faces at me. That tore it. I broke into a run and so did Joan. I did not catch up with her until we were right inside the house, fetching up against the front door, which she couldn't open fast enough. She was backed into a corner beside it, livid with rage, fright and her own disobedience. I let fly into the twirl of swift elbows with which she defended herself and landed one in her stomach, the only spot unguarded. Exactly as I did so I saw two steely eyes boring into mine, which told me I had reached the end of that method if I didn't want to be punched right back. I never touched her again.

I have always believed that one quick smack is worth a thousand words with kids and dogs. Today's alternatives for cheeky, sulky kids, of talking back and flagrant disobedience and the feeble helplessness of their weak-kneed parents leaves one quite sick. We never heard of Dr. Spock or of later permissiveness, and a good thing too. My kids never interrupted elders or made public scenes, nor did they shout and yell in public either. In fact they were damn well behaved, generally speaking. They were all spanked on occasion, but Joan had a great system when she saw it coming; she would sit on the floor and make herself very heavy and often won out. My children like to tell stories about me now, but I don't notice any real grudges.

Soon after that Joan decided not to be beholden. She was taken on in the kitchen of the Cariboo Lodge by the owner, who one day was to become more than a nodding acquaintance. His name was Fred Hoad. After a while he let her go. Determined not to look like a mother with feathers up, I didn't ask the man until a year or two later why he had fired her. Grinning with all his teeth he made motions of drying a dish like a slow windshield wiper. He was not altogether fair. Joan's desire for cleanliness—usually evinced by kids away from home—made her seem slower and the housekeeper had given her a lot of extra jobs.

At one time the kitchen staff played a trick on her. One last lot of guests remained in the dining room that night and the kitchen was closing down. They invited her to finish off a nearly empty barrel of ice cream and encouraged her to sit up on a counter out of the way. While she was swinging her legs and scooping away, they held open the dining room door deliberately to expose her to the guests. The person Joan saw looking at her was the movie star, Gary Cooper. He surveyed her with red eyes, being slightly boiled but lovely as ever, far too busy with his companions to notice an embarrassed kid.

When she got over that shock she did have the grace to tell me my idol was present. From Lilac Time onwards I had wept sheets of tears at his war movies and I was his slave. This time, for the love I bore Coop, I couldn't bring myself to go into the hotel and gawp at him, to my own fury later.

Eight years after that Cooper died, and the news came over the radio at the same time that the phone rang to say I had become a grandmother. Henry had been presented with a son. When Mark saw the state I was in he went out and made a dandelion chain with which he crowned me. And a friend plied me with rye as I cried and cried wonderfully for dear old Coop and my new old ladyhood. But all that is a different story.

Bombs Away

The new life was too good to be true. Something was going on but I was not to hear about it until the last of the snow had gone and the willows in the swamp were turning green. All our mail came to General Delivery and, as Bob usually picked it up, I did not see the official letter that changed our lives.

One Sunday morning when we had been in the house for about eight months he suddenly told me to come and sit down. The children were out, I was working at the sink and he was drinking coffee at the breakfast table. It was nothing unusual for us to have conferences like that and I suspected nothing.

It was his habit to wander about the house wearing a plaid viyella shirt with green cords belted below the hips, coffee cup in hand, while he looked at things he intended to alter or had just finished, lazing between jobs and talking things over. In so wandering he had a most sexy walk left over from navy days, a totally innocent unconscious rotten little swagger. With his red wavy hair, now fading a little, and his freckles, both highlighted by a green jacket or plaids—though he often favoured red—with his classic boyish features and merry mud pool eyes, which I told him were the colour of swamp water, he had never cured me of watching him or loving him. He was not my childhood sweetheart and the love of my life, now lost, but I did love him very, very much. He was my chum, my saviour.

He could read my thoughts, knowing me inside out, and though he did not tolerate any wimpishness—being utterly scathing—he had taught me to value myself and stick up for my rights.

"The trouble with you," he had said, "is that you're a success and don't know it." Very different to a remark made by my ex concerning Bob some time later: "At least he's put some spine into you."

So, unsuspecting, I dried my hands and sat down to hear what beautiful new idea was cooking.

"I've had it," was what he said. "I can't stand Dogpatch another minute. You know it. What is there for a man to do? I've put in for the US Forest Service at Juneau again and they've accepted me. Glad to have me back, they said."

The spring sun coming in the windows from across the swamp turned very chill.

"You'll be all right," he continued hastily. "You've got everything you need here and the kids have a good school. I'll send you money regularly..."

I jumped up. There were times when nobody needed to give me backbone.

"If you think for one minute you can leave me here you've got another think coming! If you take off I can take off! D'you think I live in this godforsaken hole just to please me? If you go to Alaska I'm going to the coast! Try and stop me!" Woe was my bedfellow. Why was woe always with me?

He had not seen this development and was visibly upset. He had no rebuttal. Then I saw the whole thing. He had settled us in this valley and gone to all the trouble of making a proper home so he could leave us with a clear conscience. Many a man is a rover but this one was a chronic nomad and I'd had to pick him.

All I felt was the pain. Hindsight would reveal to me that he would always come home. I was his lode star, his centre, but after reaching it he would always veer off again. It would not have helped to know that but it might have eased the hurt. I thought he was sick of us and wanted to get rid of us the only decent way he knew, by building a house.

"Calm down. Sit down." He was furious too. "If you're absolutely sure you won't stay here we'll pack up and I'll move you down. My father can find a house you can rent. I'm not due in Juneau until July first. We'll sell this place and you can use the money to buy a house down there. I think Ernie would like to buy this one." Ernie Ruckle was the piano tinkling son of our sawmill friends.

We spoke little for the next few days and said nothing to the kids. He was simply sick to think I would not keep his house and I was simply sick to think he could take off and leave us. Neither of us believed it was happening but he stuck to his guns.

"Look," he stated, after a day or two, "I'll make a great deal of money up there. We can never save here. Up there it is work I love doing. You can't see me on a greenchain forever, for God's sake. Someday I'll build a better log house than this; it was only practice. Maybe someday we can start up a resort but I'll never do it without a head start."

With such palliatives he covered my worst fears, and when we broke the news to the children they were not too unhappy about living on the coast again.

By mid-June 1953 we were heading for an empty house in Richmond (Brighouse) that Mr. Smith had found. The senior Smiths had moved to Richmond, near Vancouver. Joan was to remain to finish her exams and share a cabin with another girl—her first taste of freedom. She would come down by bus. The old boy was to keep an eye on us after Bob had gone north, but to start with Bob came with us. Everything was glossed over by his people as being as right as rain, which would not be the case if we were near my people, whom at that point I didn't want to face anyway.

The house was an old abandoned rectory, large, empty and echoing, save for bits of furniture around. We left behind the rustic table and chairs but brought Dingbat. Even he did not last. A taxi got him. Bob dug a hole in the back yard and plopped him in, callously I thought, in my current mood.

The inevitable day came. He just said goodbye at the house and left. Shortly after his actual flight I watched the great silver bird circling over the rectory and knew what I must do: get the hell out and go home and face the family.

CHAPTER XIV

The Prodigal's Return

Trying It for Size

The lower mainland in 1953, with its gloom and rains and flat fields and long interurban rides, was no place to spend a summer. Joan and Robert disappeared on a short visit to their father in Port Alberni, leaving me to wind things up. My in-laws invited me for a dinner or two but things went a little stiffly. I was smarting from desertion—as I saw it—and they were trying to make nothing of it. They were kind to me and possessive of Mark, keeping him for a day sometimes when I could have used his company. We lived in Brighouse less than two months, then the children returned and helped me pack for Victoria.

In the time it takes to give notice regarding one house and move into another I had done that, as well as obtained a job back in the Parliament Buildings and installed Mark in playschool. We took up life in a long upstairs apartment in an enormous old house in Oak Bay owned by a spinster of means. It was comfortable, on a bus line, all tea and crumpets, and I was right back to square one and everything I had previously avoided.

Regarding tea and crumpets, I was hideously reminded of

remarks from my friend Sandra when I wrote her a "this is the life" letter from somewhere during our ventures. She replied, "You're fighting it with a teapot in one hand and a crumpet in the other." As though that were not enough, she emphasized it with a drawing of a sailor in round rig with a teapot in one hand and a crumpet in the other.

My mother said nothing but just helped when needed. Her calm face and silence on various matters were scourge enough. My oldest friends reappeared using comments like, "My, it must have been…" Soon I began to hear, "You know So-and-So who married So-and-So?" No I did not, and never wanted to. Winifred had been right. I was turning my back on my own kind.

Not for one minute did I believe in dreams of operating a bush resort—or did I? The family noose seemed to have tightened around me with everyone pulling on it. Sardonically I felt they sensed another divorce in the offing, after which I could marry someone sensible.

The children liked their new home well enough. It was summer and we all went to the beach on my off days, doing happy things as time went along.

When advised of our move, Bob used his brains and said nothing; he simply sent his money orders to our new address. His letters were like those of his bachelor days: funny, brief, and telling me nothing of his friends or social life of which I had the worst suspicions.

One Saturday morning, towards the end of summer I was at home writing letters when I heard footsteps coming along the echoing boards of the grand old attic, looked up, and there was this vision: red hair, Harris tweed jacket, knife pleat slacks and Scottish brogues. He came in without a word and sat down beside me. In his hand was a little packet that he opened carefully for me.

I found an exquisite gold Bulova watch with diamond chips at each quarter and diamonds in the works, being slipped over my wrist by means of an expansion bracelet made of little rhinestone butterflies with gold fittings. It was all his love and contrition.

And so he came back.

After just a few months in Alaska, he was rich by our standards and now we were to buy a house. First he took up residence with us and went to look for work. We would get a house, any house, and then he'd build a log one. Here? Sure, why not? Do them good. He'd be the first in town to do it. And he was.

Everything hit the fan though at first. Bob and my mother did not exactly click. Her face told her thoughts and his pride did not permit him to be placatory. At gatherings he was forced to attend she remained stilted with him, or stiff and shy at best, and when he had had enough of her atmosphere he'd simply get up and walk out of her house. Such conduct she had never seen in all her life.

Logs in Suburbia

Troubles blew over. We remained in Victoria for three years and three months as one work contract after another kept Bob from taking off. We bought an ordinary stucco house at the corner of Oregon Avenue and Bay Street, which my father said was "on the wrong side of the tracks," but strangely my mother, who was astute in business matters, saw it for the financial stopgap it was. The house is gone now, a park in its place.

Bob became involved with a construction company and made friends of the owners, considering future partnership. Then he put his mind to building a log house in spare time on Ten-Mile Point, a very desirable site near the sea. We had put down a deposit and, in a deal with the adjoining lot owner, had cleared his forest in return for keeping his logs. At that point the developer got cold feet at the idea of slow building, and with logs at that, and reneged on the whole thing.

With logs going nowhere, Bob coerced his parents into hiring him to build them a house in Victoria. Thus I lost my new log home. A year later the developer, who had refused to hear of anyone building a house after work and on weekends, not on Ten-Mile-Point, could have seen a photo of the log bungalow and a long article in the Sunday newspaper about the lovely result. (As of 2011, it was still there, on high Quadra Street in Victoria.)

Meanwhile I continued working. Mark attended a little private school, and we had a housekeeper in the afternoons whom Mark teased when she was looking after him. Finally he acquired some colourful language from children nearby and was sitting on the chopping block outside, calling picturesque things to Robert in the field beside us, when his father chanced by and overheard. So he got frog-marched, spanked occasionally, made some little friends, and we had more pets. Robert fetched Mark after school, read books, played football with friends in the field, and cut grass.

The cat we acquired is worth mention. Smokey lived for twenty-two years, knew when anyone was coming home, met cars and buses, and tapped on windows to be let in. He was trained to "do his business" outdoors. He slept on Bob's chest, and would not get off. When forced to get off with a good swat, he would not cross the threshold of our room for a week.

Hattie

In the spring of our first year in a city, as though it were Cariboo time again, a letter reached us from the ranger's wife up the North Thompson. We knew what it would mean.

It seemed Hattie had committed some bravery that had done her in.

> She was fighting the village again. She was broadcasting about the morals of some girl she saw going into a barn with a boy. The girl's mother appealed to the welfare woman, the one who called on you, and they went to see Hattie and got thrown out. Her eyes had seen what they had seen and she told the welfare worker that government busybodies were not going to get all her property and lock her up, so both of them kindly get off her land.
>
> What happened next was that two young boys were playing around her place, getting cookies. She wasn't so bad with kids, you know. Instead of going home they went

around the side of her place where the well was. The rotten coaming gave way and one of them fell in. All the screaming brought her on the run. She threw down the well bucket on its rope and got the kid to hang on and put his foot in it. Then all by herself she winched him up.

She always had a back like an old tree and muscles like a wrangler's. She dumped the kid on the grass and went indoors to lie down saying she had 'wind around the heart.'

The boys ran home with the story and the mothers went quickly over to Hattie's. Everyone was feeling a bit cheap. She had locked up behind her but they found her crowbar on the porch and jimmied the kitchen door. Your dog was barking madly inside.

They said she was cold on the living room floor, looking cross but noble. They said she had so loved her home and that she had not needed anyone.

Mrs. Travers took the dog. Look us up if you're ever back this way. Just thought you'd like to know about Mrs. Davis.

Bonnie Jean

There were some amusing incidents in our lives at this time. Mark was getting to be a handful, running away. At first he started to meet my homecoming bus, breaking away from the housekeeper around five o'clock. I would see this little figure waiting on a stop, dressed in his little uniform of brown pants, brown blazer and gold-crested cap, representing a little school called Westerham, or by Bob, "Westerh'mm." Once when I did not get off the bus Mark thought I was on, he got on and told the driver I was aboard. After driving him around the city with no one claiming him, the bus driver took him to the police station. After a long neighbourhood search we phoned the police and I opened our door later to a big blue knight standing there with Mark in his arms.

Whenever this happened, I would first phone Sandra because he used to run away to her house to get cookies, but more than once there was a policeman on the doorstep. He was a good little boy though, which amazed his father, who expected much worse. "What I can't get over is that he's such a good little kid," he said, remembering his own pranks. He would read Thornton Burgess's *Mother West Wind Bedtime Stories* to Mark after supper, lying on the couch and creating great inflections and drama while the boy sat cross-legged near him. All was manly.

Occasionally I had run-ins with Sandra over differences in outlook, and we would sometimes cease to be on speaking terms for a while. At the same hairdresser's we would eye each other surreptitiously from under the shelter of our hairdryers or from under large hat brims on the street. Meanwhile, Bob and her husband Alec were meeting for beers downtown. These spats probably lasted a week; the men laughed at us.

My father took to coming over when he was at loose ends and would sit with Bob having tea and making "rollings." They would have played a game together but Bob didn't play "draughts" (checkers) and Dad didn't play chess, so they made do.

The star performer was Joan. She had been living with her father in Port Alberni for another school year after a dust up with her stepfather not long after his return when we had our attic suite. He was used to going to bed early, lights out, and she wanted lights on to do homework she could have done much sooner. Because of the tension I asked her father to have her for a weekend and teach her sense. His reply was to appear with her stepmother and a steamer trunk and Bob came out and helped him carry it in. All three so-called parents sat together deciding to rob me of my kid. I couldn't stop them. My last sight of her was a face full of cold pride through their car's back window, as though to say, "See?" Years later she told me, "But I was expecting you to rescue me."

By July of 1954, that first year when we had our house, Joan came home, or was sent back as she put it, "the minute the ink was dry on my exams." She had been given a nice piece of luggage for her birthday that month. "Here's your bag. What's your hurry?" was her comment.

The year following she graduated from Victoria High

School with her father and my father attending. She dressed at my mother's house for some reason and they all went off to the event together. It was assumed by all that I would not go under the circumstances, that of course meaning sitting next to my ex. I couldn't bear it and did sneak away to the ceremony finally, but missed her turn on stage and her father and grandfather in the audience. Then I saw her in the crush waving to me merrily from among her friends. I came home stricken and heavy-hearted for more than one reason (HE was there; and this was *our* kid) and crawled up the back steps.

Bob was sitting at the kitchen table when I went in. Instead of being accused of hobnobbing with the enemy, which I expected, Bob took one look and handed me a beer. He knew. He was no fool. I realized how lucky I was after all.

Henry had enlisted with the UNTD (University Naval Training Division) at UBC as a naval officer in training. Soon he brought over his fiancée for a ball at Royal Roads Naval College and produced a date for his sister. From then on the house seemed to be full of sighs and corsages. Bob took the young company in his stride or went into the basement.

Things came to a head when it was mandatory for Joan to find work. After some false starts she joined up as an ordinary airwoman in an RCAF summer scheme. Her father wrote, "You'll be nothing but a hewer of wood and a drawer of water," but he was not prepared or able to send her to college or training school to make an officer of her. Her recruiting sergeant was a snappy redheaded female who told her, "You'll be no good to yourself or the Air force until you get that monkey off your back." Poor Joan. It must have been visible. She couldn't hide her resentment at all her elders for her strange upbringing and consequent contempt for authority.

But she stayed on with the RCAF when her first enlistment was over, did not hew wood, and for three years became what they call a Recreation Specialist, and a very good one.

CHAPTER • XV

The Red Lamp

The elders' log home was now completed, subject to cabinet-work inside being finished. Again, almost the entire home was filled with built-ins. It was as if Bob could not stop making them. Tom did appear, from off a ranch he was managing, to help at the roofing stage and to speed things up.

Eventually their parents moved in and Bob went back to his contractor friend, practicing how to get a sound house up quickly, until he was ready to solo on the market. He had no patience with unions and working for his unorganized friend led him from the idea of partnership to the goal of becoming independent.

A new dream began to form and he thought we might start again and gradually build a lodge and cabins somewhere near Quesnel Lake, wilderness country then with a vengeance. The map indicated we would have headquarters in Quesnel. Moving between schools did not bother Bob's conscience because he said Robert was so smart he'd land on his feet no matter what school he attended and Mark was too young to worry about. Quesnel was an established place. I began to hope.

Bob always became pale and sickly in a town life and I knew he wouldn't last unless some move was made. He was too confined and wages were too unspectacular for accumulating a nest egg. In May of 1956, our third year on the coast, he went to Kitimat to build houses that were going up in rows in the new town. Then he came home for a break and took off again for 100 Mile House where more houses were going up.

He rented a cabin beside a small lake at 108 Mile and it was there that Mark and I joined him for a week of my holidays. The site is now a valuable exclusive waterfront estate, an expensive resort area, the picture of rolling green mounds and a lake or two, commercialized. While he was at work I explored as far as Mark's legs would carry him and when Bob came home for supper we'd spend a good deal of time in the water while he showed off with jack-knife dives. He was quite a sight in the early sunset as he shook the water out of his red hair and rubbed down with a red towel. It was one of our nicest times together. He also encouraged me to develop a hobby.

"You don't need a gun. You've got a camera. It's more of a triumph to sneak up on an animal and get a picture than to shoot from a distance." This from him.

He was having weird fits of melancholy though, which alarmed me. There were crazy accusations that I didn't love him enough and he went so far as to say I'd married him for security. That did it.

"If I'd wanted to marry for security I'd have stayed in Oak Bay and I wouldn't have picked a goddamned trapper!" That settled him for awhile.

He took us for a ride with friends of his in our green boat, up the lake to see an ancient mansion built around 1908 by an eccentric nobleman. Too late I realized his friends were drunk and that once more the water was nearly over the gunwales. Nothing happened but I was scared to death. Then he took us for a truck ride and kept flirting with the shoulder of the road, though stone sober. It felt as if he wanted us to go over the edge. I began to think he was concussed. He had met our bus wearing dark glasses to conceal bruises and I found a door off his truck after he'd rolled it and survived. During the war he had received head injuries that we all forgot about. He'd been attacked by some sailors outside Halifax and beaten about the head with a bottle, which netted him three days unconscious in hospital. Something was not adding up; but he would pull himself together after one of his unaccountable gloomy fits and laugh and that kept me fooled.

Our holiday came to an end and he saw us onto the bus with one of those haunted looks that seemed as if he was memorizing our faces. He wanted to come with us and he wanted to be free; that was the crux of it, I thought. My only defence against fear was anger. There was nothing to put a finger on.

Once I told my father-in-law of my fear of being abandoned and he said, "I don't think so. What we need here is time, time and more time." Miserable at work and worried sick, I needed advice from someone unbiased. My government boss, Barry Gault, had always been approachable; he listened to me privately when I really feared desertion.

"Is he sending you money regularly? Does he keep up the money for the bills?" I assured him there was no trouble there.

"Well then," stated my friend, "as long as the money is on the barrel head every month there is nothing to worry about." He brought out his own boyhood scout knife for me to give to Mark.

Shortly afterwards Bob wrote to say he was moving up to Williams Lake to build a 100,000-dollar log house for a wealthy Chinese man, but first he must see to cutting the logs.

Home from work and getting supper one evening in September the phone rang with a call from Williams Lake. It was not Bob on the line but a doctor in Williams Lake hospital.

"Am sorry to tell you but there's been a serious accident and your husband is in serious condition. We would have told you before but he didn't want you or his parents to be worried. We had to respect that." The voice went on with details that chilled me to the bone.

"Shot himself! In the stomach?"

A roar came from the boys' room. "No, no, NO!"

"How fast do you think you can get up here? He's in poor shape and doesn't want to get better. Maybe you can turn the tide."

Tom answered his parent's phone. Within half an hour he

had me racing to the airport to a small plane on which he had managed to get me a seat and had, like lightning, arranged a passage right through to the Kamloops airfield and thence to Williams Lake. He still had air force friends in the flying world.

The flight to Kamloops hit air pockets all the way. I was airsick and sat in frozen nausea until it was all over. I do not remember changing planes at any place, only being in them. At Williams Lake I deplaned onto a field of grass with a fence beside it. I went over to the fence and was violently sick. Someone put me into a cab and directed it to the hospital.

The place was packed, beds in corridors, and nurses run off their feet. At the end of a narrow corridor lined with beds was a sort of utility cupboard space with a small window. They had put him in there.

The very first thing that met me was the smell of gangrene. His voice was far away and non-committal. "Oh, hello." His nose was dead already, snow-white, but he was in there, mind turning over, voice like gravel. A couple of times he rolled his eyes right back.

I ran out and asked for a clergyman. "Please! Please!" Tiresome questions. "Protestant. Any!" Then I went back in to sit.

Though delirious he turned on his side and spoke to me semiconsciously but sensibly. "Mother. Where's Mother? Is she coming?"

"She'll be here soon. Very soon." They'd be down around Hope because they'd started to pack immediately.

"Have a cigarette," he said, pulling out one of his plastic drains from the wound and pretending to smoke it. Conversationally he spoke of the nurses "doing the best they can." He knew of the overcrowding.

His doctor came in and beckoned me out. "He's nuttier than a fruit cake. He's schizophrenic. Picked up a staph bug and thinks he's got VD. That's why he doesn't want to live now. Maybe. See if you can talk him out of it. Try anything. Promise anything. We did the best we could to sew him up and he's young enough and healthy enough to pull through but he's not cooperating. Keeps taking off his dressings and pulling out the drains. We tried tying him down but he went berserk."

Bob spoke to me from behind eyes that could not see or were too dark. It was probably that the pupils were wide open.

"You'll bring the boys up to this country, won't you? Make men of them." I promised. I told him his mother would be here soon with his father and Tom.

"I love you," I said.

"Of course you do," he snapped.

A young man in a clerical collar walked in just then and said he was Todd Lee. "You'd better go and get some rest. I'll sit with him. I came through something like this myself once. It's surprising what you can recover from. It's going to be a long night for you and you're done in."

Relief knew no bounds for I felt that Bob was in safe hands, and in God's hands at that with a preacher praying beside him. I leaned over the bed.

On the metal table beside the bed in this broom cupboard of a room was a glass milk bottle that was his water carafe, with a bent straw in it. With sudden energy and a look full of deadly intent, or hate, I'll never know which, he reached out and seized the bottle and smashed me with it full in the face.

Todd Lee grabbed me. "Did he hurt you? You must go. You seem to excite him." For weeks I carried the bruise on my chin.

There was nowhere to sit. The waiting room was full. I found a nurse and begged for a spot in which to lie down.

"You can't have a bed. Come in here. You can be alone in here." The tiny windowless room was a sort of linen room with bedspreads and other articles around. I took a long spread and folded it into a pad and lay down on the floor like an animal. My fear was black.

"You can't stay here," another voice said roughly. "You'll have to go out into the waiting room." Somehow I found a seat on a short white bench affair, which I shared with an Indian kid and his mother. They went, after half the night it seemed, and I curled up on the short white plank. I could not risk going into Bob's room before dawn and knew he'd be quiet with the young, self-assured clergyman. I longed for others to come—anyone—someone to share this. Then I fell asleep.

Todd and the doctor woke me, a white-coated figure holding a glass of something. Todd knelt and held my shoulder.

"Bob has gone, Mrs. Smith."

Gone. Gone?

"Drink this," said the doctor, pushing it down me before I had time to register.

"You must come with me," ordered Todd. "You can't stay here. My wife will look after you." Between the two men I was led, stunned, to the main hospital door and marched swiftly out as I tried to look down that long corridor. I wanted to see him, I should see him, but I couldn't, couldn't. They pushed me ahead.

Outside was warm daybreak showing a trace of coral above the trees, merging upward from blue into midnight blue, in which a few stars shone uncertainly.

But low on the horizon, hanging like a lamp, nearer to earth than I had ever seen it, burning red with contempt and satisfaction, red with the vile deed done, was the planet Mars.

||||||||||||||||||||||||||||||||||||||||||||||||||||||||||||||||||||||||||||||||||||||||||||||||||||||||||||||||||||||||||||||

In August of 1956, the orbit of Mars placed it in perihelic opposition and unusually close to the earth. It was prominent on the western horizon at sunrise.

CHAPTER · XVI

Packing the Torch

Bandaging

Halfway up Jackass Mountain in the Fraser Canyon traffic was stalled for about one hour. Sun poured down into the rock defile and the temperature outside the Chev, for which I had traded Bob's truck, was at least 90° Fahrenheit and going up. All the metal on the car was blistering. Inside on the back seat atop a load of luggage was the budgie in his cage and he was not doing too well. There was nothing we could do about it. But Smokey the cat beside him accepted anything and was going to his new home without demur as long as he was with his people.

Robert and Mark sat on the front seat with me, feeling as I did that it was useless to get out of the car and be hotter still. The wait was interminable. Ahead of us in the northbound line-up was our moving van, which we were at pains to keep in sight. Eventually the traffic warden let northbound traffic trickle through singly, and we inched forward hoping that our van would not get revved up too quickly.

My thoughts were a jumble: fear, tension and fatigue, and yet a feeling of high triumph in bringing off our holy cause. Another winter and spring had gone by and soon I would be in Bob's country where I could cry my eyes out without exciting comment. Let my hair down. Wallow. What effect that would have on the boys never crossed my mind because their role was to become men.

At home a month before, when my mother-in-law telephoned my mother for details I was not supplying, a very revealing role reversal had taken place.

"Why on earth does she want to take those kids all the way up there?" cried the mother of heroes, herself no mean hand with a salmon line and at climbing mountains in days gone by. "No comforts. All that heat and ice and snow and mosquitoes."

"I think," replied my mother quietly, "that she has the spirit of Bob in her." Little lights were going on all over the place in my mother's mind.

To recap events, I had gone back to work exactly one week after Bob's death—a week of solid morbid action.

The exceptional clergyman from Bob's bedside had taken me, well doped, home to his wife. They put me to sleep in their own bed. Horror struck when I awoke, but I dressed and felt as if my head and ears were being pressed in. I wandered into the young mother's kitchen and was made to sit down while she got coffee. I could not help seeing on the table at my elbow a half-written letter. Words arose willy nilly.

"And now," after a torrid description of Williams Lake, "Todd has brought home this woman whose husband has managed to…"

Bringing coffee my hostess said, "There is someone to see you." Standing two steps down in the September sunlight was Tom.

"I knew he was gone. I knew it last night."

Instead of piling into their car the minute my plane had taken off, his parents had taken time to gather food and be practical and had stayed the night at Hope. He could not budge them. If they had driven all night as Tom had urged them to they might have made it. He had to stay with them.

Tom and I now had some mopping up to do, Williams Lake style. The morgue was a tiny disused chapel right up against the hospital wall. It was another little dog kennel with a cross over the door. I yearned toward it but Tom was rough and pushed on. Our business was with the RCMP who were waiting for us with Bob's valuables and to tell us there had to be an inquest into the accident.

"But get him underground as soon as possible in this heat," the big corporal told me callously.

Bob had always said never to waste money on a funeral. "Just dump me into a packing case and drop me into the nearest cemetery." Tom had surveyed the Williams Lake facility and had announced, "There's no way we're putting him in there."

"Of course not," I said. "Boot Hill in Clinton is where he is going. That's where he said he'd wind up. The view is good and he belongs there." Back at the parents' motel all three agreed with me.

Tom and I spent the rest of the day driving down to Clinton and breaking the news to anyone who knew Bob, seeing the cemetery curator and arranging for diggers immediately. His friend Amos Fowler struck his knee on hearing about Bob and promised to go around getting pallbearers. He was always there when local emergencies occurred.

No one would do for the service but my benefactor Todd Lee, who consented readily. I washed my hair three times and didn't know I had done it before. Tom had made all arrangements by phone to Kamloops.

By now Bob's mother was showing the stuff of which she was made, doing what I was doing, saving herself for later. I slept in a twin bed beside her in their Williams Lake motel while the old man and Tom had cots in the kitchen.

Next morning we were all in the parental car going down to Clinton. Tom and I sat in the back. Conversation was nil as we hugged our individual grief. Suddenly Bob's mother flipped.

"Bobbie is coming home with us, isn't he Frank?" she said gaily to her suffering husband, whose knuckles, like Bob's, showed up white on the wheel. She turned around to look at me.

"And you!" she shouted. "YOU can't have him anymore!"

"MOTHER!" roared Tom, leaning forward at her.

"Leave her alone," ordered his father quietly.

Bob had died on his father's birthday, September 14, 1956, just eleven days before his own thirty-fourth birthday.

There was Clinton. There was the little church, doors wide open. Amos had kept his word and a knot of men Bob had known were waiting at the door, among them old Chris. It nearly finished me to think a frail old man thought enough to come and give a hand.

As I greeted everyone a station wagon brushed by me and parked under a nearby tree. Glancing casually into it I saw it contained a long grey box.

"Here we are," I said brightly, as if the host had arrived.

And no flowers. While people watched as if I'd gone mad I scrabbled about the roadside and pulled up flowers like those that had graced our days before: yellow daisies with brown hearts and wild mauve Michaelmass. Always and always they would be his.

The men surged forward and took him inside. Wooden chairs served as pews and immediately his parents moved to crouch near the casket. I had to sit beside them, third in the row.

Afterwards, as they carried him out, Chris stumbled on the doorsill and the other bearers took more weight to ease him. As I followed behind him I heard someone say, "He'll be next, I'm afraid."

The place Tom and I had chosen was just was just over the brow of Boot Hill and near the far left corner, facing a sweep of rangeland and belts of trees. Beyond were the mountains. Sweet airs blew over the ground.

Committal was hardest. Throwing in my little lump of earth, I cried. "Goodbye, Hon." Then I ran to lean over the wire fence and sob my heart out. His parents were standing far off, stunned. The old man led Bob's mother away. An arm around me proved to be that of the clergyman.

"We are going to take you back to Williams Lake," he said. "We think it best his parents be left alone and you don't need them either, just now."

"Come on, Stella," said Tom. "We've still got work to do."

As I looked out of the rear window of Todd's car towards the receding hill, the last sight I saw upon the round of the mound was a silhouette of the two diggers. Spades and earth were flying rhythmically.

Rebounding

By now it was Tom's turn to become a little wingy. The crippled musketeer alliance had to be put back in shape.

"What we are going to do when we hit town is have some hot rums and a steak. Do you realize you have eaten almost nothing for three days? And we'll go back to the same motel. I fixed it up. Are you going to join me in a steak?"

You bet. Anywhere a musketeer was going I was going. The spirit of the three of us on a new highway. Anywhere but by myself. The torch had to be carried, Bob-style, forever and ever more.

Todd dropped us off near Bob's cabin where we rescued the truck for our transportation. Steak and rum at a cafe restored courage. I knew backbone was expected of me, for already I was getting funny nudges, or believed so. A folder of Bob's matches was on the floor of the truck and I took it surreptitiously into the palm of my hand. When I glanced at the front of it I read KEEP SMILING. That omen was the beginning of a wild hunch that I would never be alone.

At the motel, exhausted, Tom got into his father's cot in the kitchen and I went into the other room, shut the door and went to bed. In the middle of the night I sensed a presence and awoke to see a figure outlined by the moonlight that was coming through the window. For a moment I believed...

"Move over," said a voice. I shot over the end of the bed with a wild obscenity, taking my clothes with me into the bathroom. I dressed and stayed looking out of the window for a long time. When I went out he was making coffee.

"You didn't need to do that, Stella," he said with quiet dignity. "I wouldn't have touched you." It was some years before I felt philosophical enough to ask him what had got into him.

"I was cold. I have never been so cold in all my life. I just needed to be next to another human being."

Of course. Damon and Pythias, those inseparable friends. Tom had looked after me and his parents, done all his duty and no one, especially me, had taken into account his own grief. In other words, to my mind he had been spending the night in that ice pit, six feet down, prostrate by his brother. I had failed him in comfort. It was all a bit much. As he said when we were discussing it, "I think we were all a bit crazy at that time."

Certainly I was, for when together, welded in pain, we got to work loading the old tin trunk and kit bag and Tom suggested I burn the Stetson, I packed things around it when he wasn't looking and hid the ski cap. I was completely batty and enjoyed it.

The motel bill read "Peace be with you." After paying them we had little left for the trip to the coast. Unless we wanted to drive all night or sleep in the truck it meant sharing a hotel room. His idea. I was trying not to think.

"Don't worry, I won't touch you," he bantered, grinning evilly. Though I did not relax all night the snores from the next bed and socks on the floor were familiar and comforting. He was to be my deliverer many times after that, and a buffer between his mother and myself.

A belt of pines along the highway reminded him of something.

"As soon as I can I'm going to make a cross out of pine and get it out there. He wouldn't want any other crap."

We caught the CPR (Canadian Pacific Railway) night boat for Vancouver Island and sat up in the lounge. I had notified my parents by phone of our loss. Mother answered. She just said, "Oh, Billy!" which was my father's nickname for me. She stayed stunned and couldn't say more. I asked her then to tell the kids.

||||||||||||||||||||||||||||||||||||||||||||||||||||||||||||

Canadian Pacific Railway operated ferries between Vancouver, Seattle and Victoria until 1959, the first year of operation for BC Ferries. *Princess Patricia* and *Princess Margueurite II* would load late at night in Vancouver and deliver their passengers five hours later, early the following morning. Vehicles disembarking had to drive through the quayside warehouse to exit the property.

As we drove off next morning I saw a familiar figure wearing a homburg and standing in the sun beside the exit of the quayside warehouse.

"Hello, Bob," my father said to Tom, having seen me beside him in Bob's truck. "Oh gosh, I'm sorry," he added, realizing what he had done.

"You couldn't have paid me a higher compliment," replied the stricken brother, as we made room for Dad to climb in.

Mother threw her arms around me and over her shoulder I saw thirteen-year-old Robert being fed brandy by my sister. He had only just been told. He had kept hoping. Mark, just six, was merry as a cricket and knew nothing.

"We thought we'd better leave him to you."

Somebody took the children home and I stayed with Mother that afternoon and night, doped with brandy, letting it hit me, lying in a back bedroom with my face to the wall. The next morning it was "Now then. Your kids need you," and I went home.

Numbness

All five children were at the house. Joan must have had compassionate leave. Henry was painting the trim on the porch and the others had a roaring fire going inside.

Sandra came over bearing food and to help break the news to Mark. We sat him between us on the couch and he was awhile taking in the bit about heaven. Sandra told him of a comfy bed with satin pillows. He burst into tears and Sandra told me years later, scandalized, that I had said, "Stop that. Daddy wouldn't like it."

They all bustled. Dishes clattered, fires got banked, the radio played. Lying on my bed from sheer exhaustion I got used to the slap, slap of cards as they all sat around and played black jack in order to put up with me. The budgie escaped from its cage later and flew around the room. It alighted on my hair and somebody grabbed a camera and preserved that sight.

Mark sat up in my bed next morning saying his daddy was

never, never coming back, as he pounded the quilt. He was just a frozen little block and never mentioned it again. What did make him cry was having his porridge served by mistake in the cat's dish by the older children. He burst into wails and left the table, assuming in his pathetic rage that they had done it deliberately because they didn't care about his dad as much as he did and now he was an outcast and they were in power. A little of his maternal grandmother there; the kids stood around in consternation, as he meant them to.

I was not much better. I kept bashing the icebox.

Thoughts swirled in my mind as I sought to define my own loss, accept it and find a way out.

> An icebox was a vertical chest with an upper box large enough to hold a single fifty-pound block of ice. The bottom food compartment was chilled by cold air circulating downward, with the melt water caught in a pan underneath. Ice was delivered weekly, carried by the iceman on his shoulder padded with a gunnysack, or using a huge set of tongs.

Home they brought her warrior dead:
She nor swooned, nor uttered cry:
All her maidens, watching, said,
'She must weep or she will die.'

Then they praised him, soft and low,
Called him worthy to be loved,
Truest friend and noblest foe;
Yet she neither spoke nor moved.

Stole a maiden from her place,
Lightly to the warrior stepped,
Took the face-cloth from the face;
Yet she neither moved nor wept.

Rose a nurse of ninety years,
Set his child upon her knee—
Like summer tempest came her tears—
'Sweet my child, I live for thee.'

—ALFRED, LORD TENNYSON

Grief is like a warm cloak to roll up in and lets us stand apart awhile to look at our own lunacy.

Not Adieu

Back at work, on being questioned solicitously, I complained to my boss, Mr. Gault, about the uproar my children had made when I needed peace, having no understanding myself of the dilemmas they were in.

"Yes," he said, "and if they hadn't come you would be the first to cry, "Where are they?"

The chief clerk went whistling by into the vaults singing "John Brown's body lies a-mouldering in the grave," probably from sheer nerves at my presence. When I went back to work I had worn black, which the next day Mr. Gault asked me not to do for fear of making the others uncomfortable.

Oh, those were the days. Legal affairs occupied my off hours. The registrar came to inquire of my health. I complained about the dreariness of handling lawyers.

"Just look at it that all annoyances keep your mind off your loss." Hmm. Any little thing helped.

Winter wore on. One day, like Hattie, I got my guidance, for my love came back to me.

My office desk was placed within a bay window on the ground floor and I sat with my back to the street. In other times when Bob had picked me up after work, he had sometimes tiptoed across the grass boulevard and had tapped gently on the glass or had flattened his nose against it when no one was looking. Then one afternoon in my widowhood when the sun was warming my back I heard a gentle tap, tap. Nothing there of course. But as I turned to my work freshly stricken, a tune started playing very strongly in my head. "Come and sit by my side if you love me. Do not hasten to bid me adieu." *Red River Valley* was one of his specials and I was getting my marching orders.

From then on, swelling with love and relief, I knew what I had to do: keep my bedside promise.

Those who believe in survival after death stand apart from

those who don't. Those who do not believe, or do not believe in post mortem contact, pull down the blind, close their eyes and minds, put the past behind them and try to build new lives. Pragmatic souls. Those who are drawn by love with their antennae up have innumerable experiences and guideposts and find that death has no victory, but rather brings a companionship that could never have been there before.

Keeping my promise to Bob was easy. Everything clicked. The first person I phoned was my friendly handler in the personnel office, Merle, who had engineered my leave for Smithers in 1949 and all my subsequent government placements. She was not out of patience with me yet, in view of the circumstances. I asked if there was any, any chance of filling a vacancy in the government agency up in Clinton. She hedged around and consulted records.

"They do have a certain turnover when girls get fed up with that life. I'll keep it in mind."

Next I wrote to our friend Ernie to see if he wanted to sell back our house and he replied sure, but he had just put in plumbing and a lot of improvements and named his modest price. He was quite interested in our return and wished us luck. No hurry about the sale on his part.

The big stickler was whether or not we could sell our present house. A new job and a house sale would have to coincide. And they did.

One day the personnel supervisor phoned me excitedly about a vacancy at the agency. It seemed that the government agent was unhappy with a certain clerk and when he found he need not keep her, he had her transferred tactfully to Williams Lake. "You have two months to apply, give notice and wind up your affairs here."

It was no time to dance jigs. A real estate friend found a buyer for our house if I would settle for nineteen hundred dollars after paying off the mortgage and her commission. It was just enough for a down payment to Ernie. Would he accept that sum with mortgage payments to follow in lieu of the rent he'd been getting? He would. The log house was becoming a bit of a lemon for him in any case.

This time family and friends knew better than to hold me back. My widow's woes were not an asset to them and the trivia of their everyday lives did not amuse me at all.

"Laugh and the world laughs with you. Cry and you cry alone. You'll have to brace up." That was the best that my mother could do, anxious though she was.

My sister was not much better. "You were never that much in love with him. I don't see why you want to go on building shrines." It was one of those unfortunate remarks we make that we wish to God we had not, because it catapulted me out of there quicker than any other.

And here we were in the canyon in the heat.

CHAPTER XVII

Tuning In

Margaret

The boys were ecstatic. Running water was in the kitchen with good chrome fixtures, there was a bigger wood stove that heated the hot water tank, and Bob's great big wood box with the lid making a seat was there between stove and wall. There was a three-piece bathroom and some of the upstairs had been finished to make the second bedroom. Otherwise all was as we left it, the rustic dinette table and chairs, bookcase and gun rack. Tenants had been a little rough and Robert set to work at once to repair the sliding overhead garage door that Bob had installed. The furnace was our old one, the huge oil barrel on concrete.

At this point Robert, at fourteen, became the man of the family and took his position over-seriously. He would go about with a pained authoritative air, his eyebrows making a tent that pointed upwards over his nose. There was a family of boys just below our meadow lot and he lost no time in seeing how they had turned out in his absence. Evidently satisfied, he was quick to get thick with them and I soon found out the Pugsley boys were geniuses at thinking up trouble, especially Ronnie. But before I knew it Robert and his childhood friend were laying linoleum throughout the house with the expertise of grown men.

On arrival I checked in at the agency. My predecessor was not long gone and they were short-handed. I was to start at once. Next morning I reported for duty at 8:00 a.m. and was greeted by the deputy government agent who was unlocking the agency door.

She was civil but frosty and I thought, "Oh no! Not another Brünhilde." Oh yes. This one was just as tall, big and commanding but I could not figure what ailed the woman in being so cool with me. What had I done? Oh Lord! Could it be something to do with the former clerk? The frostiness continued.

"The first thing we do is run up the flag. You might as well do it now and learn how." I was shown.

Then I was taken to my desk and given an hour of instruction intermingled with questions. During this time the government agent had appeared and made my acquaintance warmly before going into his office. William MacLean was a spare, serious, distinguished-looking very quiet gentle man with a moustache and a faintly military bearing. His smile and handshake did not go over well with his cohort and gradually, as I sat there among the previous girl's erasers and clips I began to piece things together.

This woman thought I had engineered the transfer of the other one. It took the deputy three days to thaw out and realize my innocence, while I realized finally that the other girl had been her protégé. All I had done was to wait for a vacancy. They had not been asked to create one.

My desk was in good daylight by a window and I discarded my glasses, acquired under neon conditions. I typed letters, searched titles, took the counter and all the variety it brought, and at motor vehicle time did the banking, carrying all that cash down the street accompanied by a Mountie. It was gloriously important.

I was never to learn so many skills at once in my life. They were everything: lands, mines, vehicles, courthouse, anything governmental within a radius of several hundred miles.

Across the hall was the land inspector and beyond him the courtroom; the police were down the road a trifle. The forestry office was beside us and the rangers popped in and out of the main room, leaving the connecting door open through which came forest fire details and other illuminating messages over the squawk box.

Most of the time I was directly under the aegis of the deputy agent. Her name was Margaret St. Laurent and she was married to a forest ranger of that name, whose headquarters were in the office next door and who happened to be the nephew of Canada's twelfth prime minister. He'd been sent to work outdoors for reasons of health.

The rangers were a story in themselves in their fights with the locals about stumpage, encroachments, slash burning, fire watches from tall towers over miles of landscape, and the conscription of local able-bodied men for fighting fires. They were also closely allied with the land inspector and the game warden. They would all turn out at meetings when locals closed their waterfront properties all around some small lake to keep the fish to themselves. Whatever such meetings dealt with, it was always "government" versus them, and fun to watch. Locals did exactly anything they wanted any time they could.

Margaret, however, was a real local gal of German extraction. She would say of her maiden name, "I have a name like a sneeze." Hinsche. She was a gold mine in herself. She knew everyone in the valley and everything about them. She had the most tremendous sense of humour, delivered with a poker face, and she loved a crummy joke if it was truly funny. That was what she missed when my office predecessor moved off. The agent could not tolerate unladylike behaviour in his office, or the typing of smutty little limericks to pass around, the giggles and so forth. Offhand I felt the girls' life was none of his business, but he was responsible for the office image.

In any case it had all come to a head one day when the agent, who wore a hearing aid, was at the counter with this girl beside him. He always kept it turned off to avoid crackle unless he was addressed directly.

Counting on this being the case and being annoyed because he was in her way at the counter, the girl had turned back to Margaret with her complaint.

"If he doesn't get out of the way I'm going to shut his balls in the drawer."

He heard every word. It was that remark, and that alone, that got the boys and me back to Clinton.

Flying Solo

Once back in the Cariboo my main difficulty was in facing down loneliness. Margaret became aware of this and was kindness itself, giving me jobs to do when I stared out of the window, making me smile with witty little remarks. One day she put a rose on my desk. One suggestion I treasured after realizing the inevitable gossip about widows that goes on in a village.

"Make your home your refuge. Make it somewhere you can go into and shut the door on the world outside."

She was the most wonderful mixture of spite, love, caring and competence to all who came up to her counter. She ran the place. The agent had enough to do dealing with court work and Victoria-Cariboo relations. She was his despair, though, at times. Margaret had developed a very real throat allergy to smoke and when uninitiated persons came to the counter she might eventually say, "and d'you mind taking that damn cigarette out of your mouth."

When the weekends came the boys and I would set out in the old Chev. We would take the guns and go into the hills and I would try to find him again while they learned how to hunt. I would see again his dusty boots tramping around the side hills. "Side hill gouger!" I'd called to him. Or else I would walk up to Boot Hill and sit on his stone, recalling the fight I'd had with his mother over that. We were still in Victoria then, about six months after the September funeral. She had phoned just before we took his memorial up to the Cariboo after the following Easter spring thaw. "I hear you have had a stone made for Bob's grave. How dare you do such a thing without consulting us!" I hung up.

316

When consulted, the stonemason swore. "We get this sort of thing all the time. The body is yours. The stone is yours. You do what you like in these matters."

Tom had tried in vain to patch us up. Then one day, after the gravestone was in place, the boys and I were invited to dinner and Mrs. Smith hugged me and whispered, "Sorry." I said, "Same here." Months later they screwed up the courage to drive up and look. "We have just seen the stone you put in there. It's beautiful. Just beautiful."

So that's what I sat on, having a cigarette, or "having a smoke" as he'd called it, feeling him beside me. It was not morbid. It was a good rendezvous spot. But such equanimity was not arrived at easily.

Contact!

Right after Bob's passing I had made a point of doing any grieving in the basement away from the boys. One day I was having a glorious go, my face a sheet of slime, when there was an enormous crash over on Bob's workbench. A batch of tools had fallen over unaided and a spiral of dust was writhing upwards as I watched. Christ, I thought, you don't like me doing this do you? There was absolutely nothing that could have triggered that. No earth tremors, dynamite or rumbling truck.

Then one Sunday morning as I was bundled under the quilt in our bedroom, hidden away, I felt someone nudging knees into the edge of the mattress, a habit Bob had developed Sunday mornings when he didn't want to wake me too quickly. Suddenly there he was. I "saw" him through closed eyes as he gently raised a corner of the quilt and peered in at me.

"What are you doing?" he said. He was as ever, dressed in his town tweeds, but seemingly in a sort of golden haze. I knew if I opened my eyes he'd be gone; I did and he went.

Then Bob's mother caught flu and she tried her hardest to turn it into pneumonia and die. Her husband and Tom were frantic and phoned me. At the height of her illness, before they could call an ambulance, she saw Bob appear in her doorway, in the same golden light.

"Mother," he said sternly, "I can't come back. I can't ever come back," as though to say she must stop bugging him. Only then did she remember her mother doing the same thing over a lost son. After that she became a model of fortitude.

Added to Tom's loss was remorse that he had not picked up a signal that his brother was in trouble; usually he sensed it. Though at the time of the accident he had thrown up unaccountably, he did not register alarm or drive north to investigate. He had something to tell me when I saw him next.

"I was walking along this road toward Anahim Lake," he said of a dream, "and there Bob was coming along the road towards me. 'But we just buried you,' I said. He threw back his head and laughed in my face. 'You never buried me,' he said. Then he laughed himself sick."

Back in Clinton, I got up the nerve one Sunday to go back into the little church. I crept in to the left side of the aisle. During that service a shaft of sunlight, as it seemed to me, came from a window near me to fall upon the spot where the casket had been. Later I realized the left side was the north side of the church and the sun never enters from that angle. From eleven to noon it is high overhead but eventually when it shines in it is from the right or south. It was a comfort, and I soon joined the congregation.

At another time I was having a wonderful relapse at home in Clinton in the woodbox corner. The children were outside. I was curled up in the warmth of the stove with my soggy-paged Bible on my knees, seeking sustenance and sniffling away. Beside me on the stove was our breakfast frying pan with the lifter still in it. Suddenly right in my ear this instrument seemed to lift itself and bang a tattoo on the rim with its handle. It was a hell of noise. I wish the kids had seen and heard it. It was the second time I'd been made to leap out of my skin. Was I supposed to dance a fandango? Happiness made me feel guilty.

Little by little the spirit of Bob, or the influence of his mind, coaxed me back into common sense. Once when I went for a walk along a local lake road a little dog ran out of a garden and started running ahead of me. Every once in awhile it would stop, turn around, sit up, look at me and beg. This seemed somehow familiar. Then a memory broke of how Bob, to be funny or make a point, would sit upright with his hands dangling from upraised wrists like forepaws and I'd say, "You look like a gopher that's popped out of its hole." The dog did this several times, running ahead and then sitting with its paws up and panting at me (another Bob trick) before I got the message, which was, "Okay. You know you're not alone. I know what the boys and you are doing so get on with it. Don't make me work so hard to prove it."

Birds flew from bush to bush ahead of me, chittering and chattering. I remembered the budgie that had landed on my head. There was no end to the between world, but this one had to go on.

Norwegian Salmon

Old Chris was glad to see us. He needed thanking for his job as pallbearer if nothing else. I took Mark out there after our arrival.

His loneliness, which we all took for granted and expected him to be used to, was very apparent. In we went and sat about and Mark had his chocolate and pop from under the trap door. It was the first time I had seen it lifted by the ring bolt in the floor and we watched him go down its little set of stairs.

He asked how we did and I said very well except for the loneliness, that you think you can cope with it but you can't. He shook his head.

"People don't know the meaning of the word."

I sat on his black leather couch and he sat on a chair beside it. There were facets of his nature I had never taken in before— his quiet perception of people and acceptance of them. I began to say there was only one thing that bothered me now. We had not got the wooden cross ready to erect that Tom was going to make because he and Bob liked rustic things.

"Ah, you gotta forget all that. Start living. 'Minds me one time I was going through the bush where it was pretty dense when I came upon a mound that suddenly give me the shivers because it had to be somebody's grave. Hidden far from anything and no marker. So I went home and made up my mind to make a marker and go back with it and put stones around. But when I went back I couldn't find the place. Tried and tried. It haunted me that I couldn't do it. I dreamed and dreamed about it. Seemed as if it was me in that grave. My one fear is to be in an unmarked grave."

There we sat in a pall of melancholy. His understanding was anodyne.

"Stay for supper," he asked abruptly. "I'll make you some Norwegian salmon. Ever had that?"

Mark, who had been coming in and out meanwhile, was all for it. I hesitated, not knowing whether we should impose or what to expect. Bush sense won and I said we'd love to.

He went under the trap door again and came up with two cans of salmon and some spuds. As he busied himself Mark—old enough to trust now, with warnings—went off to look at the dam. Chris and I talked about the village folk, news of the van Horlicks, and anecdotes about the agency. He knew Margaret, it seemed. Pretty soon the potatoes were boiling and the tins were opened. Then he came to lay the table, refusing help. I had been bidden: "Just sit there and talk to me."

Having put out the knives and forks he came over to the couch, talking companionably, and sat down on the curved head of it. Before I knew what had happened an arm slid behind me and a big, rather wet kiss was implanted on my cheek. My consternation showed. He shot up and stalked over to the stove again.

"Too old! Too old!" he muttered to himself, rattling stove lids with his back to me. "Too late and too old." I felt awful but I just couldn't...It never occurred to either of us to blame my reluctance on bereavement. And I was sorry he worried about age. When I thought of it later, I guessed he was the first one in all that village of raunchy males to try to unveil the widow.

Norwegian salmon had turned out to be heated canned salmon with a white sauce mixed with nutmeg and poured over it. It had been delicious.

"Come again," he called as we drove off.

We did go back several times but I kept the boys with me, mostly as if en route for somewhere else. Everything was as if that startling embrace had never been.

The deadpan face, with the nonchalance of manner, became a role model for me.

CHAPTER XVIII

The Making of Men

Manly Arts

Out in the back lot Robert had been teaching Mark how to cast a fishing line with a fly rod. Mark was also shown much about guns though at the age of seven not entrusted with them. It astounded me to see a friend of Mark's, his own age, being allowed by his rancher parents to carry a rifle while on horseback.

Then there was the business of driving cars. Not yet sixteen, Robert had no business on the roads and I was adamant about that. Mounties or no, kids in the country got away with murder in faking adulthood. Some families bred like rabbits and seemed not to bother controlling their children. The cemetery was full of them. Mostly they would go joy riding in their father's cars to shoot the hills and wind up crashing into an underpass, the average age of such a youth being fifteen and, as noted before, being considerably grown up and almost ripe for marriage.

One day Mark and I were roving the ranges looking for future game sites when, from up on a ridge, I espied the Chev going round and round in circles on the plain below.

Defiance, by God. Yet Robert was safe enough and he had

to learn. The only way to be a man around Mother was to ignore her and to be one. At fifteen Robert was fully grown up inside his head and bowed down with the cares of the world. He did some research and informed me statistically how many widows there were in the United States.

Our peak triumph as a self-sufficient unit came with the fishing derby held locally. This was where I rubbed my hands and showed the local males, who behaved as if I had smallpox, what a dumb woman and her kids could do. Words cannot express how much we missed those old expeditions to the lakes and woods.

Cars and more cars and trailers, from Clinton and surrounding ranches, bumped over the rutted roads to the chosen lake. The so-called parking lot was ringed with boat trailers when we got there.

Some of these men were supposed to be Bob's friends. They looked at our trio in surprise and said nothing as Robert helped me get the duck skiff off the roof of the car to slide into the water. Into it we all climbed, with the little kicker outboard so ideal for trolling, and set out our fishing tackle. We were well equipped with sporting gear and Robert had been taking care of every piece, as well as keeping our guns oiled.

It was a great day. We got sunburned and caught a couple of rainbow trout of unspectacular size, but it brought the existence of the boys to the attention of the local men. Not that these men would do anything about it. A widow with kids? Too dangerous. As a family we were making our mark.

Another expedition might be better kept under wraps. We had started to explore Bonaparte country, rich in game. Thickly forested Crown land. Showing off our hunting prowess ended with an extremely dangerous downhill drop on the only road in. It looked far too risky for the heavy old Chev as I backed away. Then there came driving up the hill towards us a churchy, frail real estate lady. To come up it she would have had to gone down it first, there was no other road into that country. I was bit mad at myself for chickening out.

The next sortie brought another steep hill on the road to Horsefly. This we headed down, but just then the Chev pigeon-toed to a stop. We were right in the middle of the narrow gravel road with a big truck behind us; with thick forest on either side, it could not pass. Luckily, the men in the truck were able to identify the problem—a cotter pin had sheared and allowed a nut to fall off the tie rod— and they had tools to fix it. They set to work replacing the missing nut and then then they jury-rigged a new cotter pin from one of my steel bobby pins. It was hot work and I had no money to pay them except by cheque.

"*We* could write a cheque," they said disdainfully. Fortunately there was a case of beer in the trunk. Bob had taught me never to travel without a six-pack at least, for unforeseen moments. They were delighted.

We had a dear old neighbour on one side of us who owned a small house and garage with a neat little vegetable plot at the back. His name was Leo Lloyd. He was a spunky, crusty old beggar who had seen better days and had once been somebody. That is, he had once owned a fairly large sawmill, not to mention a big yacht. The boys chose to torment him because he was always watching them with suspicion and his threats and tirades were such fun. By "boys" I mean Robert's friends, happily accompanied by him. Those friends were highly original and had a father, Mr. Pugsley, who taught at the high school. Cleverness inherited needs somewhere to go. In winter the boys plagued old Pop Lloyd with snowballs on his corrugated metal roof and in summer they played Bugs Bunny among his carrots. He was ready to load up with rock salt by the time he appealed to me. I'd had no knowledge of these goings on. My tirades when I found out just added to the fun.

But teasing Mr. Lloyd was nothing compared with their next brainwave. Robert did something that brought attention I could have done without. He had been a painfully square and law-abiding boy until then.

"Hoosegowed"—Frontier Justice

The time-honoured way for children to make money in Clinton was to rove the edges of the highway and pick up beer bottles to sell for two cents each. They dragged sleds or wagons and sold their load to the junkman. It was quite profitable because by Sunday morning the highway verges were well stocked.

This was kid stuff to our young worthies who one day discovered a cache of empties in a shed down a back lane. Here was vast profit indeed and the guy was finished with the bottles; they were saving him trouble in fact.

In a small village everyone has an eye on certain youths and when you phone a policeman he has only to step around the corner to nab any culprits. As the boys got busy, a window shot up and someone yelled "Hey!" The other boys scattered but Robert was not fast enough and was recognized.

Coming into the agency almost every day was a nice Mountie, Sgt. van Nostrand, whom the children called van Nasty. I came home late one afternoon to find a police car outside our front door with the lights swivelling. Sick with terror at the idea of an accident, I bounded over only to find Robert sitting very small in the back seat.

"Come on in the house a minute," ordered Van, "I want a word with you and old Pop here has long ears."

What the policeman had done was to apprehend Robert and throw him into prison behind bars and had then gone pompously into the cell with pad and pencil to take down his statement. All of it was illegal, Robert being a minor without being given a chance to make a phone call or have a legal guardian present. But Van only told me that they detained him while looking for me. He made the mistake of telling Margaret the whole story.

I was too furious at Robert bringing such dishonour to us to consider what the policeman might have been up to. My rage at the boy made the copper blench and he tiptoed out with his collar up. Robert was to be arraigned and tried by the magistrate. Next day at the agency they were all having a ball at my expense because I had to ask for time off to attend in the courthouse down the hall.

At this particular time I was running a CGIT (Canadian Girls in Training) pack of girls connected with the United Church. A more restless, rangy lot of maidens to handle I had never seen and their ringleader, a real minx, unfortunately saw me with Robert as we were going up the steps into the courthouse. She followed me up.

"What are you doing going into the courthouse? Why are you and your son going into the courthouse?"

I shooed her off. The little devil had given me no end of trouble in Kamloops when I had taken the pack to a rally and had to house the girls there overnight. It had been a hot sultry evening and the hotel had given them a long dormitory room right over the pub door below. They demanded a pyjama party and dropped their pop bottles off the windowsill onto the sidewalk outside the pub as they leaned out to look at the customers. Having quelled that, I found out why this girl had wheedled our stay to be at this particular hotel. She had something going with the bellhop. I caught them dallying and I was responsible. You needed eyes in the back of your head.

When we went into the courtroom van Nostrand was in full scarlet regalia and the accused was put into the dock. I was told to be an audience of one. They did have the decency to keep it a closed session.

After Van had bidden "All stand," the local magistrate came in wearing a long black robe and a long face. Robert looked as if the world was going to cave in, but he stiffened and toughed it out. Van Nasty read the charges slowly and loudly and then the magistrate cross-examined the prisoner and asked him if he pleaded guilty or not guilty.

"Guilty," said Robert, then suddenly rallying, "Of course!"

"That will do, young man," snapped the black-robed figure most of the agency people had coffee with. "I don't like your attitude."

Van was standing at full attention meanwhile and sentence was being pronounced, not a lawyer in sight. I trembled in my boots at the fine they'd likely want. There followed a long dressing down, figuratively up one side of Robert's frame and down the other, in which he was adjured to consider the disgrace to his mother, the likelihood of where his habits would lead him, the trial and worry he was to me. The latter was a bit thick considering he was such a help to me. The other boys were the ones needing the blast.

During this performance Robert sat with his chin up, not enough to look arrogant but just enough to be able to look at the ceiling. Suddenly I knew what he was doing during the lecture: counting the holes in the acoustic tiles.

"I am remanding you into the care of your mother. Case dismissed."

Over the counter next morning Van leaned at me, all smiles. "All I wanted to do was to scare the hell out of him. Nip that stuff in the bud. He shouldn't be running around with those boys. Christ! If you knew what some of the kids in this town get up to you'd get yours out of here!"

Deputy Agent Margaret had heard my side of the story. Apart from giggles at the show put on by Van and her magistrate friend, she was very cross.

"You know you had no business to put Robert in a cell at his age and take statements."

"So what? It worked, didn't it? We didn't put him down on the blotter."

I felt it would have worked just as well with a good police flaying and a warning, without the pageantry.

When he'd gone, Margaret said, "You know why he did that, don't you? He did it for you. He has had no end of trouble with his own kids. Policemen's kids are always the worst in town." This was true—thirty years later, in Dawson City, it happened that Mark met his son Dick, who happily corroborated with a long list of mischievous things he had been up to as a boy in Clinton.

Dogpatch Unincorporated

Clinton was really an unincorporated village. There were three hotels, a general store, some small stores, a couple of cafes, two or three gas stations and garages, a motel or so, a bank or so—very small—and the government agency with its courthouse and flag. Believe it or not, there was a row of elms along the main street. Markedly along that street in front of the agent's residence was a white picket fence. Finally there were the drug store, telephone office and post office. The postmistress teased Mark about letters from a little girl aged eight who had moved to Kamloops.

Almost all these merchants and business people had to approach the agency at some time and I got to know everybody. Margaret saw that I did, for the good of the agency and my own welfare. In the end I had quite a few friends, but most of them turned out to be men. It was rather odd, but I was not cut out for hen parties and always liked to pick over my women friends. The women here were a rum lot, generally much more outgoing than I was; the men were often much more reasonable because they didn't ask as many questions.

My choice of women friends ran to the churchy real estate woman, Beth Crothers, who got me into CGIT work; a rather mannish quiet efficient woman accountant; a female taxi driver who chain-smoked; and a dizzy blonde. The blonde took exception to my knowing the last two women and warned, "You'll have the whole town saying you are going around with Frannie-Man and Peggy-Man." I didn't know what on earth she was talking about. She wanted to get me going socially again, to blind date with her.

At her insistence I tried it, and because I'd moved my wedding ring to my right hand the blind date, Dan, thought I was a married woman trying to pass and have a good time. I was trying to look like a single woman so that nobody would think I was married and fooling around. It was weird. And the blonde sang all the way to our destination.

"He's got the whole worruld in His hand. He's got the whole wide worruld in His hand...It's you and me, baby..." giving me a thump. I knew the girl was alone and rootless and that she was not singing for fun only. She kept thumping my knee to keep time. I loved her for it. There were strings of local males after her stacked curves but she wasn't interested in them.

"I take myself and I sit myself down and I talk to myself good. And I say 'Is this what you really want? Is this where you are heading?' You do that," she advised me, "if you don't know what to do next, then ask for guidance and you'll get your answer."

At one time I went on an overnight camping trip with "Frannie-Man," a gentle, wise soul in stout clothing named Frances Engemann. We were on our way to Anahim Lake country on one of my eternal sentimental journeys and when we tented down Frances opened up under my questions out of sympathy for me and admitted to a love lost.

"What did you do? How did you get over it?"

"Oh," came the matter-of-fact voice from the sleeping bag, "it leaves a great hole but you just throw a plank over it and keep going."

The taxi driver I did not see much. She was competent, intrepid on rural roads and a going concern. We did have some drinks together. In this place of all places I wouldn't try going into the pub alone.

And then there was Walter Adams, the man who brought the stove oil. He came from Saltspring Island, the son of a clergyman. He was a big, tall man, part owner of the Cariboo Lodge with Fred Hoad and quite a friend. He remembered Bob and made the remark to me when the prospect of my dating came up, "If you could handle him you could handle anyone."

Fred, the one who had fired Joan, was even more my friend. A bachelor who never dated, he was regarded as "fruity" by the local wags, but he wasn't. When these wags were drunk they teased him unmercifully and he put up with them loftily for the sake of business and because of his philosophical nature. Once, when his smugness became unbearable, they threw him into his own fireplace.

Friendship with him came about slowly. Their hotel had a coffee shop and I was always in there during my coffee breaks with one or another of the agency staff. Or by myself; I stayed alone as much as possible. God knows why. Really I was criminally shy and saved myself from extinction with a ready wit and by being very articulate when pushed.

At any rate Fred Hoad, the active hotel owner, took an interest in my children, in fact in all the decent town children, and even more oddly defended some of the queerer characters who patronized his establishment. He knew how to turn a buck, to the chagrin of many, and how to keep customer good will, but he was genuine in all his beliefs. Town gossip died on his counter and he heard it all. He was also a good digesting machine for what was going on in town or was likely to transpire. He gave me many a warning, and my kids also.

One of the people he defended, the last person you'd think this proper little man would want to rescue, was a woman who came from one of the copious bush families around there. "The woods are full of them," people said. She was a real wrangler by trade and looked exactly like Pansy Yokum of the comic strip *L'il Abner*. She was dressed from head to foot in blue denim in an age when women felt jeans were men's work clothes only. She wore a Stetson and smoked a pipe just like Pansy. Her legs were saddle-bent and she walked like a cowboy. Louise Grinder was truly a real wrangler with a reputation for being able to reel off a very lengthy stream of scandalous epithets that would never once repeat the same word.

"That's a lot of rot," cried Fred indignantly. "I've had her in our cafe lots of times and I've never heard her swear once." Be that as it may, the poor woman died as roughly as she had lived. We heard she had her head kicked in by a horse.

Wild things happened to others too. On May 15, 1958, a fire in a shed ignited the old Clinton Hotel, which burned to the ground, killing one family of three who had gone back to sleep again after being roused. Robert and I went up to see the smoking ruins and suddenly he turned me around saying, "Don't look! Don't look!" Skulls among the bed springs, likely. Amos Fowler had cried the alarm at all doors and thought the building clear. Of course he got the dirty job of taking the remains into Kamloops. The whole town had turned out with a bucket brigade and sandwiches for the workers later, but I had slept through the entire commotion. "Where were *you*?" asked Margaret pointedly when I dragged to the scene.

Then Walter Adams blew up his great oil truck. One day during winter he could not get the engine started and tried to warm it by building a small fire under it. He wasn't stupid; he was taking a calculated risk and lost. Another thing he did was to bring down his little Piper Cub too close to a fence. It tipped him ass-over-teakettle and he simply walked away.

The daughter of one of the motel owners had been given her own open sports car on her sixteenth birthday. She was one of my CGIT girls and not a bad kid, but very sexy. On one of her joyrides she had come down the long hill just north of town and failed to clear the underpass, which she hit at some speed. Her death and the lesson learned were soon forgotten by the other young people.

Apart from his hair going grey over the Clinton children, van Nostrand and his cohorts had a thing about the provincial government highways minister, Phil Gaglardi. Going into Kamloops once I saw dust plumes flying up as a small tornado crossed the sagebrush fields. Shortly afterwards he passed me on the double line going downhill into town, at ninety miles an hour. The Mounties hoped the underpass would get him too.

"One of these days," savoured Van, "I'm going to scoop that guy's brains off the road with a teaspoon."

Phil Gaglardi was the minister of highways for BC's Social Credit government from 1952 to 1968, as well as being Pentecostal minister. Known as Flyin' Phil, he was renowned for his disregard of his department's own speed limit postings. He resigned from government in 1968 after a scandal involving allegations he used the government jet for his family.

Van made Robert's acquaintance again in a very different way from the court scene. I had accepted an invitation from my previous blind date who offered to provide an outing to Lytton in the late summer. It became late afternoon then early evening as we had supper in that town and a great moon was up. I had to be getting back but I wasn't successful in bringing it off. My date was not one to be denied and he suggested that instead of going home via the highway we take the back road out of Lytton, which went through the mountains. "No traffic, a beautiful moonlight night and the scenery is gorgeous." He had wanted to do it for a long time and hoped I wasn't chicken. It took twice as long to go home that way and was not especially terrifying. But I crept into my house in the very early hours of the morning, after being effectively kidnapped.

Van Nasty came into the office that same morning, leaning at me as usual with grins of delight. "Where were *you* last night?"

"What's that to you?" I retorted, alarmed.

"Only that your boy phoned me. He wanted me to go searching for you. I calmed him down and said never mind, mothers have to have some fun too, and if you weren't home in the morning I'd do something about it." He went off chuckling and I realized how constricted I was if I didn't want to strike terror into my children. Margaret smiled and said softly, "You want to be careful whom you pick next time."

On the other hand there was a clique of serious, respectable old-timers who maintained a steady gait. They seemed to be mostly United Church people with a Methodist viewpoint, who lived modestly but were solid with land. As a matter of fact they, and the general store owners and the long-term ranger, owned the entire valley along with the ranchers. At a Fish and Game meeting they could manage to control everything and could shut down access to lakes or open up access, as they saw fit. Outsiders stormed and ranted but the landowners could not be moved. The same thing applied to Cattle Association meetings. The cattlemen owned land even further afield. These settled locals were priceless folk, I felt. They were decent and interesting. An illustration of their worth was their devotion to their church—except during hunting season.

One Sunday at the very beginning of the season the church was empty, almost. This minister and his wife would drive up from Ashcroft no matter what the weather and on this occasion they had opened the church themselves and the lady was seated at the small organ. Only one member of the congregation was there as I went in and he an usher. When no one else came he solemnly closed the doors, the minister began the service, we sang hymns—all four of us—then at the appointed time this gentleman passed me the collection plate and we had our sermon.

After that Sunday whenever I ran into that man and his poker face he would give me a small smile and wink. There was not one of his respectable lot who did not know about life in the raw in that valley or who had not experienced it. They just appeared starchy and puritanical.

Ranchers were in and out of the office all the time and so were miners. Claims were issued for sites in the surrounding hills and some prospectors were working quietly for big companies. They would come in to lay claims or to show they had proved up.

There was one prospector, a French Canadian named Lawrence Frenier, who lived in town but was seldom home. He called himself a rock hound for, as a sideline, he tumbled quite fine jewellery. For some reason I seemed to attract him, although he had girlfriends enough. His English was a little broken and his reputation with women a touch tarnished, but he was quite an endearing character in his dusty canvas clothes.

One day McLean said, "What is that guy coming in again for now? He keeps coming in and he was here only yesterday."

"That," said Margaret, pointing at me, "is the reason."

"Oh I see," said our boss, not seeing. He seemed perplexed.

Lawrence began to ask me to do some typing in return for a bit of jewellery. It was a good bargain. It went on apace with me keeping things strictly businesslike until one day he asked me if he could take me to see an outdoor movie. The drive-in was twenty-five miles away, in Cache Creek, and I sometimes took the boys there.

"Go ahead," said Margaret, in front of Lawrence whom she loved to tease. "Give the town a treat. You'll have old Mrs. Lloyd in fits." This was Pop's wife, Martha, a spry friendly woman, but as nosey as he was.

We went to the movie but when he drove me home sedately in his dusty jeep the curtains at Mrs. Lloyd's window were quivering. What a wigging I got from old Lloyd about the company I was keeping!

Once, however, Lawrence stood at the counter with no excuse. I thought I'd better get up and attend to him.

"This is for you," he explained, bringing out a pendant of moss agate mounted in silver. "It's just for you. Not for typing and you don't have to pay me. One day I'm going into those hills and I'm not coming out. I want to think someone will remember me."

Yes, I have always. He had a heart condition and did seem to disappear eventually. I have the pendant and a funny little valentine card when most memorabilia from those days have been destroyed.

The Lloyds were as good an example of "indignants" — leave-me-alone, self-sufficient old people—as one would find. He was all of seventy-five or older and she was about seventy. It must be realized that few people then lived into their nineties or much beyond eighty, at least not under the rugged conditions in the region. A person of seventy-five then was the equivalent of an eighty-five year old today.

Each fall they went off in their truck, which would be seen driving along the edges of fields, to some unknown destination. That meant they were getting their winter moose and knew secret places to go. They never failed to get one, dismember it then drag it into the truck somehow. The local butcher cut it up and kept it in a rented storage locker. Nobody their age went hunting and nobody with moose meat would dream of offering some to them. They just went on looking after themselves.

Old Pop Lloyd was my self-appointed guardian and sometimes was a darned nuisance. Nobody could visit me without him or his wife checking on me and making comments next day. It was useless to get angry. The thing about the Lloyds was that they wanted me to socialize but not see any man privately. So I did make friends.

Fledgling Flights

In time my social needs were turning outwards instead of pining inwards, a healthy sign, and I judged it time to entertain if I wanted to be asked out. My error was in jumping in too directly instead of obliquely.

The only person who had called on us after our arrival back in town was Bob's friend Amos, whom he had respected so much. He was stocky and fair and not too tall, which fit my image of whom it might be nice to have around. In view of his friendship with Bob, I thought that if he would bring his boss and a lady of their choice to dinner we could have a nice evening. I sent a formal little invitation to the sawmill, setting the date. All these people had known Bob, and I wanted to get back in.

There was no reply. I couldn't believe it. My blood ran hot and cold with embarrassment. One day I saw Amos in the distance and I knew we'd have to pass on the sidewalk. We didn't. He stayed where he was, disappeared, and then I saw a green whipcord jacket sticking out from behind a telephone pole. That fixed it. In a bank line-up next day or so he told me he was sorry he had not contacted me sooner but his partner could not come and he himself wasn't much of a one for parties. I was to see him partying his head off in some cabins just down the road from us.

In retrospect, I may have sunk my own boat that first time he had visited after we'd settled in. He'd been friendly enough, but in the ensuing conversation I was trying to find a subject that would interest him. Thoroughly disarmed and with never a thought that his might be more than a social call, I'd discussed Bob with a recital of his prowess in walking around BC and mentioned the Telegraph Trail.

"That's nothing," he said churlishly, "I've walked all over the country myself."

I then realized that, like most men, he did not like women talking about other men when he paid a call.

I wrote to my mother about what had happened when I tried to entertain. "Really," she wrote back, "I thought you had learned wisdom and good judgment. How could you be such a goose?" Indeed.

That was not the last of Amos. Early summer became time for the annual Clinton Ball and this time my services were required at the hall. Helping was an excuse, for without a partner I could not otherwise have gone. The music, noise and good fellowship had almost succeeded in doing me in with sadness when I saw Amos coming towards me to do his duty.

As we got onto the floor the band started to play the *Tennessee Waltz*, Bob's absolute favourite. Amos said he liked waltzing best and I said yes, meekly, my heart bursting. How appropriate to be dancing it with Bob's friend. With lips tight and eyes stinging—and some mixed feelings, I admit—I must have made Amos's worst partner that night.

Late that summer my parents came up and I took them to the local skeet shoot to watch me perform. "There they are," I told Mother, pointing out Amos and his friend, Harold Shiefke, since she had taken an interest in my fiasco. She thought they looked nice but pursed her lips.

"Just pray I don't miss," I told my parents as my turn at the skeet came up. I didn't. First shot out of the barrel. "But I'm quitting while I'm ahead." By this time, in Clinton, I'd do absolutely anything to prove I was the equal of all the damn men.

That urge reached its zenith at 4:00 a.m. one pearly dawn when the boys and I, carrying shotgun and rifle, were to be found atop a mound some miles north of town in our own special game preserve, one discovered by Bob. Blood was in my eye. By then I had acquired a man friend who said he was going to take me hunting at the very first opportunity but on the eve of the big day, the first day of hunting, he forgot and went off with his friends. I would teach them a lesson. These men did not know about Bob's prolific spot where the boys and I were now.

Time passed and then we heard the celestial caterwauling of geese flying low. Next we saw them coming right at us.

At first I had carried the 12-gauge while Robert grudgingly made do with the small rifle, clip loaded with .22 long bullets. The little rifle would have been useless. The shotgun, a full-choke Winchester Model 1897, was the kind you pumped before firing—Bob's old "Betsy." Its scatter area was dead sure for a long distance and the .410 could not touch it for power.

Robert had insisted that we switch guns and I had just yielded when the geese came right over the rise I was on, flying very low. I could not miss. All I had was the .22 and I let fly, thinking I saw a ruffled feather fall, but the geese did not falter and Robert, much further down the slope, was too far away and the geese veered just as the old gun roared. I could have screamed with disappointment. The various men went home with deer and ducks but not one goose. If we hadn't switched guns we would have been heroes; or at least I could have put paid to certain patronizing remarks.

For further socializing there was a curling rink up the road from us; Mrs. Lloyd introduced me there. It was of natural ice roofed over and stayed frozen all winter. Once a week somebody would hose it and scrape it down. There I learned to curl and overcome my shyness.

There was an anteroom with a red-hot heater beside the rink where people stamped their feet and drank cocoa. Sometimes they came down to my house for drinks and coffee after a game: Frances, Walter the oil man, and others, and we had a great time.

But one night I fixed Pop Lloyd by having two men to dinner together.

That morning an auditor from the Parliament Buildings at home in Victoria had stopped at my desk to bid me hello from an old friend. I had heard of this auditor fellow from other girls and my father had known his mother. In chatting by my desk the man discovered I knew an old friend and schoolmate of his, Harley Hawes, who happened to be the mill manager who had not taken me hunting. Harley was a tall, fair gyrating monkey with a cookie duster moustache and a cheeky manner, an English sort from the Okanagan. The auditor was quite a dish himself. That was not the point though when I invited him to have dinner with his friend at my house. He was ecstatic. Meals on the road were the bane of his life and fun nonexistent.

The most frightful old home week went on when they met, and to top it all they nearly collapsed when they saw the oil painting on our living room wall. It was a large portrait of Bob in his sheepskin jacket, painted posthumously from photographs, by the well-known Victoria artist, Peggy Walton Packard, an old schoolmate of mine. They peered at the signature.

"God, I don't believe it!" said the mill man to the auditor, "She was my first girlfriend. I gave her up because she could throw rocks across the quarry further than I could."

When I was nine Peggy had saved me from a gang of little girls at St. Margaret's who were beating me up because I wouldn't join their dirty little club and help them shoplift from the local confectioner. She tore strips off broom bushes and flailed about her until they ran away yelling.

By the time we drank to all that and had dinner it was quite a night; they had got into a lot of scotch. When I worried about old Pop hearing them, my saucy friend pressed his face flat against the window next to Lloyd's and made gestures.

"That should give him something to talk about for awhile."

When they left they said, "What a day of surprises!"

The evening had to last me for some time. And it did give Pop Lloyd something to talk about. "Out on the tiles" was the sort of comment floating up from his woodpile beside our driveway. I ticked him off, but it didn't stop him. Besides, it was handy to have a "watchdog" next door.

Inspections Again

When my parents came and my mother ascended the staircase inside the house she saw the height and sweep of the logs and was very impressed.

"If I'd known he was capable of this I'd have understood him. I wouldn't have bucked you the way I did. I thought you were living in a hovel." I just hope he heard her. There has to be justice somewhere.

It was very hot, and apart from going to the local skeet shoot, we went to a lake nearby where I swam and Mother watched from an upturned rowboat. Into this heat one day my father disappeared; he was seventy-eight and not allowed out in the boiling sun.

The boys said he had gone to "look around." We were getting very anxious and thinking of scouting the area when he came back. He had gone, cane and all, up the red-hot street through town and up the highway to Boot Hill. He had wanted to pay his respects, having determined on it before leaving home, without saying a word. He stayed on Boot Hill, combing the whole place, until he found what he was looking for.

Then Sandra and husband came and left their son, who was Robert's age, with us for a week and the boys got on very well. We took him into the Pavilion Mountains one day, following a narrow dusty road that wound around cliffs of earth and gravel with no room to pass. Blocking our way was a huge longhorn steer that looked intent on getting his horns, each a yard long, in through a car window. While we were negotiating past him marmots whistled at us from their burrows above. Big fat marmots.

The longhorn episode reminded us of a day the boys and I had been traversing a tiny lake that the land inspector wanted me to look at; before waterfront alienation closed down I could buy a marshy lot for two hundred dollars if I had it. We were walking single file along a dust path between the water's edge and a hedge-like growth when a great face extruded through the brush, a face with three feet of horn on each side of it. Robert and I couldn't turn around without tottering into the water, especially with a skittish Mark behind us, and had to back up single file while the face just stared.

While the shorthorn Hereford breed is now predominant in the BC cattle industry, many ranchers in the 1950s raised longhorn cattle instead because they were hardy in the elements and resistant to disease. They were a common sight.

We also took Sandra's boy to see the blue, emerald and turquoise lakes among the Marble Mountains. Visitors made a good excuse for excursions.

My friends returned for their son. They stayed at Fred's hotel and were not impressed by the housekeeping. As he didn't allow pets they'd had to smuggle in their little Boston terrier and it had snuffled under the bed to emerge triumphantly waving a used article of female necessity. They dared not complain. Next day the same inquisitive little dog earned a nose full of porcupine quills.

When alone between visitors on a hot evening we would drive down the highway to the drive-in theatre, being careful not to park near the fence because the next field was full of rattlesnakes. The boys loved these trips, and we'd make it an event by going to Hungry Herbie's Drive-In for burgers before the movie.

Late that summer Tom reappeared with a lady in tow. He was going to get married again. Molly was an Albertan nurse of hardy competence who was used to farm life and the country.

As he mixed us all hot rums and came to join us at the old rustic table, Mark, trying to be devilish like his father, quietly slipped Tom's chair out from under him. His uncle did not see this but as he lowered himself, talking away, he became aware of the lack too late to stop the sitting position but went down gracefully on one bent knee with the other stretched out as balance, didn't spill a drop of rum, and quietly retrieved his chair and went on talking as if nothing had happened.

Giggles came from behind him. He ignored them. Mark got closer, full of his own funniness. Too close. Without glancing at him, Tom shot out a hand and grabbed a handful of shirt, then rising and putting down his glass he frog-marched Mark to the porch and hung him by the collar over the void. I was on the point of screaming, as it was a leg-breaking drop.

"Do not," said Tom, replacing the miscreant, "ever do that to anyone again. You might break their back." His face was purple with the sustained fury he had smoothly contained. Mark was scared spitless, but the lesson worked—throughout his life he has lectured others on the perils of surprising others or pulling chairs out.

Tom then took his bride up into Chilcotin country where they raised cabins at Fletcher Lake and took on big game hunting. Everything Bob and I had been aiming to do. Quoth the raven, nevermore. It was quite useless to feel black or jealous about it. I could only wish them well. Tracts of land on a beautiful lake. Before long Tom was blessed with another son, Frank.

A bright note came for the boys when I said they could have a dog and we went to Kelowna to get her. A charming little springer spaniel that Robert christened Phoebe, who slept on the boys' quilts. We knew nothing of female dogs at all and of course our puppy came into heat. I came home from work on a hot evening to see a cloud of dust and clamour in front of our house where Robert, amid a sea of dogs, was doing a most horrible wrenching job of getting Phoebe away from some big brute. She had been locked in the basement while the boys were in school and nobody realized what would happen if the floor were made of earth. Every dog in the town helped to dig her out and she soon sailed forth like a little queen to her doom. Fortunately, Robert's timing was good and no pups ensued. This time.

Black Ice

In October of the second year on our own there, when her term of duty with the RCAF was finished, Joan came home to us.

Now twenty-one, there was not much for her to do socially. As she said, "All my friends married each other while I was away." She stayed with us through Christmas and beyond, managing somehow to fill in her time. She worked for Fred for a while. As she had no prospects of any import in sight she spent a fair time putting in applications by mail for jobs of one sort or another.

We still had a lot of gramophone records and revved up our memories with those saved from the sojourn before. The machine in use was my old girlhood wind-up portable, which Joan had brought to replace the highway one. The kids loved the *Flying Eagle Polka*. Our *Wrong Highway* was gone, but it had no significance for Joan. *Scarlet Ribbons* was one of her favourites and we had a lot of Chet Atkins and Johnny Cash. The bare log walls echoed with old wails and sweet sadness and I fought half-heartedly against the strong surge of life coming back to me from those sounds. For my part I was apt to play *My Prayer* by the Ink Spots, and weep buckets. How Bob would have hated it. He had been interested in Doris Day though.

Once he said to me, "If I died would you marry again?" I replied "Certainly not," and meant it.

"Of course you would. Look at Dottie," the widow with sons. "It's much too lonely."

Thus I had his blessing, and his presence I was sure, until

I was safely settled with someone else. In fact I had the funny feeling he was sifting them out, though in that first year remarriage was the furthest thing from my thoughts. Some people should have known that. I simply wanted to get back where we'd been before and to go on with the same people in the same way, but of course they would not let me. I had learned that with Amos.

One day Pop Lloyd said to me, "You watch yourself. Do you know what they are saying up at the garage?" That garage was his hangout where there was also a mechanic dressed always in black coveralls, his old schoolmate and the brother of a well known RCN admiral. A lot of people in Clinton were like that. The whole north was incognito, I sometimes thought.

"They said 'The widow Smith would marry anyone who threw his pants at her,' Pop continued. "I told them 'No she would not! She's just being friendly, that's all. And you cut out that talk!' You watch it," he said, "I'm telling you!" Dear old soul. He had put up a fight for me. I was grateful, little suspecting he would later prove to have his own ulterior motive.

While Joan was with us the four of us went on good trips while the fall lasted and we left no back roads unexplored. Sometimes we drove down to the coast but always at night. I liked to see the oncoming headlights rounding curves far, far away with time to pick a pulloff. It was quite exhilarating to hop into the Chev on a Friday night and be back at the same time on Sunday.

With Christmas, disaster struck.

After mailing small gifts to the coast we had taken what money we had to go on to Kamloops to get our own gifts and supplies. It was to be such a joyous junket. Joan sat in the front with me and the two boys sat in the back. I was used to driving locally in the snow and our snow tires were studded with nail heads for better traction. Chains are pointless on a bare windswept highway.

Near Walhachin the blacktop was seemingly dry and bare but was a sheet of black ice, which had filled the pores to the surface without showing. I was doing about twenty miles an hour with extreme caution but didn't see the ice until we started to fishtail. Instinctively I started to brake as Robert shouted, "No Mum, no! No! NO!" We did one sickening pendulum slide after another.

To our right was a dropping slope, but luckily we headed into a deep sandy ditch on our left while the rear of the car slowly rose behind us and over our heads. I came to, suspended over the steering wheel and looking down on the roof of the car, across which Phoebe was crawling, while blood dripped onto her back. Mine.

Joan had been thrown clear into the rear of the car on top of the boys. A seatbelt would have killed her as the roof post was crumpled on her side. She got out and with a grand gesture swept the car door wide for my exit, whereas I crawled through the windshield instead and picked up a lot of glass.

At first Joan did an RCAF job of waving traffic on, then used her head and stopped a couple of cars, east and westbound. Mark had crawled out and was found sitting in a snow bank with no shoes on. Robert was tearing out wires around the engine to stop the terrible noise of the horn. Aware I was injured, he slowly turned me around to look at my face and slowly turned me back again.

Though first offered as options by Nash in 1949 and by Ford in 1955, seatbelts were not introduced as standard until 1959. The two Chevrolet cars described in this book were a 1948 four-door sedan and a 1951 two-door Fleetline with a "torpedo back," neither with seatbelts. Seatbelt use only became mandatory in BC in 1977.

The eastbound car took Mark and me into hospital in Kamloops while the westbound turned around and took the others the short distance to Savona where Della and Cec Ruckle now lived. They kept the dog for us and drove Joan and Robert to the hospital.

Joan was appalled at our neglected state. I had lain trembling and uncovered on a gurney for an hour, while Mark sat on a high stool shivering and waiting. The kids wiped the blood off me and found a sheet as cover, then had nowhere to sit themselves. In due course all heads were x-rayed and my nose stitched up. They left a piece of black paper sewn into it from the backing behind the rear view mirror. It was not removed until I broke my nose again twenty years later in the same way on another rear view mirror. They got the job right that time.

The hospital insisted we phone somebody and the only person we knew was my rather rambunctious mill friend, Harley, who was doing business in town. The last person I wanted to see with my two black eyes and bashed-in nose.

He took charge over the phone, told Joan to take a cab, and we found ourselves installed in two rooms in his hotel. When he saw me by dint of throwing open my door and surveying my face against the pillows he roared with glee and shut the door again. Later he came back to say the children were all being fed down in the dining room.

"I've prepaid the bill. Robert didn't like that. He made noises. Doesn't want to be beholden. Don't worry," he told me wickedly, "I've run into this sort of thing before (as in toying with other mothers) and when I left I noticed he was tucking in handily." The SOB, as he called himself, had been very humane and kind.

Christmas was ruined and the agency let me stay within walls until my face could be shown. The car was fetched and lay crumpled and bashed in the basement. In fact it was Tom who fetched it, leaving work up country to come and help. With a friend towing the wreck he sat steering in the glassless front seat and got windburn.

"When are you going to marry again, Stella, so I can stop worrying about you?"

In early spring of 1959 my former brother-in-law Jack, the Cab Calloway one, indeed the uncle of Joan and Robert, came down from the Yukon with his wife Diana and paid us a visit enroute to the coast. He went downstairs to look at the wreck, was down there a long time, and came up looking thoughtful.

"You can't survive in this country without a car. It's still in running order and the chassis is okay. You just need to straighten out all the dents."

He saw money written on my face. "Look. I'm going to give you two hundred dollars and you find someone to do the job."

That was a lot of money then. He said he would work it in as a business expense, but afterwards I felt his domestic budget had absorbed it. He was continually helping lame ducks in the Yukon and BC, often with his wife's money and her consent, and they were always broke. I could scarcely feed my boys properly. Fourteen years later I had a cottage to sell and paid him back. He phoned from Whitehorse, close to tears. No one ever, ever paid them back.

His was not the only offer I received to pay for our Chev.

Old Pop would appear on our porch from time to time with a bunch of carrots or a great head of cabbage which he knew we could use and which gave him an excuse to be invited inside.

On our long refectory table—maple to match the logs—was a small ceramic keg in a holder that bore eight small glasses. We kept the keg filled with rum almost exclusively for him; a glass of rum for a cabbage. But he would follow me to the sink and stand beside me while I washed it, laying a friendly arm across my shoulders. As the arm slipped off it would manage to slide slowly past my bottom. I always ignored such gestures as if they had not taken place, but I told Robert I was fed up with his little liberties.

One spring day after the accident I was out at the back of our lot trying to dig. Pop came over to talk to me, well out of earshot of his house and ours, and looking conspiratorial. "What are you doing with that car of yours? You can't go on like that."

"Well I'll have to, won't I?"

"I'm going to give you the money to fix it up. Yes, yes I am."

"What on earth would Mrs. Lloyd say?" I was horror struck.

"She doesn't need to know," crowed her husband, "I'll never tell her."

My voice had been pretty well raised and a thundering came from our house of Robert's feet coming down the stairs inside and onto the porch, from where he surveyed us with breathless ferocity.

"Mum, is he bothering you? Because if he is I'll deal with him." Pop gave him a practiced unfazed look and walked off. Thundering downstairs when he thought his mother might be getting the worst of something was one of Robert's specials. Poor Robert. He really did have a lot on his young mind. At first he went about with his forehead creased in worry as if Mark and I were the biggest burdens a man ever had, though you could count my visitors, male or female, on one hand. But he was respected for it, and his "tented eyebrows" earned him the sobriquet "Crowbar" from Harley.

He spent his days teaching all the tricks of the bush that his stepfather had taught him to the son who had no father any more. In short, Robert kept faith.

Soon after Jack and Diana's visit, Joan left us. Through the help of a local woman's connections she found herself in a small match factory in Vancouver and living at the YWCA. With her Air Force references she applied for a job looking after the recreational needs of inmates at Essondale, a psychiatric hospital in Coquitlam now known as Riverview, but heard nothing. She went all the way out to the mental establishment, desperately, to inquire what the job entailed, got talking to those concerned and was hired, almost on the spot. From then on she never looked back.

It was time for us to move on too. Before we left Clinton a chapter closed. There were some regrets. One day in July of 1958, young Bobby van Horlick had gone over to Chris's place to tell him dinner was ready. He pushed open the door and found him sitting bolt upright against the goathide in his rocker, quite dead. His shoelaces were undone as if he had been trying to tie them.

I was back where I came in, at the cemetery. As they brought Chris onto Boot Hill some of us stood around the yawning pit. Mark was with me. I felt he owed this to Chris, no matter what people thought. Near us were the van Horlicks, Una and I standing at the foot during committal. Nobody seemed very perturbed by Chris's passing—more curious than anything. Una was sobbing quietly. Then came the time to throw the first clod of earth. Nobody came forward. No next of kin.

"You do it, Una," I said loudly, getting startled dirty looks.

"But I'm not a relative," she whispered.

"Yes you are. You're his next of kin."

Shaking, she stepped forward as if expecting the whole town to fall on her, picked up a clump and threw it in.

"Goodbye Chris!" she called loudly, as with my arm around her I led her away.

Returning to the office I pulled myself together by relating to Margaret all that had happened. While I was doing it our lanky cowboy friend with the small ranch came in sputtering. "Guess what. That asshole…"

"Who?" said Margaret.

"Buster. Buster van Horlick of course. He thanked me, thanked me for going to Chris's funeral. Who does he think he is!"

Everything was back to normal. The town was itself again.

CHAPTER · XIX

The Point of It All

There had to be a reason for us staying on in this country outside of pure cussedness. One was my promise to return. The boys had proved up and were wise and dependable, heading for manhood with the groundwork laid.

The other was my reluctance to leave our old happy places. Of course I would have to take the boys "outside" eventually to give them a chance.

During our second year in Clinton I'd been told by teachers and friends to get the boys out of there and to where they would learn something. I called Merle Campbell, my personnel friend in Victoria, and once again she came through: there was an opening in Kamloops, only seventy-five miles away; the teachers had told me the schools there were excellent, and it was still close to the bush.

There had been no trouble in selling the log house as my real estate friend found a couple with a "solid gold" credit rating. There was no trouble with the job transfer either and another life opened up. Bill McLean in Clinton said, "They'll give me some knothead when you go," which put paid to the parting shot about my shorthand from the Smithers engineer. For my part, leaving Clinton had been a lukewarm thing. I had not wanted to stay and I had not wanted to go. I didn't know what I wanted.

Robert lasted only six months in Kamloops, he felt he didn't fit in. At seventeen he said he wanted to go and live with his father, where he was welcomed and taken in to his father's seafaring life.

After his brother left, I watched in tears as ten-year-old Mark went out into the park alone. The stalwart little figure hid behind a tree and surveyed all the children playing. Then he walked in a straight line towards some boys playing marbles and he was in. Like his sister, he had found himself and never looked back either.

A camping trip nowadays up the Alaska Highway shows that the old one is purest history. It has heritage status, peeking out in places from under the new one. Symbolically it convinces me that the wrong highway was the right one. Some long-range plan that I came to recognize involved us all. In the years that followed I was to realize that the move to Smithers, taken in such fear and defiance, had ultimately been the best thing for my kids.

The effect of bush living and Bob's influence on their lives came out in many ways. Joan for one might have remained an insular girl in the Oak Bay of those times. Had it not been for Bob, that cocky little stepfather, Joan would have never known how the other half lived. And the bush skills he passed on to Robert stayed with him through his career as a geologist and public servant.

As my five children astounded me with one achievement after another, I became convinced that Bob had somehow helped the three youngest kids every inch of the way to get to their feet, and no doubt watched over the older boys for my sake too, from "there" as well as here. So many things they undertook turned out too pat, too like him and his rampant sense of social justice and what he would have hoped to attain for himself later on: "prestige," as he said more than once. Also, I know he helped me.

Atonement for being a nomad? It must have been a great relief for Bob at his watching post to see the job of upbringing finished and to get off the hook.

And to say to himself, "It takes me!"

Epilogue

In May of 1961 I transferred from the Land Registry Office in Kamloops to Victoria where, to my joy, I spent my last twelve years as assistant librarian to the BC Forest Service, and stayed in touch with all that I thought I had lost. I dabbled sporadically in university courses, did some writing, and devoted my off hours to amateur theatre. And I did marry again.

After two or three false starts at finding love again, as men usually don't like readymade families, I said, "To hell with them," and bought a little cottage. Then I found myself besieged by Allan, a man of three careers: journalist, RCN information officer (retired), and finally a writer for the BC Minister of Lands and Forests.

Lt. R.A.V. Jenkins was the Canadian Navy (RCN) publicity officer for the Far East during the Korean War, serving aboard HMCS *Cayuga*. He wrote a press release about the remarkable surgery performed by ship's doctor Surgeon-Lieutenant Cyr, who actually was the imposter Ferdinand Waldo Demara. The real Dr. Cyr was in fact practicing medicine in New Brunswick. Demara was exposed and removed. He later sold his fascinating story of a lifetime of deception to *Life* magazine; it became a movie, *The Great Impostor,* starring Tony Curtis.

Our marriage in 1972 was the third time around for both of us—we had eleven adult kids between us!

I never lost my interest in paranormal matters, in spiritualism. My curiosity made me want to know more, so I researched the subject and wrote a book about it, which I titled *Mind the Gap*. A few years ago, with all three of my husbands now gone (Bob in 1956, George in 1980 and Allan in 1991), I asked a medium to contact them. The medium told me that Bob and my first husband, George, had come to see me together, with great hilarity at the situation, and that they were "the best of friends, like peas in a pod." I'd always known they'd like each other with me out of the way, both having an appetite for engaging with life. But when I asked what had happened to Allan I was told that he would have nothing to do with those two degenerates and had come with my mother!

All these events are still with me, although they happened more than a lifetime ago. I never expected to live as long as I have. With all the twists and turns on the roads I've traveled, even heading down the wrong highway, I am ready to think that I got it right.

Index

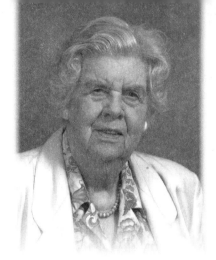

About the author

Stella Jenkins, née Cuming, was born in Victoria, BC to parents who had emigrated from London, England. The Cuming family was part of the "Victoria 400" society set. Following her graduation from St. Margaret's School in 1933 she married George McCandless, whose family was close friends with her parents, and with whom she had four children. By 1945 the marriage was failing and the couple finally separated in 1948.

By this time Stella had met the six-years-younger, peripatetic trapper and outdoorsman, Bob Smith, who—much to the chagrin of her family and friends in Victoria—she married in 1949. The couple had one son, Mark. *Wrong Highway* is the story of their relationship.

Bob died in 1956. Stella remained a widow until 1972, when she married Allan Jenkins, a provincial government employee and former navy officer. She was widowed again early in 1991.

Over her working life, Stella held various office positions in the provincial government, eventually retiring from the office of the BC Forest Service in Victoria. She has had an enduring interest in the paranormal and spiritualism, and in 2007 published *Mind the Gap: Bridging Here with the Hereafter*.

Stella, now in her 90s, resides in Delta, BC.